Grashey
(1876-1950)

Dandy
(1886-1946)

Sweet
(1860-1926)

Law
(1875-1947)

Caldwell
(1870-1918)

Béclère, A.
(1856-1939)

Graham
(1883-1957)

Scholten B. Jones

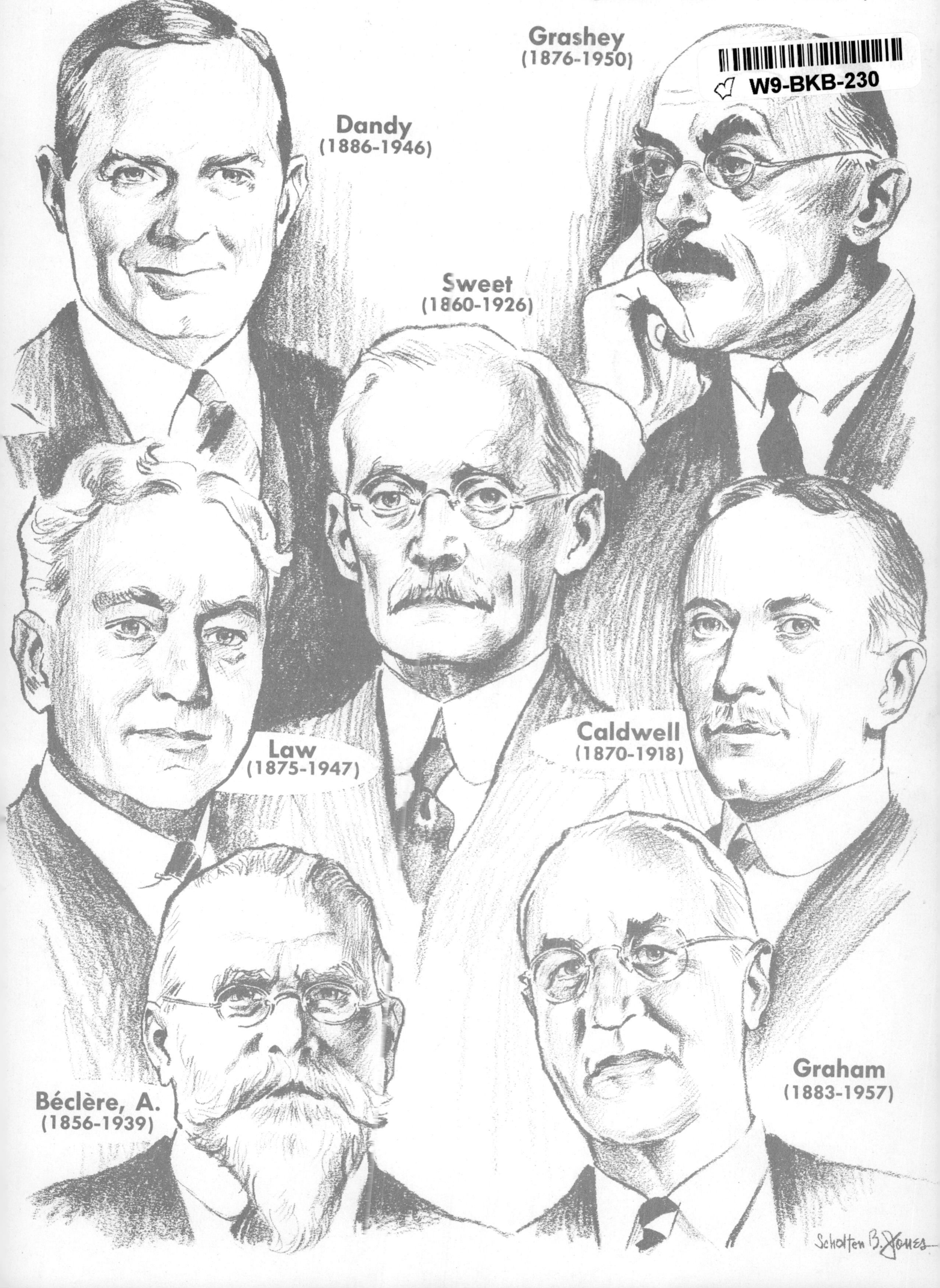

Atlas of
Roentgenographic positions

Volume one

Atlas of
Roentgenographic
positions

Vinita Merrill

Volume one of three volumes

Third edition

Saint Louis

The C. V. Mosby Company

1967

Third edition

Copyright © 1967 by
The C. V. Mosby Company

Fourth printing

Previous editions copyrighted 1949, 1959

Printed in the United States of America

Standard Book Number 8016-3407-5

Library of Congress Catalog Card Number 67-31012

Distributed in Great Britain by Henry Kimpton,
London

In gratitude to our
Pioneers
a few of whom are shown on
the endpapers

Preface to third edition

The purpose of this edition is that stated in the Introduction and in the Preface to each of the two previous editions. Extensive research, which again involved many months devoted to surveying the ever-increasing volume of medical literature and many consultations with numerous experts in this field, has been carried out in selecting and assembling additional roentgenographic positions and specialized roentgeno-graphic procedures for presentation in the present completely reset edition.

Each of the various chapters has been carefully revised, and some of them have been partially or completely rewritten for the inclusion of more information or to bring them up to date. Certain of the roentgeno-graphic positions have been rearranged, some to face each other for ready comparison and others for the purpose of placing them in more logical sequence. Many valuable roentgenographic positions and specialized roentgenographic procedures, some old and some of comparatively recent development, have been added. Further anatomic information has been added where needed. Numerous new illustrations have been added and a large number of the older illustrations have been replaced or otherwise improved.

For the benefit of instructors, and of technologists and students who desire more information about a subject than is presented in this text, the original works to which direct references have been made are appropriately footnoted throughout the three volumes, and, conveniently set up chronologically under the respective anatomic or procedure headings, an extensive listing of bibliographic references is given at the close of each volume. In addition to these references, and the further original papers to which their bibliographies will lead him, the reader is urged to take advantage of the excellent abstracts of international literature presented in *Radiology*, in the *American Journal of Roentgenology*, and in *Excerpta Medica*.

Because of the amount of material added to the book, it has been divided into three volumes; this has the advantage of placing the skull positions and other procedures usually performed in the skull unit in a separate volume as well as providing greater ease in handling.

To each user of this text the author desires to extend her grateful appreciation and to express the hope that he will find the present edition a practical and useful one.

V. M.
New York, 1967

Preface to second edition

A survey of the relevant literature of the decade which has passed since this work was published and a review of much of the older literature were made preparative to revising the material for a second edition. Some valuable positions have been developed in the past ten years, but the literature of this period revealed comparatively few new positions, a finding which can be interpreted only as a tribute to the thorough work of our pioneer roentgenologists. This period has seen great advances in the development of improved opaque media, and, as a result of this, in the investigation of the structures which depend upon opacification for visualization. The basic roentgenographic positions have thus far proved adequate for the demonstration of these structures throughout the various regions of the body. The review of the older literature was rewarded not only with the discovery of several excellent positions, but also with the discovery of a few more originators of positions long familiar to us.

Over forty positions, including a number of time-tested old ones as well as the selection of new ones, have been added to this compilation of roentgenographic positions. Many new illustrations have been added, and a number of the older ones have been replaced. Several sections have been partially or completely rewritten.

In an effort to use more uniform and more informative terminology for the purpose, fairly extensive changes have been made in the titles employed to designate various positions. Where the term *oblique* appears in the title of a position described in this text, it indicates part rotation and not central ray angulation. An oblique view can unquestionably be obtained by angulating either the part or the central ray, but a comparison of the resultant projections shows a difference great enough to make it desirable to differentiate between the two methods used to produce them. The oblique view obtained with part rotation shows no distortion, whereas that obtained with central ray angulation shows distortion in proportion to the degree of angulation.

Longitudinal angulation of the central ray, when it coincides with or parallels the long axis of the part, is herein designated in the position title as *axial* or *semiaxial* angulation, or, more specifically, as *superoinferior* or *inferosuperior* angulation. *Transverse angulation* of the central ray, when it parallels the transverse axis of the part, is designated in the position title as *mediolateral* or *lateromedial* angulation where it is employed with a frontal or near frontal position and as *anterior* or *posterior* angulation where it is employed with a lateral or near lateral position. The anatomic points of entrance and emergence are, in accordance with custom, used as position titles without regard to the direction of central ray angulation. *Eccentric angulation* of the central ray is designated only according to the anatomic points of entrance and exit because, being the result of a double angle, that is, a combination of longitudinal and transverse angulation, it parallels neither the longitudinal nor the transverse axis of the part.

The orbitomeatal line is generally known as the *radiographic base line*, with the result that different authors frequently designate it nonspecifically as the *base line*, a term usually reserved for the *base line of the cranium*. In order to eliminate doubt as to which localization line is indicated, the brief term has been deleted from the instructions and the base line of the cranium designated as the *infraorbitomeatal line*. All references to the backbone have been changed from the older term spinal column to the preferred term *vertebral column*. Since contrast media stain nothing, the misnomer *dye* and its derivatives, *dye-laden* and *dye-impregnated*, have been deleted in favor of the correct terms.

Other misnomers which ought to be deleted from the language of our profession are *plate* and *picture*. Glass plates have not been available for roentgenography since the early days of the first world war, an era which predates a majority of present-day radiologists and technologists. Plate is, however, a misnomer of small importance. Picture is a misnomer of more serious proportions. A radiograph is not a picture: it is a permanent roentgen record of a fairly complicated medical examination, the technical phase of which is performed by a medical technologist and the diagnostic phase by a qualified doctor of medicine. To call a radiograph a picture is to imply that radiologists as well as technologists are photographers, an implication made by dictionaries, and, unfortunately, by many members of the medical profession. Unless this impression is to be perpetuated, an accurate definition for the terms *radiograph* and *roentgenogram* should be submitted to the respective publishers for future editions of their dictionaries and to individuals as the occasion arises.

It seems appropriate at this point to consider a few other terms idiomatic to the language of our profession. As applied in roentgenography, the terms *projection* and *position* are synonyms and convey a meaning *exactly opposite* to that of the term *view*. Projection and position apply to the *tube side* of the part from which position we *face the film*, while view applies to the *film side* of the part from which position we *face the tube*. Projection and position are the terms used to indicate the direction in which the central ray traverses a part in casting its shadow on the film. The surface of entrance and the surface of exit, that is, the surface facing the tube and the surface facing the film, are designated in that order in the title of the position, except in lateral projections, where only the side adjacent to the film is designated. Oblique projections are designated by the *side adjacent to the film* and the *surface facing the tube,* as left anterior oblique, left posterior oblique. View is the term used to describe the projected image as it is seen from the position of the recording medium (film or radioscopic screen), from which position the above-listed designations are described in reverse and the surface facing the film is mentioned first. A posteroanterior projection thus becomes an anteroposterior view; a left lateral projection, a left lateral view; and a left posterior oblique projection, a left anterior oblique view.

Doctors usually think in terms of the resultant image and not in terms of the process by which the image is obtained, so they frequently use view as if it were synonymous with projection and position. Experienced technologists are aware of this line of thought and rarely, if ever, misinterpret an incorrectly stated order, but it is often misleading to students and less experienced technologists until they realize that while they are accustomed to *visualizing* the image from the tube side of the part, the doctor is accustomed to *viewing* it from the film side.

The field of roentgenography has grown to such proportions that the many subjects involved in the work can no longer be given adequate coverage in one book. The present-day technologist needs more than a smattering of information about or a nodding acquaintance with each subject embraced by his profession. For two reasons the material presented in this text has been restricted to positioning and to those subjects having direct bearing on positioning. First, the allied subjects are considered too important to be presented in a perfunctory way in a few chapters of a book professedly devoted to another subject. Second, a text dealing with the factual subject of roentgenographic positions should not be consigned to early obsolescence by the inclusion of data pertaining to changing factors. Whatever the changes in contrast media, films, screens, processing solutions, exposure techniques, localization devices, specialized and standard equipment, it is not likely that established body positions will change. An effort has been made, therefore, to avoid, in so far as possible, the demonstration or discussion of those topics which are undergoing constant change. It is the belief of the author that a reasonably complete reference work of roentgenographic positions should be as permanent as a standard dictionary—that it should not, at this stage of development, need frequent revision. It is hoped that the material presented in the *Atlas of Roentgenographic Positions* has now been brought, if not to, at least near, this goal.

V. M.
New York, 1959

Preface to first edition

The purpose of this work is to provide a practical reference book for x-ray technologists by:

1. Describing many roentgenographic positions and procedures, the unusual or specialized positions not used as part of a routine examination and not ordinarily included in general textbooks, as well as the standard positions.
2. Presenting information pertaining to anatomy and physiology.
3. Presenting the definitions of the more usual terms used in roentgenography.
4. Providing a bibliography to facilitate further detailed study.

The selection and preparation of the material presented in these volumes resulted from a survey of the relevant literature of all countries covering the past fifty-two years. While the survey was extensive, it was not the intent to include everything in the literature. The review of so vast an amount of material was not an easy task; and for several years, due to wartime restrictions, the current literature of several countries was not available.

An effort has been made to illustrate each procedure and to describe it as briefly as is consistent with clarity, to include only those facts and principles which the x-ray technologist needs to know, and know well, in order to work with understanding and intelligence. The drawings were, for the most part, prepared from actual anatomical specimens, from radiographs, or from the related photographs. A number were adapted from the illustrations published by the authors of certain positions, credit being given for each of these in the respective legend. Considerable effort has also been expended on the layout of the material to present it in a form convenient for quick reference.

V. M.
New York, 1949

Acknowledgments to third edition

The most truly enjoyable part of assembling the material for this text has always been derived from the contacts, by correspondence, by telephone, or in person, with many long-time friends and with many new ones, all of whom graciously responded to every request for assistance. Second only to that pleasure is the pleasure I take in recording my sincere appreciation and full gratitude for the valuable assistance so freely given me.

For permission to reproduce copyrighted material, grateful acknowledgment is made to the respective publishers of (1) *American Journal of Roentgenology,* for the five photographs appearing on pages 116 and 117, the two foreign body studies on page 537, the two radiographs on page 621, the six illustrations appearing on pages 670 and 671, the ten illustrations appearing on pages 746 to 749, the upper photograph on page 802, both photographs on page 803, and for several of the radiographs appearing in the section on diskography; (2) *Radiologic Technology,* for the photographs and radiographs appearing on pages 532, 533, and 649; (3) *Annals of Surgery,* for the drawing and composite photograph-radiograph on page 802; (4) *Medical Radiography and Photography,* for the radiographs appearing on page 720; and (5) *Radiology,* for the drawing appearing on page 839.

For the excellent new art work added to this edition, sincere thanks are extended to Mr. Scholten B. Jones for the end paper drawings, to Mr. Neil O. Hardy for a number of the figure drawings, and to Miss Harriet E. Phillips for the beautiful anatomic drawings and for a majority of the figure drawings.

It has again been my good fortune to be able to place the photographic work in the capable hands of Mr. Don Allen, to whom I extend my sincere thanks for the excellent quality of the new radiographic reproductions and for the new photographs.

A special word of thanks is also extended to Miss Agnes Craig, to Mr. Frank Gisondo, and to Mr. Mark Katz, fellow technologists who posed for a majority of the new photographs.

For valuable assistance in testing the practicality of numerous roentgenographic positions, their addition to the text being determined by the ease with which they can be performed and duplicated, and for taking many of the final radiographs, I extend special thanks to Mr. Anthony Antinoro, Mr. Roy B. Boone, Mr. Thomas T. Christenberry, Miss Agnes Craig, Mr. Vito L. Fodera, Mr. Frank Gisondo, and Mr. Jonothan E. Hough.

For making the facilities of their offices available to me for radiographic work, I am deeply grateful to Dr. Herbert F. Hempel, Dr. Lawson E. Miller, Jr., and Dr. Judah Zizmor.

For making the facilities of the radiology departments available to me for both radiographic and photographic work, I am profoundly grateful to Dr. Richard G. Lester, Duke University Medical Center, Durham, North Carolina; to Dr. Alex Norman, Hospital for Joint Diseases and Medical Center, New York City; to Dr. Robert L. Pinck, Long Island College Hospital, Brooklyn, New York; to Dr. William H. Shehadi, United Hospital, Port Chester, New York; and to Dr. Judah Zizmor, Manhattan Eye, Ear and Throat Hospital New York City.

Special thanks are extended to the many physicians and several technologists who so generously loaned drawings and/or radiographs, individual acknowledgment for which is being made under the respective illustrations.

To Mr. John B. Cahoon, Jr., and to Miss Kaethe Fengler, good friends and fellow technologists, sincere thanks and full gratitude are extended for their reading of the entire text and for their excellent criticisms and suggestions.

For reading certain sections of the manuscript, for valuable criticisms and suggestions, and for loaning numerous illustrations for the respective sections, I gratefully acknowledge my indebtedness to Dr. Joshua A. Becker, Dr. Walter E. Berdon, Dr. Kuo-York Chynn, Miss Barbara Curcio, Dr. John A. Evans, Dr. Robert H. Freiberger, Dr. J. Gershon-Cohen, Dr.

Roger W. Lambie, Dr. Robert S. Sherman, Dr. Ruth E. Snyder, Dr. M. A. Worth, Jr., and Dr. Judah Zizmor.

A special acknowledgment of gratitude and thanks is due to Dr. John A. Goree for his valuable criticisms and suggestions for the sections on cerebral pneumography and cerebral angiography, for supervising the taking of the related photographs, and for supplying a majority of the radiographs for these two sections.

It is again my pleasure and my privilege to record my great indebtedness and profound gratitude to Dr. Henry K. Taylor, not only for the many excellent suggestions made during his critical reading of the new and revised material for this edition, but for similar guidance in the preparation of the two previous editions.

For significant contributions that have greatly enriched this text, I extend my deepest gratitude to:

Dr. David L. Benninghoff, for supervising the preparation of the anatomic drawing of the lymphatic system and for writing and illustrating the section on lymphography.

Dr. William H. Shehadi, for his critical reading of and many helpful suggestions for various sections, particularly the section on the biliary tract, for always so willingly being at the other end of a telephone for consultation, and for writing the section on protection against ionizing radiation.

Dr. Richard G. Lester, for reading the entire manuscript, for innumerable helpful criticisms and suggestions for its improvement, and for writing and illustrating the section on visceral and peripheral angiography.

V. M.
New York, 1967

Acknowledgments to second edition

Grateful acknowledgment is made to the Eastman Kodak Company for permission to use the copyrighted chart appearing on page 403, for which proper credit is given in the legend.

To Mr. Don Allen, photographer par excellence, I extend my appreciation for the fine quality of the photographic reproductions of the new roentgenograms.

It is my pleasure to express my thanks to Mr. Alfred Feinberg for illustrating the second as well as the first edition of this work, and, most particularly, for the gratifying experience of working with him.

To Mr. Harry Blumenthal, Chief Technician, Department of Urology, New York Hospital, grateful acknowledgment is made for his careful reading of the section on the urinary system and for his several excellent suggestions.

An expression of appreciation is extended to Dr. Berten C. Bean for permitting me to use his Chart of the Intracerebral Circulation, and to the many doctors who so kindly loaned roentgenograms, for all of which acknowledgment is made in the respective legends.

I take considerable pleasure in recording my indebtedness and profound gratitude to Mr. Ivor David Bennett, Vice President of the Picker X-Ray Corporation, for his wise counsel and encouragement, for his meticulous reading of both the original and revised manuscripts, and for his constructive criticisms and innumerable helpful suggestions.

There is a great obligation indeed to be acknowledged to Miss Lisbeth M. Sass, good friend, former student, and later colleague. Miss Sass worked with me in surveying the literature not only in preparation for the second edition of this work, but also for the first edition from 1936, when I started this compilation of positions while Technical Director to the Department of Radiology and Instructor in the School of Radiography at the New York Hospital, until 1948, when I brought it to completion while Director of the Educational Department of the Picker X-Ray Corporation. No expression of gratitude is adequate for such faithful and tireless assistance.

Especial thanks are extended to Dr. William H. Shehadi for his careful review of the section on cholecystocholangiography and for the constructive and valuable criticisms and suggestions he made for the improvement of this section.

I am heavily indebted to Dr. Henry K. Taylor, and I am deeply grateful to him for his careful reading of all the new and revised material and for his discerning criticisms and excellent suggestions which have done much to improve this work.

Dr. Ramsay Spillman, my chief, I cannot thank sufficiently for granting me the time necessary for part of the writing, the free use of the facilities of his office for the radiographic work, for valuable assistance during the survey, for carefully reading the revised manuscript, and for his many fine criticisms and suggestions.

V. M.

New York, 1959

Acknowledgments to first edition

For permission to use copyrighted material, grateful acknowledgment is made to: The Eastman Kodak Company for the radiographs appearing on pages 195, 215, 219, 370, 373, 604, 605, and for the photographs on page 456; The C. V. Mosby Company for the drawings on pages 624 and 625; The Charles C Thomas Company for the chart on page 19, the photographs on pages 626 and 627, and for the top drawing appearing on page 630; the Thomas Nelson & Sons Company for the lower drawing on page 630; and The Yale Journal of Biology and Medicine for the drawings on page 621.

Grateful acknowledgment is also made to Miss Agnes Goodwin for the compilation of the index; to Mr. Saul L. Bell for his assistance with the photographic work; to Miss Sophie Rakowska for her assistance with the correlation of the material, and for her capable handling of the many secretarial details; and to Mr. Alfred Feinberg for the drawings used to illustrate anatomy and positioning.

Appreciation is expressed to Miss Kaethe Fengler who made a majority of the radiographs appearing in Volume I, and part of those in Volume II. Also to Miss Lisbeth M. Sass who compiled the bibliography, translated from several languages during the survey, and made part of the radiographs appearing in Volume II.

Especial thanks are due to Mr. William F. Bruning of Picker X-Ray Corporation for his cooperation and wise counsel in the design, and for his assistance in the production of both volumes.

The help given by the many doctors who so generously loaned drawings and radiographs for the special procedures is gratefully acknowledged, and individual acknowledgment is being made under the respective illustrations.

Grateful acknowledgment is made to the following doctors for reviewing the procedures devised by them, and, in most instances, for loaning the respective illustrations: Dr. Robert P. Ball; Dr. Charles W. Blackett; Dr. W. Edward Chamberlain; Dr. Albert B. Ferguson; Dr. Howard C. Moloy; Dr. Herbert Thoms; and Dr. A. Justin Williams.

The many courtesies, constructive criticisms, and valuable suggestions extended by Dr. Robert P. Ball, who reviewed the section on the female reproductive system, and Dr. Henry K. Taylor, who reviewed the entire section on the visceral organs, are deeply appreciated.

Grateful thanks are due to Dr. Marcy L. Sussman and the governing body of the Mount Sinai Hospital, New York City, for making available the facilities of their X-Ray Department, and for the many kindnesses extended at all times.

An especial acknowledgment is made to Dr. Ramsey Spillman, Dr. William H. Shehadi, and Mr. Arthur W. Fuchs for their careful review of the entire text, and for their constructive criticisms and many valuable suggestions.

I wish to express to the Picker X-Ray Corporation my deep appreciation for their help and encouragement and for having provided the facilities and finances without which this work would not have been possible.

V. M.
New York, 1949

Contents

Volume I

Introduction, 3

Preliminary steps in roentgenography, 4
  Radiograph, 5
  Clinical history needed by the technologist, 5
  Initial examination, 5
  Diagnosis and the technologist, 5
  Ethics in radiologic technology, 5
  Care of radiographic examining room 6,
  Ventilation, 6
  Aseptic technique, 6
  Isolation unit, 7
  Disinfectant solutions, 7
  Operating room, 7
  Minor surgical procedure in radiology department, 8
  Procedure book, 8
  Cleansing enema, 8
  Motion—its control, 8
  Structural relationship in positioning, 9
  Preparation instructions, 10
  Patient's dress, ornaments, surgical dressings, 10
  Lifting and handling patients, 10
  Preexposure instructions, 11
  Foundation exposure technique, 11
  Adaptation of exposure technique to patient, 11
  Identification, 12
  Film placement, 12
  Direction of central ray, 12
  Focal-film distance, 13
  Delimitation of x-ray beam, 13

Protection against ionizing radiation (William H. Shehadi, M. D.), 14

General anatomy and anatomic terms, 19
  General anatomy, 20
    Skeleton, 20
    Epiphyseal chart, 21
    Body planes and positions, 23
    Joints, 24
  Anatomic terms, 24
    Anatomic projections and depressions, 24
    Part location and position, 25
    Body positions, 25

Upper extremity, 27
  Anatomy, 28
    Hand, 28
    Wrist, 29
    Forearm, 29
    Arm, 31
  Positioning, 32
    Hand, 32
    Fingers, 36
    First carpometacarpal joint, 39
    Wrist, 40
    Carpal canal, 45
    Carpal bridge, 46
    Forearm, 47
    Elbow, 48
    Distal humerus and olecranon process, 54
    Humerus, 56

Lower extremity, 59
  Anatomy, 60
    Foot, 60
    Leg, 62
    Thigh, 63
  Positioning, 64
    Toes, 64
    Sesamoids, 68
    Foot, 70
    Ankle, 80
    Leg, 92
    Knee, 94
    Patella, 102
    Femur, 106

Long bone measurement, 108
  Orthoroentgenographic method, 109
  Slit scanography, 110
  Spot scanography, 111
  Measurement of differences of leg length, 112

Contrast arthrography, 114

Shoulder girdle, 119
  Anatomy, 120
    Clavicle, 120
    Scapula, 120
    Humerus, 122
    Shoulder joint, 123

Positioning, 124
  Shoulder girdle, 124
    Teres minor insertion, 126
    Subscapularis insertion, 127
    Coracoid process, 128
    Glenoid fossa, 129
    Bicipital groove, 130
    Shoulder joint, 131
    Acromioclavicular articulations, 136
    Clavicle, 138
    Scapula, 144
    Scapular spine, 148

Bony thorax (sternum and ribs), 151
  Bony thorax, anatomy, 152
    Sternum, 152
    Sternoclavicular joints, 153
  Sternum, positioning, 154
  Sternoclavicular articulations, 160
  Ribs, 164
    Anatomy, 164
    Positioning, 165
    Radiography of ribs, 166
    Wide-angle technique, 172
    Costal joints, 173

Pelvic girdle and upper femora, 175
  Anatomy of pelvis, 176
    Hip, 176
    Femur, 177
    Hip joint, 179
  Positioning, 182
    Pelvic girdle and upper femora, 182
    Hip, 189
    Acetabulum, 200
    Anterior pelvic bones, 202
    Ilium, 206

Vertebral column, 207
  Anatomy, 208
    Cervical vertebrae, 210
    Thoracic vertebrae, 212
    Lumbar vertebrae, 214
    Sacrum and coccyx, 216
  Positioning, 218
    Occipitocervical articulations, 218
    Upper cervical vertebrae, 220
    Lower cervical vertebrae, 226
    Cervicothoracic region, 238
    Thoracic vertebrae, 240
    Lumbar-lumbosacral vertebrae, 246
    Lumbosacral junction and sacroiliac joints, 248
    Lumbosacral junction, 252
    Last lumbar intervertebral foramina, 253
    Lumbar-lumbosacral apophysial joints, 254
    Lumbar intervertebral disks, 257
    Sacroiliac joints, 258
    Sacrum and coccyx, 262
    Sacral canal—sacroiliac joints, 264
    Scoliosis series, 266
    Spinal fusion series, 268

Glossary (anatomic and medical terms), 271

Volume I Bibliography, 289

Volume II

Skull, 311
  Anatomy of skull, 312
    Cranial bones, 314
    Organs of hearing, 322
    Facial bones, 324
  Radiography of skull, 327
  Positioning, 332
    Cranium, 332
    Sella turcica, 346
    Orbit, anatomy, 351
    Optic foramen, 352
    Optic foramen, superior orbital fissure, and anterior clinoid process, 358
    Sphenoid strut, 359
    Superior orbital fissures, 360
    Inferior orbital fissures, 361
  Eye anatomy, 362
  Localization of foreign bodies within orbit or eye, 365
  Nasolacrimal drainage system, 376
    Anatomy, 376
    Examination procedure, 377
  Temporal bone, 378
    Mastoid process, 380
    Mastoid and petrous regions, 390
    Petrous portions, 392
    Temporal styloid processes, 410
  Jugular foramina, 414
  Hypoglossal canal, 418

Paranasal sinuses, 419
  Anatomy, 420
  Positioning, 424

Positioning of facial bones, 439
  Lateral, frontal, and oblique positions, 440
  Nasal bones, 446
  Zygomatic arches, 450
  Maxillae, 458
  Mandible, 461
  Temporomandibular articulations, 476

Mouth (salivary glands and teeth), 485
  Anatomy of mouth, 486
  Salivary glands, 488
    Anatomy, 488
    Positioning, 489
      Parotid gland, 490
      Parotid and submaxillary glands, 492
      Submaxillary and sublingual glands, 493
  Dental arches and teeth, 494
  Anatomy, 494
  Dental radiography, 496
    Periapical projections, 497
    Interproximal projections, 510

Volume II Bibliography, 513

Volume III

Anterior part of neck (soft palate, pharynx, and larynx), 527
  Anatomy, 528
  Methods of examination, 530
  Deglutition studies of pharynx, 532
  Positioning, 534

Pharynx and larynx, 534
    Soft palate, pharynx, and larynx, 536

Body cavities, surface markings of abdomen, and habitus, 539
    Body cavities, 540
    Surface markings of abdomen, 541
    Bodily habitus, 542

Thoracic viscera (respiratory system and mediastinal structures), 545
    Anatomy, 546
        Respiratory system, 546
        Mediastinal structures, 550
    Radiography, 551
    Positioning, 555
        Trachea, 555
        Trachea and superior mediastinum, 556
        Trachea and pulmonary apex, 557
        Pulmonary apices, 558
        Chest—lungs and heart, 560
        Lungs, 568
        Lungs and pleurae, decubitus projections, 570
    Bronchography, 572

Digestive system, 577
    Anatomy, 578
    Radiography, 586
        Abdomen, 586
            Body positions and specialized procedures, 590
            Abdominal pneumoradiography, 592
        Liver and spleen, specialized procedures, 594
            Liver, 596
            Spleen, 597
        Biliary tract, 598
            Examination procedures, 598
            Oral cholegraphy, 604
            Intravenous cholegraphy, 606
            Positioning, 612
                Gallbladder, 612
                Extrahepatic bile ducts, 616
            Percutaneous transhepatic cholangiography, 617
            Operative (or immediate) cholangiography, 618
            Postoperative (or T tube) cholangiography, 620
            Operative pancreatography, 622
            Simultaneous cholegraphy and urography, 624
        Alimentary tract, 626
        Examination procedures, 626
        Esophagus, 632
        Gastrointestinal tract, 634
            G. I. series, 634
                Examination procedures, 636
                Serial and mucosal studies, 638
                Retrogastric soft tissues, 641
                Routine positions, stomach and duodenum, 642
                Stomach and duodenum and diaphragmatic hernias, 646
                Minimal hiatal hernias, 646

Motility studies, 650
Small intestine, 652
    Oral methods of examination, 652
    Intubation methods of examination, 654
Large intestine, 656
    Examination procedures, 656
    Administration of opaque enema, 662
        Radiography of opacified colon, 664
    Administration of gas enema, 668
        Radiography of insufflated colon, 669
    Examination procedure with disposable enema apparatus, 670
    Diagnostic enema via colostomies, 672

Urinary system, 677
    Anatomy, 678
    Radiography, 684
        Retroperitoneal pneumoradiography, 696
        Bolus injection nephrotomography, 698
        Infusion nephrotomography and nephropylelography, 700
        Excretory (intravenous) pyelography, 702
        Retrograde urography, 706
        Retrograde cystography, 710
        Female cystourethrography, 714
        Male cystourethrography, 716

Male reproductive system, 717
    Anatomy, 718
    Examination procedures and positioning, 720

Breast, 723
    Anatomy, 724
    Mammography, 726
    Positioning, 730

Female reproductive system, 735
    Anatomy, 736
    Nongravid female patient, 742
        Hysterosalpingography, 744
        Pelvic pneumography, 746
        Vaginography, 750
    Gravid female patient, 752
        Fetography, 754
        Placentography, 756
        Roentgen pelvimetry, 758

Central nervous system, 773
    Anatomy, 774
    Cerebral pneumography, 778
    Myelography, 795
    Diskography, 801
    Cerebral angiography, 805

Circulatory system, 821
    Anatomy, 822
    Visceral and peripheral angiography (Richard G. Lester, M.D.), 830
    Lymphography (David L. Benninghoff, M.D.), 839

Volume III Bibliography, 845

Atlas of
Roentgenographic positions

Volume one

Introduction

The aim of this work is assembly of material: first, the compilation of a reference book of positions, giving all of the standard positions and as many of the more unusual or specialized positions as seems practical, and, second, the inclusion of an extensive bibliography for the purpose of further study. The references given, particularly the more recent ones, should be studied for a complete understanding of the more complicated examinations. While the main emphasis in this book is placed on positioning, consideration has also been given to the anatomic information necessary to technologists, and to numerous preparatory steps in roentgenographic procedure.

A survey of the literature available from the date of the discovery of roentgen rays has been made in the preparation of this text. The descriptions of the positions are scattered through hundreds of articles and books in many languages; however, a vast majority of the original work was written in English, German, French, Swedish, Spanish, and Italian. The technique of positioning recommended by the respective authors for obtaining some of the projections is involved, complicated, and in several instances quite vague. This fact may account for the lack of common usage of some of the projections.

With no pretense of complete coverage of material, every effort has been put forth to compile a bibliography that will make the complete data available to technologists without the difficulties they have heretofore encountered. In addition to the bibliography, a list of general textbooks is included, as well as a list of medical journals that may be followed to keep abreast of the developments set forth in the literature of other countries as well as of this country. These books and journals are usually obtainable through the medical societies where there is not a conveniently located medical library.

No claim to originality is made in any of the methods described in this text. All of the material is based on information obtained from the literature, from lectures, and from information gathered during thirty-seven years of experience as a medical x-ray technologist, both in hospital and office practice.

The positions that have been established for the numerous projections of the body structures have each been worked out according to the shape and position of the organ involved, and its relationship to adjacent organs as to size, shape, angulation, and tissue density. The respective focal spot-part-film positions were determined by these anatomic relationships, the part being adjusted and the central ray angled accordingly to avoid the confusing shadows cast by the surrounding structures, or the superimposition of denser ones. The aim is always to project each structure in such a way that it will be as free as possible from superimposition and from distortion. The rules, therefore, are, first, to adjust the part so that it will be, depending upon the view desired, either parallel with or at right angles to the film, and, second, to adjust the central ray so that it will be directed at the desired angle to the structure.

Many organs are so situated in the body that positioning for their radiographic demonstration requires only that the part be placed against the film in one of the anatomic positions, that is, anterior, posterior, or lateral surface to the film. Where the position necessary for the visualization of a given structure has required accurate calculation in the adjustment of the part, film, and central ray, every effort has been made to trace the origin of the projection in order to give credit to the author of the position. Many of the positions that seem so logical and easy to us now, required considerable research before they were reduced to their present simplicity. The handicap of primitive equipment (slow x-ray sensitive emulsions, lack of intensifying screens and Potter-Bucky diaphragms, to name a few of the drawbacks) retarded the progress of the pioneers in establishing positions for certain regions of the body because of the impossibility of obtaining a suitable exposure technique for those regions.

While a large number of the positions recommended in the literature on a given organ are only modifications in focal spot-part-film relationship that produce the identical projection, or only minor variations in the projection, many of them were worked out independently at about the same time. This has made it difficult to trace some of the positions to their origin, and in certain instances impossible.

Where several similar positions for obtaining an identical projection have been recommended, the least complicated one has been selected for illustration. In many instances, however, several methods for obtaining similar projections are illustrated to aid in selecting the one most adaptable to the individual patient.

Since standard projections for each part have not been adopted by the radiologic profession, it is advisable for technologists to familiarize themselves with the positioning of as many projections as possible. By so doing, they will be prepared to carry out not only the routine positions selected by the radiologist but also a reasonable number of the less frequently required specialized positions.

There is no uniformity regarding the terminology applied to projections. Any given projection may be referred to by either the originator's name, the structure shown, the angulation of the central ray, the anatomic points where the central ray enters and emerges, or the anatomic points of contact with the film. For example, the position used to demonstrate the maxillary sinuses is variously called the Waters position, the maxillary position, the verticomental position, the occipitomental position, and the nose-chin position. While this lack of uniformity is sometimes confusing, the complexity of the factors involved makes it difficult to establish a standard nomenclature. The similarity of position, of central ray angulation, and of the points of entrance and emergence of the central ray in so many projections makes these terms unsatisfactory. It would seem that either the originator-name or the structure-view would be more satisfactory terms.

The author, having been a technologist for many years, fully realizes that all patients do not fit into textbook illustrations of positions as do the models shown. The foundation from which we work in positioning atypical cases is the individual of so-called normal or average form. The aim in each position can be demonstrated quite clearly with the normal, whereas it would be difficult, if not impossible, to show the aim with an obese model. Normally formed models are selected for this reason. It is believed that if the *aim* in each position is clearly illustrated and described on the normal person, the technologist will be better able to adapt the position to atypical patients.

Preliminary steps in roentgenography

1. The radiograph
2. Clinical history needed by the technologist
3. Initial examination
4. Diagnosis and the technologist
5. Ethics in radiologic technology
6. Care of radiographic examining room
7. Ventilation
8. Aseptic technique
9. Isolation unit
10. Disinfectant solutions
11. Operating room
12. Minor surgical procedure in the radiology department
13. Procedure book
14. Cleansing enema
15. Motion—its control
16. Structural relationship in positioning
17. Preparation instructions
18. Patient's dress, ornaments, surgical dressings
19. Lifting and handling patients
20. Preexposure instructions
21. Foundation exposure technique
22. Adaptation of exposure technique to patient
23. Identification
24. Film placement
25. Direction of central ray
26. Focal-film distance
27. Delimitation of x-ray beam

1. THE RADIOGRAPH

A radiograph is the end result of an exacting technical procedure. Each phase of this procedure must be carried out with care in order to obtain the greatest possible information concerning the anatomic details of the structures for the purpose of demonstrating the absence of, or the presence and extent of, traumatic or pathologic changes. There is no examination in radiology where accuracy and attention to detail are not essential, be it of a finger or a brain.

The technologist should be thoroughly familiar with the radiographic shadows cast by normal structures. In order to develop the ability to analyze films correctly, and to correct or prevent errors in technique, the technologist should study radiographs from the following standpoints:

a. The relationship of the structural shadows as to size, shape, position, and angulation.

b. The degree of detail in each structure as compared with that of adjacent structures, such as the head of the humerus as compared with the glenoid fossa and the acromion process.

c. The comparative detail obtained with tubes of different focal-spot sizes.

d. The coarsening effect of magnification on detail at different focal-spot-film distances.

e. The blurring effect of magnification on detail at different part-film distances, as in an anteroposterior projection compared with a posteroanterior projection of a given region.

f. The fuzzing effect caused by (1) slight motion, both voluntary and involuntary, (2) poor screen-contact, and (3) a pitted focal-spot. The effects produced by the last two of these factors are sufficiently characteristic that the experienced technologist seldom needs to make a screen-contact test or a focal-spot test.

g. The degree of structural distortion obtained at different central ray angulations, and, depending upon the part-film distance, how far a structure will be projected by different central ray angulations.

By familiarizing himself with these effects, the technologist will know just how much magnification and distortion to expect of each body structure under the particular circumstances, and, as a result, will be readily able to determine the cause for any deviation from the detail expected.

A sound knowledge of anatomy and the ability to analyze radiographs correctly are of particular importance to technologists who work where the radiologist is not in constant attendance. Under this condition, the radiologist must be able to depend upon the technologist to perform the technical phase of the examinations without aid.

2. CLINICAL HISTORY NEEDED BY THE TECHNOLOGIST

The radiologist, after establishing a standard procedure for each region of the body, usually places the responsibility of carrying out the technical phase of the examinations on the technologist. With more and more of the radiologist's time being consumed by the diagnostic and therapeutic phases of radiology, he has less and less time to devote to the technical phase. This circumstance makes it necessary for him to depend upon the technologist to a great extent in carrying out this phase of the patient's care for him, just as the physician and surgeon must depend

upon the nurse to carry out certain phases of the patient's care for them. This places a grave responsibility upon the technologist and makes it necessary for him to know, first, normal anatomy and normal anatomic variations so that he can position the patient accurately; and, second, the radiographic characteristics of numerous pathologic conditions, that is, their effect upon the normal radiopacity of structures, so that he can select the exposure factors accordingly. The technologist is not concerned with the causation, diagnosis, or treatment of disease, but he must know what to do about its radiographic demonstration if he is to be expected to do more than "push a button."

When the radiologist cannot see the patient, he depends upon the technologist to take the necessary history and observe any apparent abnormality that might affect the radiographic result, such as jaundice in gallbladder examinations, and surface masses which might cast shadows that could be mistaken for internal changes. When it is necessary for the technologist to assume this responsibility, the radiologist will give specific instructions as to the information he desires.

The requisition received by the technologist should state both the exact region desired and the condition present or suspected. The patient must be positioned and the exposure factors selected according to both the region involved and the radiographic characteristics of the existent abnormality. These factors make it necessary for the technologist to have some knowledge of the rationale behind the examination, or it will not be possible for him to produce films of the greatest possible diagnostic value. Having the information in advance saves both the delay and the expense of reexamination, not to mention the inconvenience and, of far greater importance, the unnecessary radiation dosage, to the patient.

3. INITIAL EXAMINATION

The views the radiologist lists for the initial, or general survey, examination of each body part are based upon the anatomy and/or function of the part, and upon the nature of the abnormality indicated by the clinical history. The views utilized for the exploratory examination are usually held to the minimum number required to detect any demonstrable abnormality in the particular region. Supplemental studies for further investigation are then made as indicated. This method or routine of performing each examination is timesaving, eliminates the necessity of taking unrequired views, and at the same time reduces radiation exposure to the patient.

4. DIAGNOSIS AND THE TECHNOLOGIST

It is quite natural for the patient to be anxious about the result of his examination, and quite natural for him to ask questions. The technologist should tactfully advise him that his doctor will receive the report as soon as the radiologist has interpreted the films. Referring physicians are also prone to ask questions of the technologist. Again, do not discuss diagnostic problems; refer them to the radiologist. The technologist who tries to make diagnoses succeeds only in informing his audience that he is pretending to be what he obviously is not—a doctor.

5. ETHICS IN RADIOLOGIC TECHNOLOGY

Ethics is the term applied to the science of duty and right conduct toward others. The nature of the work requires that the rules of conduct in the medical profession be strict. The doctor, being responsible for the welfare of the patient, must be able to depend upon absolute honesty in his lay assistants in carrying out his orders, and in reporting any mistake immediately. The fundamental rules governing the conduct of lay assistants in the medical profession may be grouped under (a) conduct toward the patient, (b) conduct toward the doctor, and (c) conduct toward co-workers.

a. The technologist must keep the safety and comfort of the patient ever before him. He should avoid any display of irritation, no matter what the provocation; such displays merely lessen the technologist's influence with the patient. By remembering that a difficult patient's mental condition is probably such that he is not responsible for his actions, little effort will be required to handle him with tact and kindness. The technologist should at all times conduct himself with the dignity becoming a professional person. A well-modulated voice and a quiet manner create confidence and gain the patient's respect and cooperation. While the technologist must be pleasant and cheerful with his patients, he should do as little talking as possible without appearing to be unsympathetic or disinterested. It is impossible to keep up a running conversation and concentrate on the work being done.

b. The technologist must be loyal to his radiologist at all times, and carry out his instructions accurately, promptly, and courteously. He must be honest, conscientious, and obedient in performing the duties assigned to him. He should take care of the equipment, use supplies economically, and conduct himself in such a way that he will be an asset to the radiologist or the hospital employing him.

c. The technologist must extend his full cooperation to his fellow technologists, nurses, and other co-workers in performing the day's work. He should be cheerful and friendly with co-workers, but not familiar with them. No unnecessary conversation should be held within hearing of a patient, and certainly no discussion pertaining to another patient should take place.

6. CARE OF RADIOGRAPHIC EXAMINING ROOM

There is every reason why the radiographic examining room should be as scrupulously clean as any other room used for medical purposes. The mechanical parts of the x-ray machine, such as the table and tube stand, should be dusted with a clean, damp (not wet) cloth every day. The metal parts should be cleaned periodically with benzine and then polished with any good metal polish to protect the finish and keep it looking well. The overhead system, x-ray tube, and other parts that conduct electricity, should be cleaned with alcohol or a clean, dry cloth. Never use water to clean electrical parts.

Cones, compression devices, and other accessories should receive daily cleaning. The gummy substance left on cassettes and cassette stands by adhesive tape should be dissolved with benzine and then washed with alcohol or warm soapsuds. The film holders, cassettes and cardboards, should be protected from bleeding, ulcerated, or other exudative lesions by using waxed paper or plastic covers. Stained holders are both revolting and inexcusable.

Have the radiographic room prepared for the examination before bringing the patient into the room. Put fresh linen on the table and pillow, and have everything in its place so that the room will look clean and fresh, not disarranged from the previous examination. Select the accessories to be used with the examination and have them nearby. These duties require only a few minutes' time, but they create a lasting impression on the patient.

7. VENTILATION

In order to prevent air vitiation, keep the rooms well ventilated. There should be a change of air in the room two or three times an hour. Unless there is a mechanical ventilation system, arrange the windows and doors so there will be cross ventilation, but be careful not to have a draft. Open the windows from the top in very cold weather. An inch or two will be sufficient. The rooms must nevertheless be kept warm, and since patients must be lightly clad, the room temperature should be about 75° F. If the room cannot be kept warm enough with constant ventilation, take every opportunity to air it between patients. This is more important for the protection of the technologist's well-being than that of the patient, since the technologist is breathing the room air all day. Radioscopic rooms that are used for prolonged periods of time should be opened up and aired as often as possible, preferably every hour. Electrical ionization is added to the air-vitiating factors in these rooms.

8. ASEPTIC TECHNIQUE

Technologists are engaged in caring for the sick and should, therefore, be thoroughly familiar with aseptic technique. They should know how to handle patients who are on precaution or isolation without contaminating their hands, clothing, or apparatus, and should know how to disinfect these things when they do become contaminated. As one of the first steps in aseptic technique, the technologist should keep his hands smooth, free from roughness or chapping, by the frequent use of soothing lotions. Any abrasion should be protected by collodion or a bandage to prevent the entrance of bacteria. The hands should be washed frequently, after each patient if possible, and should be kept away from the face and head.

For the protection of the health of the technologist as well as that of the patient, the laws of asepsis and prophylaxis must be obeyed. Use scrupulous cleanliness in handling all patients whether they are known to have an infectious disease or not. If the patient's head, face, or teeth are to be examined, let him see you wash your hands. If this is not possible, at least do so and enter the room drying your hands on a fresh towel. Let the patient see you clean the cassette front with alcohol if his face is to come in contact with it, or cover it with a suitable paper.

Keep a sufficient supply of gowns and rubber or disposable plastic gloves in the radiology department to care for infectious patients, and, particularly when examining their teeth, wear gloves. When examining the teeth of an infectious patient, either wrap the film packets in waxed paper before placing them in the patient's mouth, or lay them on a paper towel as they are exposed and then wipe them with an alcohol sponge before taking them out of the room. After known or suspected infectious cases, the technologist should wash his hands in running warm water and soapsuds, immerce them in a disinfectant solution for two or three minutes, rinse them, dry them thoroughly, and then apply a soothing lotion. Where the washbasin is not equipped with a knee control for the water supply, the valve of the faucet should be opened through a paper towel when the hands are contaminated.

Before bringing isolation patients to the radiology department, the nurse drapes the stretcher or wheelchair with a clean sheet to prevent contamination of anything they might touch. When it is necessary to transfer these patients to the radiographic table, first drape it with a sheet. The edges of the sheet may then be folded back over the patient so that the technologist can position him through the clean side without becoming contaminated.

For the protection of the cassettes when using a non-Bucky technique, place a folded sheet over the end of the stretcher or table. The cassette is then placed between the clean fold of the sheet, and, with his hands between the clean fold, the technologist can position the patient through the sheet. If it is necessary for the technologist to handle the patient directly, an assistant should position the tube and operate the equipment to prevent contamination.

When the examination is finished, the contaminated linen should be folded with the clean side out and returned to the unit with the patient, where it will receive the special attention given to linen used for these patients. If this is not possible, place it in a "precaution hamper." If an infectious patient has been examined in an office, soak the contaminated linen in a 4% solution of carbolic acid for one hour before sending it to the laundry.

When pus, sputum, or other body discharge has been expressed, saturate the deposit with a 2% solution of phenol for thirty minutes and then wipe it up with disposable toweling or rags that can be burned.

9. ISOLATION UNIT

When doing bedside work in an isolation unit, report to the nurses' desk and obtain a gown, cap, mask, and, if necessary, rubber gloves. If more than one film is to be used, stand the additional cassettes on paper towels outside the patient's room. Take the machine into the room and manipulate it into position, being careful not to let it touch the bed. Put the cassette in a clean pillowcase (a clean case for each film used), and either have an assistant technologist who can do the contamination work of adjusting the cassette and patient, or ask for the assistance of a nurse who can do this work under direction. If it is not possible to have an experienced technologist to assist where the position is an exacting one, make the necessary adjustments on the control panel and tube, and operate the machine through a clean cloth, being careful not to let the contaminated side of the cloth come in contact with the equipment.

When the exposures have been finished, remove the mask, cap, and gown, place them in the precaution hamper, and wash and disinfect the hands before leaving the room. The cable of the x-ray machine, which has of necessity been on the floor, must be wiped with a disinfectant solution.

10. DISINFECTANT SOLUTIONS

Chemical substances that will kill pathogenic bacteria are classified as *germicides* or *disinfectants*. Chemical substances that inhibit the growth of, without necessarily killing, pathogenic germs, are called *antiseptics*. *Sterilization*, which is usually performed by means of heat, is the destruction of all germ life. Thus, sterilization calls for the killing of all microorganisms, while disinfection calls for the killing of only those that are pathogenic. The objection to many chemical disinfectants is that, in order to be effective, they must be used in solutions so strong that they damage the material being disinfected. The antiseptics and disinfectants commonly used in radiology departments are alcohol, bichloride of mercury, phenol, and Lysol. Alcohol has antiseptic but not disinfectant properties.

Bichloride of mercury (corrosive sublimate). Bichloride of mercury is an effective germicide, but it stains fabrics and wood and corrodes metals. Its use is therefore limited, for us, to the disinfection of glass, enamelware, and the hands. It will not penetrate through any fatty substance, so the hands must be clean and free of soap before being immersed in bichloride of mercury solution. A solution of 1:2,000 is the preferable strength; weaker solutions are only antiseptic. Bichloride of mercury usually comes in tablets of 7½ grains each. To make a 1:2,000 (1/20%) solution, use one tablet to one quart of water.

Phenol (carbolic acid). In solutions of a strength usually used, 2 to 5%, carbolic acid is not injurious to color, fabric, wood, or metal, and thus can be used safely to disinfect these things. Phenol usually comes in an 88% solution, which is exceedingly corrosive. In making weaker solutions, hot water should be added to the phenol a little at a time, and the bottle should be well shaken between additions so that the oily globules will be thoroughly dissolved. If they are not dissolved, they will burn any tissue with which they come in contact. If any of the crude carbolic acid should come in contact with the hands, pour alcohol over the areas at once. To make a 4% solution of phenol, use one part of phenol (88%) to twenty parts of water.

Lysol. The cresols, Creolin and Lysol, are less corrosive than carbolic acid and are more powerful germicides. They can be used for the disinfection of the same objects. Lysol is not only a very effective disinfectant, but also an excellent cleansing agent and deodorant. It is usually used in solutions of ½ of 1% to 2%. In making up cresol solutions, pour the water into the bottle first, and do not have it over 100° F. or it will weaken the strength of the solution. To make up to a 2% solution of Lysol, use 20 ml. of the 95% solution to 1 quart of water.

11. OPERATING ROOM

Carrying out aseptic technique is a fixed habit with nurses, but technologists who have not had nursing training must exercise constant watchfulness to avoid doing anything that will contaminate sterile objects in the operating room. It is advisable, after putting on a gown, cap, and mask, to step into the operating room to survey the particular setup before taking the x-ray machine in. By taking this precaution, the technologist can make sure that he will have sufficient room to bring the machine in and do his work without danger of contaminating anything. If necessary, ask the circulating nurse to move such items as the sterile-bowl stand. Because of the danger of contamination of the sterile field, of sterile supplies, or of persons who are scrubbed for the operation, the technologist should at no time approach the operative side of the table.

After the setup has been checked, take the x-ray machine in on the free side of the operating table, that is, the side opposite the surgeon, scrub nurse, and sterile layout. Maneuver the machine into a position that will make the final adjustments easy when the surgeon is ready for the filming. Needless to say, the x-ray machine should be thoroughly dusted with a damp (not wet) cloth before taking it into the operating room. The film holder is placed in a sterile pillowcase or in a sterile rubber glove, depending upon the type of examination to be done. The surgeon or one of his assistants will hold the sterile case open while the technologist gently drops the film holder into it, being careful not to touch the sterile case. The technologist may then give directions for placing, adjusting, and holding the film for the exposure.

The technologist should make the necessary arrangements with the operating room supervisor when doing work in the operating room that requires the use of a tunnel or a portable Potter-Bucky diaphragm. The cassette tunnel or grid should be placed on the table when it is being prepared for the patient, with the tray opening to the free side of the table. With the cooperation of the surgeons and operating room supervisor, a system can be worked out whereby radiographic examinations can be performed in the operating room accurately and quickly, without moving the patient and without endangering the sterile field. The technologist should be present when the patient is placed on the table for hip-pinning to see that the tunnel is properly adjusted and that the perineal post of the table will not interfere with the lateral projection when this type table is being used. The Danelius-Miller method of obtaining a lateral view of the hip is the most adaptable one in fracture cases, particularly in the operating room.

In radiographic examinations of an exposed kidney, the film should be cut to the size and shape of a kidney and wrapped in black paper held by a small tab of adhesive or cellophane tape. Here the work can be speeded up by the use of a small processing unit. Three 5-inch by 7-inch specimen jars fitted into a suitable container, and a flashlight covered with red or green waxed paper, work well. Any nearby closet can be used as a darkroom.

In most radiographic examinations in the operating room, because of the necessarily limited electrical output of mobile x-ray machines, it is advisable to sacrifice a fair amount of photographic contrast to speed by overexposing and underdeveloping standard films. For example, in hip-pinning work the surgeon is looking for structural outline and is not interested in great intrastructural detail. The films are being used as a guide in surgical procedure where speed is of greater importance than contrast. Where polaroid equipment is available, the films are ready for viewing in less than one minute.

12. MINOR SURGICAL PROCEDURE IN THE RADIOLOGY DEPARTMENT

Many procedures that require a rigid aseptic technique, such as cystography, intravenous kidney and gallbladder injections, spinal punctures, angiography and angiocardiography, are often carried out in the radiology department. While in certain of these procedures the radiologist needs the assistance of a nurse, the technologist can make the necessary preparations and give sufficient assistance in others. An emergency cart such as that described in the excellent article by Hunziker and Soule[1] ought to be available in every radiology department.

For the procedures that do not require a nurse, the technologist should know what surgical instruments and supplies are needed, and how to prepare and sterilize

them. It is advisable for nonnurse technologists to make arrangements with the surgical supervisor for the training necessary to equip them to carry out these procedures. Adequate training in both aseptic technique and dressings can be given in a comparatively short time. Usually six or eight hours of classwork and supervised practice are sufficient.

13. PROCEDURE BOOK

There should be a procedure book covering each specialized examination performed in the radiology department. Under the appropriate heading, each procedure should be outlined and should state the staff required and the duties of each member of the team, and there should be a listing of the sterile and nonsterile items. A copy of the sterile instruments required should be given to the supervisor of the central supply room to facilitate her preparation of the trays for each of the different procedures.

14. CLEANSING ENEMA

The cleansing enema is important in radiography in examinations of the abdominal region. In colon and gallbladder examinations it is necessary to clear the entire colon, and unless the enema is correctly administered, it will do little more than clean out the pelvic colon.

It is customary to use 1 quart of solution for an adult and about 1 pint for a child, unless otherwise ordered by the doctor. A normal saline solution, at a temperature of about 100° F., is usually used. Normal saline solution is preferred by most radiologists for radiographic purposes because, among other reasons, it is less irritating to the mucous membrane lining of the colon than soapsuds and therefore causes less lasting peristaltic action. The saline solution is prepared by using 1¾ teaspoonfuls of common table salt to 1 quart of water.

Have the patient turn on his left side and flex his knees to relax the abdominal muscles. Lubricate the rectal tube with a suitable jelly and, after running a little of the solution through the tube to clear it of air, gently insert the tip first slightly forward and then backward, following the natural curve of the rectum. Hold the enema can about 1 to 1½ feet above the patient's body and allow from ten to fifteen minutes for the solution to flow into the colon. After about half of the solution has been injected, have the patient turn onto his back for the last half of the injection, so that it will be distributed throughout the intestine. If the patient has cramps during the injection, discontinue the flow until the pain passes, and have him breathe deeply through his mouth. This helps to relax the muscles and ease the cramp. Have the patient retain the solution five or ten minutes, if possible, before expelling it. Patients who have been dehydrated frequently retain the enema, the fluid being absorbed to satisfy the needs of the body cells. In such cases, a second enema should be given.

After use, the rectal tube, tubing, and enema can should be cleansed by letting cold water run through and over them and then washing them with warm water and soapsuds before boiling them. Rubber should not be boiled for longer than three minutes. Allow the enema can and rubber tubing to drain before putting them away.

15. MOTION—ITS CONTROL

Motion plays a large role in radiography, and since motion is the result of muscle action, it is important that

[1]Hunziker, R. J., and Soule, A. Bradley: An emergency cart for the radiologic department, Amer. J. Roentgen. 78:134-136, 1957.

we know something of the function of muscles so that we can either eliminate or control motion for the period of time necessary for a satisfactory examination of the different regions of the body. There are three types of muscular tissue; smooth, cardiac, and striated. The first two types are classified as involuntary muscles, and the third as voluntary.

Involuntary muscles. The visceral muscles are composed of smooth muscular tissue and are controlled partially by their inherent characteristic of rhythmic contractility, and partially by the autonomic nervous system. By their rhythmic contraction and relaxation these muscles perform the movements of the internal organs. The rhythmic action of the muscular tissue of the alimentary tract, called peristalsis, is normally more active in the stomach (about three or four waves per minute) and gradually diminishes along the intestine. The specialized cardiac muscular tissue functions by contracting the heart to pump blood into the arteries, and by expanding or relaxing to permit the heart to receive blood from the veins. The normal rhythmic actions of cardiac muscular tissue are independent of nerve stimulus, and thus are said to be myogenic in origin, or to be an inherent characteristic of the muscle tissue. The phase of contraction is termed *systole*, and the phase of relaxation is termed *diastole*. One phase of contraction and one phase of relaxation, that is, a systole and a diastole, are called a complete cardiac cycle. The pulse rate of the heart varies with emotions, exercise, and food, as well as with size, age, and sex.

Involuntary motion is caused by the following:

Heart pulsation	Chills
Peristalsis	Tremor
Spasm	Pain

Control: Speed of exposure is the only recourse against involuntary motion.

Voluntary muscles. The voluntary, or skeletal, muscles are composed of striated muscular tissue, and are controlled by the central nervous system. These muscles perform the movements of the body initiated by the will. Each skeletal muscle has a name that was derived from either its position, shape, structure, action, direction, or points of attachment. Each muscle consists of a body, or belly, and two tendinous extremities for attachment.

The body of the muscle is made up of cylindrical fibers that are covered with a thin membrane and bound together into primary bundles called fasciculi. The covering sheaths of the individual fibers, the fasciculi, and that of the muscle are prolonged into round, fibrous cords called tendons, or into flattened tendons called aponeuroses. The tendons serve to attach the muscles to bone. When the muscle contracts, one end is moved toward the other. While most of the striated muscles can be made to act from either extremity, the less movable attachment is called the origin of the muscle, and the more movable is called the insertion. The contraction acts in the direction of the tendinous attachments.

The skeletal muscles never work singly. A combination of muscles is brought into play in any movement. One set acts as the prime movers; one set, called synergists, acts to inhibit movements not required; one set acts as fixation muscles in steadying the point from which the force is being applied; and, lastly, one set, the antagonists of the prime movers, relax to remove resistance to the action. In radiography, the patient's body must be positioned in such a way that the synergetic, antagonistic, and fixation

muscles can perform their part of the work, or the action of the prime movers will be hampered. The patient's comfort is a good index to the success of the position.

Voluntary motion due to lack of control is caused by the following:

Nervousness	Discomfort
Excitability	Mental illness
Fear	Age (child)

Control: Clear instructions, patient's comfort, and support and immobilization correctly applied and adjusted. Immobilization can often be obtained for the duration of the exposure by having the patient phonate an m–m–m sound with the mouth closed or an ah–h–h sound with the mouth open.

Note: The voluntary motion of the last two classifications, mental illness and age, can be controlled only by speed of exposure.

16. STRUCTURAL RELATIONSHIP IN POSITIONING

The position and relationship of the organs of the trunk vary considerably with the position of the body. The technologist must know not only the size, shape, position, and relationship of the organs when the body is in the anatomic position but also the change in the relationship when the body is moved from the erect to the recumbent position, and to the sitting position.

For example, the diaphragm lies in an oblique plane on a level with the sixth costal cartilage anteriorly, and with the tenth rib posteriorly when the body is erect. When the body is placed in the dorsal recumbent, or supine, position, the diaphragm is situated from 2 to 4 inches higher than when erect. The exact elevation depends upon the curvature of the spine and the pressure of the abdominal viscera and muscles. The elevation will be less in thin patients. When the body is placed in the ventral recumbent, or prone, position, the diaphragm will be from 2 to 4 inches lower than in the erect position due to relaxation of pressure from the abdominal viscera and muscles, and removal of the tilting caused by the spinal curvature. The depression of the diaphragm will be greater in thin patients.

When the body is placed in a seated position, the diaphragm assumes its lowest position due to lung pressure, relaxation of the abdominal muscles, and relaxation of pressure from the abdominal viscera. When the body is placed in a lateral recumbent position, the upper half of the diaphragm assumes a position lower than when seated, and the lower half assumes a position higher than when supine due to unequal pressure from the abdominal viscera. Here the two halves of the diaphragm cease to function in unison with breathing; the lower half has a greater excursion than the upper half. The original height of the diaphragm varies constantly during respiration. Its excursion between deep inspiration and deep expiration is approximately 1 inch, the right cupola having a slightly greater excursion than the left cupola.

The thoracic and abdominal viscera vary in location along with the diaphragm through all its movements. Likewise the anterior bony structures of the trunk vary in their relation to posterior structures as the position of the body is changed. For this reason, the surface landmark for any given body position cannot be relied upon when the body is placed in any position other than the one specified. Nor can surface landmarks be depended upon to hold for one position on all patients. Landmarks are based on the average, and while they are applicable to a majority of patients, they cannot be used where a patient's form varies considerably from the normal.

If all patients were average in size and shape, the technologist would have few problems. Since this is not the case, he must study anatomy from the standpoint of relationship and mechanics. With a reasonable knowledge of normal anatomy, the mechanics of body movement, and the usual deviations from the normal, the element of error in positioning is reduced to a minimum.

17. PREPARATION INSTRUCTIONS

When the examination is one that requires preparation, as in kidney and gallbladder examinations, instruct the patient carefully. Though the particular routine may be an "old story" to us, it is new to the patient. Frequently, apparent stupidity is really due to lack of sufficiently explicit directions. Be sure that the patient understands not only what he is to do but why he is to do it. Patients are more likely to follow instructions correctly if they see reason in them. If the instructions are complicated, write them out. Because few laymen know how to take an enema correctly, it is advisable to question the patient and, when necessary, take the time to explain the correct procedure to him. This will often save both a film and the time consumed in giving another enema in the radiology department.

18. PATIENT'S DRESS, ORNAMENTS, SURGICAL DRESSINGS

Have the patient dressed in a gown which, with the use of a sheet where necessary, will allow the region under examination to be exposed. *Never expose a patient unnecessarily.* Have only the area under examination uncovered, and be sure to cover the rest of the patient's body well enough to keep him warm. In examining parts that must be covered, be sure that the cloth used is cotton and that it is not starched; starch is somewhat radiopaque. Straighten out any folds in the cloth to prevent confusing shadows. It is well to remember that a material that will not cast a shadow on a heavy exposure, such as that used on an adult abdomen, will show clearly on a light exposure, such as that used on a child's abdomen.

Ask the patient to remove any ornament that is worn in the region to be examined or that might be projected into the region by central ray angulation. When examining the skull, be sure that *dentures, removable bridgework, earrings, and all hairpins are removed.*

Examine surgical dressings for radiopaque substances, such as metallic salves, oiled silk, and adhesive tape. If permission to remove the dressings has not been obtained, or if the technologist does not know how and the radiologist is not present, the surgeon or nurse should be asked to accompany the patient to the radiology department to remove them. When dressings are removed, always make sure that open wounds are adequately protected by a cover of sterile gauze.

19. LIFTING AND HANDLING PATIENTS

Unless the patient is an infant, a psychiatric patient or does not speak English, explain the procedure of his examination to him. See that he understands just what is expected of him, make him comfortable, and alleviate his fears if he is apprehensive about the examination. However, if the procedure is one that will hurt or be unpleasant, as in cystoscopy and intravenous injections, do not tell the patient that it will not hurt or be unpleasant. Explain the procedure calmly. Tell him that it will hurt a little or be unpleasant, as the case may be, but that since it is a necessary part of his examination his full cooperation is needed. If the patient sees that everything is being done for his comfort, he will usually respond favorably.

Because the whole procedure is new to him, the patient usually works in reverse when given more than one order at a time—that is, when he is instructed to get up on the table and lie on his abdomen, he will usually get onto the table in the most awkward possible manner and lay down on his back. Instead of asking him to get onto the table in a specific position, first have him sit on the table and then instruct him as to the position you wish him to assume. If he sits on the table first, he will be able to assume the position with less strain and with fewer awkward movements. *Never rush a patient.* If he feels hurried, he will be under a nervous strain and therefore unable to relax and cooperate. In moving and adjusting a patient into position, handle him gently but firmly. A too light touch can be quite as irritating as one that is too firm. Instruct the patient and let him do as much of the moving himself as possible.

Regardless of what part is being examined, the entire body must be adjusted in order to avoid muscle pull against the part being examined, with resultant motion or rotation. When the patient is in an oblique position, apply support and adjust it so that he is relieved of strain in holding the position. Use immobilization devices and compression bands whenever necessary, but not to a point of discomfort to the patient. Use care in releasing a compression band over the abdomen; it should be released slowly.

In making the final adjustments on a position, the technologist should stand with his eyes in line with the position of the focal spot, visualize the internal structures, and adjust the part accordingly. The rules of positioning are few and simple, and many repeat examinations can be saved by following them.

Great care must be exercised in handling casualty patients, particularly those who have skull, spinal, and long bone injuries. Because of the possibility of fragment displacement, any necessary manipulation should be performed by the surgeon or radiologist, never by the technologist. Adapt the positioning technique to the patient so that he may be moved as little as possible. If the tube-part-film *relationship* is maintained, the resultant projection will be the same regardless of their position.

When it is necessary to move a patient who is too sick to help himself, the following considerations must be kept in mind:

  a. In order to protect the patient, move him as little as possible.
  b. Never try to lift a helpless patient alone.
  c. In order to avoid straining the muscles of your back when lifting a heavy patient, flex the knees, straighten the back, and bend from the hips.
  d. When lifting a patient's shoulders, support his head. While holding the head with one hand, slide the opposite arm under the shoulders and grasp the axilla in such a way that the head can rest on the bend of the elbow when the patient is raised.
  e. When necessary to move the patient's hips, first flex his knees. In this position the patient may be able to raise himself. If not, it is easier to lift the body when the thighs are raised.

f. When a helpless patient must be transferred to the radiographic table from a stretcher or bed, he should be moved on a sheet by at least four, preferably six, people. Place the stretcher parallel to and touching the table. Two people should be stationed on the side of the stretcher, and two on the far side of the radiographic table to grasp the sheet at the shoulder and hip levels. One person should support the patient's head and another his feet. When the signal is given, all six should lift and move the patient in unison.

Many hospitals now have a specially equipped radiographic room adjoining the emergency receiving room. These units usually have a pedestal type of Potter-Bucky stand and stretchers with radioparent tops so that severely injured patients can be examined in the position in which they arrive. Where this ideal setup does not exist, the casualty patient is conveyed to the main radiology department, where he must be given precedence over non-emergency patients.

20. PREEXPOSURE INSTRUCTIONS

Instruct the patient in breathing, and practice with him until he understands exactly what he is to do. After he is in position, before leaving him to make the exposure, have him practice the breathing once more. This procedure requires a few minutes, but it saves much time and many films that would otherwise be spent on repeats. There are definite reasons for the phase of breathing used in examinations of the trunk. The correct phase and the reason for its use are given under the positioning instructions on each region within the trunk area.

Inspiration depresses the diaphragm and the abdominal viscera, lengthens and expands the lung fields, elevates the sternum and pushes it forward, and elevates the ribs and reduces their angle near the spine. Expiration elevates the diaphragm and the abdominal viscera, shortens the lung fields, depresses the sternum, and lowers the ribs and increases their angle near the spine.

Where exposures are to be made during breathing, have the patient practice slow, even breathing so that only the structures above the one being examined will move. When lung motion, but not rib motion, is desired, have the patient practice slow, deep breathing after the compression band has been applied across the chest.

21. FOUNDATION EXPOSURE TECHNIQUE

Specific exposure techniques are not included in this text. There are too many variable factors involved, not only from one department to another, but from one unit to another within the same department, for such techniques to have practical value. Only by familiarity with the characteristics of the particular equipment and accessories employed, and a knowledge of the radiologist's preference in film quality, can a satisfactory technique be established. The electrical output of the x-ray machine, the current-carrying capacity of the x-ray tube, the radiation characteristics (whether hard or soft), the filtration used, the type of films, the type of screens, the type of Potter-Bucky diaphragm, the cone sizes employed, and the type of developing solutions must all be taken into account in establishing the correct foundation technique for each unit. With these data available, the exposure factors can be selected for each region of the body and balanced in such a way that, with the least chance of motion of the patient and a reasonable latitude for conversion of exposure factors, they will produce films having the greatest possible amount of detail and a quality that meets the contrast-density standard preferred by the radiologist.

Although the quality of the radiograph depends upon many factors, the milliampere-second and kilovoltage factors primarily control contrast and density, while distance is one of the two primary factors controlling detail and magnification. The time of exposure is the primary factor controlling motion. The first step in balancing the exposure factors is the selection of the distance factor. The distance should be determined by the power output of the unit and the capacity of the tube. If the distance is too great on a unit of limited output, either the time of exposure must be long (in order to balance the factors), which will result in motion in a large percentage of cases, or the factors must be thrown out of balance. Cahoon[1] has made an exhaustive study of every phase of exposure techniques and has made his findings available in a book that is highly recommended.

22. ADAPTATION OF EXPOSURE TECHNIQUE TO PATIENT

Select the combination of exposure factors that produce the quality of film preferred by the radiologist for each region of the body on the normal, and standardize this quality. Once the standard quality is established, it is important that there be as little deviation from it as possible. The foundation factors should be adjusted to the individual patient so as to maintain uniform quality throughout the range of patients. However, correctly balanced factors cannot be expected to produce the same amount of detail on all subjects, any more than one combination of exposure factors can be expected to produce the same contrast-standard on all subjects. Just as some people are blond and others are brunet or redheaded, some patients will have fine, distinct trabecular markings and others will not. Congenital and developmental changes from the normal, age changes, and pathologic changes must all be reckoned with in judging the quality of the film.

In order to maintain uniform contrast it will be necessary to convert the exposure factors for patients who vary enough in size to require 10 kilovolts more or less than the average. The patient's ability to cooperate, his age, muscular development, excess fat, and the pathology must be considered in selecting the correct exposure factors for each subject.

The milliampere-second factor should be decreased with a comparable adjustment in kilovoltage for the following conditions:

a. Age (infants, children, and aged)
b. Emaciated adults
c. Aeration (emphysema, obstruction with distention)
d. Demineralization of bone (age, disuse, or pathology)

The milliampere-second factor should be increased with a comparable adjustment in the kilovoltage for the following conditions:

a. Excess fatty tissue
b. Edema
c. Fluid
d. Overdeveloped muscles
e. Advanced productive pathologic lesions that cause an excessive increase in the radiopacity of structures.

[1]Cahoon, John B. Jr.: Formulating x-ray techniques, ed. 6, Durham, N. C., 1965, Duke University Press.

23. IDENTIFICATION

The identification marker should include (1) the patient's name and/or history number or case number, (2) the date, and (3) the side marker, right or left. The importance of correct identification bears stressing and restressing. There is no instance where it is not important, but it becomes vital in comparison studies on follow-up examinations, and in medicolegal and compensation cases. It is well to develop the habit of rechecking the identification marker just before placing it on the film.

There are numerous methods of marking films for identification. They range all the way from the direct method of radiographing it along with the part, to "flashing" it onto the film in the darkroom before development, to writing it on the film after it has been processed and dried. The identification should be x-rayed onto the film along with the part, particularly where there is a large volume of work. This method reduces the chance of error to a minimum and eliminates the question of correct identification in medicolegal cases.

24. FILM PLACEMENT

The part is always centered to the center point of the film, or where the angulation of the central ray will project it there. The film should always be adjusted in such a way that its long axis will lie parallel with the long axis of the part being examined. Although having a long bone angled across the film does not impair its diagnostic value, such an arrangement presents a poor appearance.

Even though the lesion may be known to be at the mid-shaft area, use a film large enough to include one joint on all long bone studies. This is the only means of determining the position of the part and of localizing the lesion. Always use a film large enough to cover the region under examination, but not larger. In addition to being extravagant, large films include extraneous parts that detract from the appearance of the radiograph and, of greater importance, radiation dosage is delivered to unnecessary areas. Use a film small enough to exclude the foot on anteroposterior examinations of the ankle. When examining the abdominal area, flex the elbows and place the hands on the upper chest so that the forearms will not be in the exposure field.

The rule of "place the part as close to the film as possible" might better read "place the part as close to the film as possible for accurate anatomic projection." While there is greater magnification, less distortion is obtained by increasing the part-film distance in such examinations as lateral views of the middle and ring fingers so that the part will lie parallel with the film, and there is less structural distortion and superimposition if oblique views of the ribs are made with the injured side elevated. Magnification can be reduced in these examinations by increasing the focal-film distance to compensate for the increase in part-film distance. There are instances when gross magnification is desirable, and it is obtained by positioning and supporting the part exactly midway between the film and the focal spot of the tube. This procedure is known as *enlargement* or *magnification technique*.

For ease of comparison, bilateral examinations of small parts should be placed on one film. However, exact duplication of the location of the images on the film is difficult if the cassette or film holder is not accurately marked. Mark the holder face in half both longitudinally and transversely, and then mark the center point of each half. Where three

views are to be placed on one film, mark the holder face in half in the longitudinal direction, and in thirds in the transverse direction.

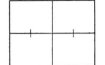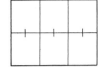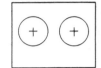

Where masks are used, it is advisable to mark the outline of the masks on the holder face. By doing this, the part can be accurately centered. After the exposures have been made, alternately covering each half of the film with a lead blocker, place the masks in position to protect the exposed areas, center the identification marker, and make an exposure just heavy enough to radiograph the marker onto the film and to blacken the background.

One word of caution on system at this point: the parts should always be placed on the film in the same manner, either facing or backing each other, according to the preference of the radiologist. The cassette should always be placed in the same manner, hinge-end to the technologist when crosswise to the part, hinge-end to the head end of the patient when lengthwise to the part. The identification marker (name or history number, date, and side indicator) should be placed so that it will read from left to right or from bottom to top of the film. For frontal projections it should face with the part; that is, it should face the tube for anteroposterior projections, and should face the film for posteroanterior projections. Even where the side markers (right and left) are radiographed onto the film with the patient, the screens should be marked in such a way that it will not be possible to make an error in side identification. Holman and Camp[1] have suggested that the letter F (lead) be mounted on the bakelite back behind the front screen so as to face the x-ray tube. The same method can be used with cardboard holders.

25. DIRECTION OF CENTRAL RAY

The central or principal beam of rays, simply referred to as the central or principal ray, is always centered to the film unless film displacement is being used for the inclusion of an adjacent area. The central ray is angled through the part:

a. When necessary to avoid the superimposition of overlying structures
b. When necessary to avoid stacking a curved structure on itself, such as the sacrum and coccyx
c. When necessary to project angled joints such as the knee joint and the lumbosacral junction
d. When necessary to project angled structures without foreshortening or elongation, such as the teeth, and a lateral view of the neck of the femur

The aim is to have the principal beam of rays at right angles to the structure, or, as in the case of the teeth, at right angles to the bisecting plane between the teeth and the film in order to project them with the least amount of distortion. Accurate positioning of the part and accurate centering of the principal ray are of equal importance in securing true structural projection.

[1]Holman, C. B., and Camp, J. D.: Identification of right and left sides in roentgenograms by a permanent cassette marker, Radiology **56**:260-263, 1951.

26. FOCAL-FILM DISTANCE

The rule of "use the greatest distance possible consistent with the electrical energy required" does not apply in all examinations. For example, in certain skull examinations, such as the mastoids and the paranasal sinuses, it is desirable to use a distance short enough to blur the detail of the opposite table of the skull in order to make the detail of the side being examined more visible. The sternum is another organ that is best demonstrated, in the oblique view, by using a short focal-film distance. A more accurate and inclusive rule to follow, therefore, might be "consistent with the electrical energy required, use the distance that will give the sharpest detail of the structure being examined."

A general rule for the placement of the tube might be "adjust the tube so that the central ray is at right angles to the structure and the focal-spot at a distance that will project the best definition of the structure."

27. DELIMITATION OF X-RAY BEAM

The beam of x-radiation must be so delimited as to irradiate only the area under examination. This restriction of the x-ray beam serves a twofold purpose. First, it minimizes the amount of radiation to the patient and reduces stray radiation toward any person who must hold the patient or who for some other reason must remain near the exposure field. Second, it serves the purpose of obtaining films showing clear structural delineation and optimal contrast, (a) by reducing stray radiation and thereby the blurring effect these rays have on structural outline, and (b) by preventing secondary radiation from being set up in unnecessarily exposed surrounding tissues, with resultant film fogging from this source.

The diameter of the beam of radiation is reduced to the required area through the use of x-ray-proof cones or of appropriately apertured sheet diaphragms or shutters that are constructed of lead or other metal that has high radiation absorption power. By so coning or diaphragming the beam, the peripheral radiation strikes and is absorbed by the intervening metal, while only the rays in line with the exit aperture are transmitted to the exposure field. Cones or diaphragms are placed immediately under the radiation window of the x-ray tube housing because their effectiveness depends upon their proximity to the tube target (the source of the divergent beam) as well as upon their power to absorb radiation.

Accurate collimation of a diverging beam of radiation depends upon adjusting its port of exit (diameter of the cone or of the diaphragm aperture) to the focal distance. The diaphragming device in radiographic collimators is in the form of rectangularly adjustable shutters, which permit close diaphragming of large areas because they coincide with the shape of the film. Rectangular diaphragms can be easily attached to circular cones, and it is important that this be done to the larger-sized cones. A further advantage of collimators is that they are equipped with a light-beam device that provides an ideal means for accurate centering and for visual restriction of the exposure field regardless of the focal-film distance.

Where cones are employed, each should bear a label listing the film area covered at each focal-film distance used. This information is calculated by dividing the focal-film distance by the sum of the focal-cone distance and the cone length and then multiplying this result by the distal diameter of the cone:

$$\frac{\text{Focal-film distance}}{\text{Focal-cone distance} + \text{Cone length}} \times \begin{array}{c} \text{Distal diameter} \\ \text{of cone} \end{array}$$

Example: With a distance of 5 inches between the focal spot and the upper aperture of the cone, the film area covered by a 3″ × 10″ cone at a focal-film distance of 36 inches $= \dfrac{36}{15\,(5+10)} = 2.4 \times 3 = 7.2$ inches.

Protection against ionizing radiation

Contributed by

William H. Shehadi, M.D., F.A.C.R.

Grasslands Hospital, Valhalla, N. Y.

There is much confusion and many unfounded beliefs in the minds of the public and among many persons in the medical profession as to the harmful effects and dangers of, as compared with the benefits derived from, the use of ionizing radiation. Judiciously and properly applied, radiation may be used to great advantage and is a source of blessing to the individual as well as to mankind as a whole. On the other hand, misguided, unintentional, or erroneous use of radiation can be a great hazard and a source of danger to the individual and to the race. No patient should be denied the great benefits derived from a radiologic examination that is needed for his or her welfare. The benefits are maximal when the examination is properly planned and carefully carried out, thus assuring the patient's safety. It is obvious, therefore, that the most important factors in maintaining high standards of radiation protection to all concerned are *good training, common sense, and experience.* Carelessness and ignorance may be the cause of serious injury. With the intelligent adoption of modern methods of protection, injury from ionizing radiation should be practically nil and the life expectancy should be normal. Thus, the average individual today enjoys a healthier and longer life because of the benefits derived from more accurate diagnosis and better treatment with the use of roentgen rays and other forms of ionizing radiation.

The standards and principles of radiation protection, the rules and regulations to be followed, and their practical application in a hospital department of radiology or the private office of a radiologist are the responsibility of the radiologist in charge, working in conjunction with a radiation physicist. On the other hand, it is the duty of the radiologic technologist to fully understand the rules and regulations pertaining to radiation protection, to be guided by them, and to follow them faithfully in his daily work.

A thorough understanding of these rules and regulations is of paramount importance, not only for the protection and safety of the technologist and of others working in the radiology department, but also for the protection of the patient. In addition, the technologist can allay the patient's unfounded fears and misconceptions and gain his confidence and wholehearted cooperation, which is of utmost importance in successfully concluding a radiologic examination or treatment.

IONIZING RADIATION

Ionizing radiation may come from natural or from man-made sources. Natural radiation is not new to man. Ionizing radiation from natural sources has surrounded— and bombarded—living matter for many thousands of years. It was part of man's normal environment long before the first appearance of man-made ionizing radiation through Roentgen's discovery of the roentgen ray in 1895.

Ionizing radiation has three natural sources. The first source is the presence of radioactive elements widely distributed in the earth, usually in small amounts but occurring in greater intensity where there are large deposits of uranium, radium, thorium, and other radioactive material. The distribution of these elements varies, and, similarly, background radiation varies from place to place. The second source is cosmic rays that originate outside the earth. These rays vary in intensity at various levels of the earth's surface, increasing at high altitudes as compared with sea level, where the intensity is lowest. The third source is the human body. Ionizing radiation from the human body (internal sources) comes from naturally existing radioactive isotopes within the body tissues, mainly potassium-40 (K^{40}) and carbon-14 (C^{14}).

Man-made, or artificial, radiation includes radiation arising from the medical uses of roentgen rays, radium, and radioactive isotopes. To this radiation is added a small additional exposure due to radioactive fallout.

Biologic effects

Ionizing radiation has a definite effect on living cells and tissues. The changes resulting from exposure to small doses may not become apparent; however, the lowest, or threshold, dose—at or below which no cell or tissue damage will occur—has not been determined and probably does not exist.

Although ionizing radiation has a definite effect on living cells and tissues, the extent of damage depends on the amount of radiation received at any one time and on whether a small or large portion of the body is exposed. A further factor is the degree of development (differentiation or nondifferentiation) of the cells. The more embryonic and less differentiated the cells, the more susceptible they are to the influence and effects of radiation. This applies particularly to the blood-forming organs and the gonads.

The effects of radiation on man are considered under somatic effects and genetic effects.

Somatic effects are of immediate importance to the individual and depend on exposure of the body tissues to ionizing radiation. The effect of small doses may be insignificant and may never become apparent. The immediate effect of large doses is cell death and tissue destruction. Over a period of time, radiation injury to the hematopoietic system results in leukopenia, anemia, and, later, leukemia. The delayed effects of radiation result in decreased resistance and increased susceptibility to disease, lowered fertility, acceleration of the process of aging, and shortening of the life-span.

Exposure of the eye to small doses of radiation may be without apparent ill effects. Exposure of the eye to large doses, as occurs in radiation therapy, may cause opacification of the lens and the development of cataract.

Genetic effects are the second important consideration. Radiation of germinal tissues results in changes in the genes, which is the heredity material contained in the chromosomes. Even small doses of radiation may produce some damage to the genes. The smallest dose of radiation that may not produce such damage is not known, and it is assumed that it does not exist. It is important to remember that such damage is irreversible and irreparable—even though it may not be overtly manifest or recognizable.

Damage to the genes may cause variations from the normal; these variations are known as mutations. The effect of small doses of radiation on the ovum or sperm is to increase the possibilities and varieties of mutations, eventually producing malformations in the offspring.

Ionizing radiation is not the only cause of mutation. Such agents as heat, chemical compounds, toxic material, and various infectious diseases, as well as factors yet unknown, can produce mutations; these agents exerted their influence in producing mutations long before the discovery and use of roentgen rays and other forms of ionizing radiation. Large doses or repeated small doses will result in decreased viability and even death of the sperm or ovum, and eventually in the absence of the sperm or ovum, with resultant sterility.

Based on knowledge so far gained, it is estimated that a total gonadal dosage of 14.3 r is allowed during the first thirty years of life. Of this dosage, it is estimated that 4.3 r come from natural background sources, 4.6 r from medical and dental sources, and 0.1 r from nuclear bomb fallout. This leaves a "safety margin" of several roentgens for future medical and dental examinations.

In pregnancy, maximum damage to the fetus occurs during the first three months. However, exposure of the fetus should be avoided throughout the period of pregnancy. Examination of the pregnant woman should be performed only when absolutely necessary.

RADIATION DOSE

The concept of a safe dose is difficult to define. Tolerance to radiation varies in different parts of the body and depends on whether a small part of the body or the entire body is exposed to a specified dose. The hand has a relatively high tolerance as compared with the gonads and the blood-forming organs.

The amount of radiation received by the parts examined, as well as by the gonads, varies with the type of procedure and the techniques used. The dosage is correspondingly increased as the examination or parts of it are repeated. This is especially true of angiographic procedures and of other examinations requiring multiple exposures, with or without radioscopy, such as examinations of the gastrointestinal tract, the urinary tract, the lumbar spine, and the pelvis. These examinations increase the gonadal dose appreciably.

Maximum permissible dose

Maximum permissible dose is considered to be the maximum dose that can be safely received by the individual over a prolonged period of time. Based on experience to date, a maximum permissible dose of 0.1 r a week, or 5 r a year, is considered safe and compatible with health,

apparent normal life, and longevity. According to our present state of knowledge, this dose is not expected to produce any appreciable genetic or somatic damage. This does not necessarily mean that a smaller dose may not prove to be injurious to the body nor that we should not strive for the smallest dose possible, thus attaining the *minimal* and not the maximal dose.

METHODS OF PROTECTION
Protection of the operator

Built-in, or fixed, factors. These factors are included in the initial planning and subsequent construction of the department. This is done in accordance with specific requirements as to the location of the department, the material used for construction, the thickness of the walls, the addition of lead lining to the walls and doors, and appropriate lead-glass windows in the doors and walls to permit observation of the patient by the operator and communication between them. The efficiency of these factors is checked by the radiation physicist, with the x-ray equipment in operation, in an attempt to detect radiation leakage due to structured defects.

Equipment. When the equipment has been newly installed, and after it has been checked by the manufacturer, a radiation physicist should calibrate the equipment and check it for radiation leakage. This check by a radiation physicist should be repeated at stated intervals during the lifetime of the equipment. Furthermore, equipment should be well taken care of and serviced frequently by the manufacturer or their representative; a so-called "preventive" service contract is indispensable.

Diagnostic procedures. The radiologist and the technologist should be outside the radiographic room while an exposure is being made. The lead-lined door should be closed during exposures.

Infants, acutely ill persons, and aged persons require special care and handling. Various commercially manufactured or homemade immobilizing devices may often be used to good advantage. Neither the radiologist nor the technologist should hold a patient or a cassette during a radiographic exposure. A member of the family, or an aide who does not work in the radiology department, should be present to hold the patient when immobilization devices cannot be used. It is important to ascertain beforehand that any woman rendering such help is not pregnant. It is preferred that such persons be past the childbearing age. These individuals should be provided with a protective lead apron and lead gloves, and it should be clearly explained to them that the dose of radiation they are likely to receive is infinitesimal and of no consequence to them. Persons rendering such help should be carefully instructed beforehand on what to do, so that the examination may be successfully completed without repeat exposures.

Lead aprons and gloves should be frequently checked by radiographic examination for the detection of any cracks or leaks.

Radioscopy. The technologist assisting the radiologist during a radioscopic examination of a patient should wear a lead apron and should stand behind the radiologist whenever possible, thus gaining the added protection of the radiologist and the apron he wears. Only persons whose help is absolutely necessary should be in the radioscopic room at the time of the examination.

Radiographic examinations in the operating room and at the bedside. The exposure switch on mobile units should be attached to a long cord so that the operator can stand at a distance that will enable him to escape scattered radiation. A cone should be attached to the tube head, and the cone (the central x-ray beam) should be directed toward the patient, away from the operator. Added protection to the operator is gained by the use of a lead apron. Technologists assigned to mobile work in the operating room and at the bedside should be rotated so that each assignment is limited to a period of two to four weeks.

Dental radiography. The same general precautions used in work with a mobile unit are applicable in dental radiography. The operator should stand away from the direction of the cone, and the unit should have a long cord so that the operator is at least 5 feet away from the patient and the x-ray tube head. It is strongly recommended that a movable lead screen be placed between the operator and the patient. Where there are several chairs in a dental clinic, the x-ray equipment should be attached to the chair nearest an outer wall and the x-ray beam aimed in that direction when an exposure is made.

Personnel monitoring. Personnel monitoring provides a reliable method of determining the radiation dose received by the worker. It is also an excellent way to determine the efficiency of the radiation safety measures used and of the working habits of the personnel.

A high reading calls for a reevaluation, careful checking and correction of the working habits of the personnel, and checking of equipment, walls, floors, etc. for radiation leakage. A record of minimal or low exposure gives the worker peace of mind and a sense of security. Personnel

Radiation received by the gonads*

Examination	Techniques		Target-film distance (in.)	Films per examination	Exposure dose per film	
	kv	ma-sec			Male (mR)	Female (mR)
Skull	65	125	36	4	0.2	0.05
Sinuses	80	100	30	4	0.2	0.05
Mastoid	70	100	30	4	0.2	0.05
Teeth						
Whole mouth	65	10	8	14	0.34	0.06
Bitewing	65	40	8	1	0.34	0.06
Others	65	10	8	1	0.34	0.06
Chest						
Straight	68	AT†	72	1	0.36	0.07
MM‡	83	24	36	1	0.25	0.15
Tomograph	62	50	48	6	6.2	0.9
Ribs, anteroposterior	65	100	36	1	0.48	0.16
Shoulder, anteroposterior	58	50	36	1	0.22	0.03
Spines						
Cervical						
Anteroposterior	58	100	36	1	0.27	0.06
Lateral	70	150	60	2	0.92	0.20
Dorsal						
Anteroposterior	62	200	36	1	8	11
Lateral	68	200	36	1	13	2.1
Lumbar						
Anteroposterior	68	200	36	1	24	227
Lateral	72	500	36	1	26.6	86
Anteroposterior	120	20	36	1	6	40
Lateral	120	60	36	1	7	16
Lumbosacral joint						
Anteroposterior	80	300	36	1	22	220
Lateral	120	350	36	1	15	800
Sacroiliac joint, anteroposterior	63	200	36	1	57	180
Pelvis, anteroposterior	65	100	36	1	1100	210
Hips, anteroposterior	68	200	36	1	710	210
Abdomen, anteroposterior	72	100	36	1	69	200
Intravenous pyelography, renal	72	100	36	3	69	200
Intravenous pyelography, bladder	72	100	36	3	93	230
Gallbladder, posteroanterior	70	150	36	3	0.6	5.2
Abdomen, obstetrics	80	150	36	1	—	260
Pelvimetry						
Oblique, anteroposterior	120	200	36	1	—	240
Lateral	120	100	36	1	—	840
Fingers, wrist, and elbow	58	25	36	2	0.13	0.026
Knee, tibia, and fibula	67	50	36	2	3	0.55
Foot and ankle	62	25	36	2	0.62	0.012
Barium meal	70	360	24		20	9
Barium enema	70	360	30		40	20

*Based on data from Stanford, R. W., and Vance, J.: Brit. J. Radiol. 28:266-273, 1955; from Braestrup, C. B., and Wyckoff, H. O.: Radiation protection, Springfield, Ill., 1958, Charles C Thomas, Publisher.
†Automatic timing.
‡Photofluorography.

monitoring is best accomplished by the use of film badges, pocket ionization chambers, or pocket dosimeters. These devices should be carried over the part of the body most likely to receive the highest radiation during the routine work, usually at the level of the left lapel of a coat. In special situations one or more monitors may be placed on different parts of the body at the same time.

Commercially available film badge service has been quite dependable. The advantages of this service are that the monitoring is done outside the department and that a permanent record is available.

The use of pocket dosimeters and ionization chambers makes it possible to obtain a direct reading at any time, but there is no permanent record. Their use is therefore best limited to special situations.

PROTECTION OF THE PATIENT

It hardly seems necessary to emphasize the importance of the technologist's gaining the patient's full cooperation and confidence and of assuring his comfort and safety. These are prerequisites for a successful examination and for obviating the necessity of repeating the examination and of giving additional radiation exposure to the patient.

The equipment used should be in good operating condition, free of structural defects, and inspected and calibrated by a radiation physicist. Modern shock-proof equipment is free of the hazards of electrical shock. Protection

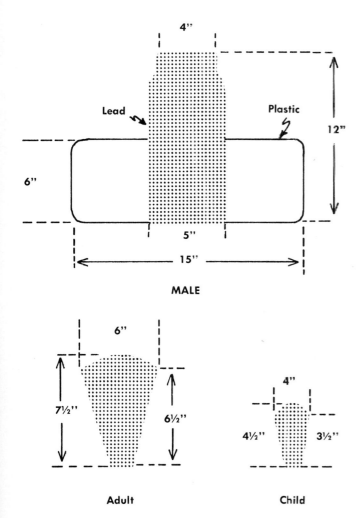

MALE

FEMALE

of the patient against radiation is best assured by observing the following:

1. Filtration. The total filtration in the path of the useful beam should be equal to at least 2 mm. Al.

2. Diaphragms, cones, and collimators. Properly attached and correctly aligned, these should be used for the purpose of limiting the useful x-ray beam to the smallest field size required to include the area of interest on the film. The size of the exposure field should be smaller than the size of the film, providing a peripheral margin of the film that is unexposed and clear.

3. Technique charts. These charts should be carefully prepared and followed so that films of optimal diagnostic quality are obtained with the first exposure. This eliminates the necessity of repeating films. Repetition of the examination doubles the radiation dose to the patient.

4. The use of high-speed screens and high-speed films.

5. The use of the maximum focal-film distance that is feasible and practical for the examination.

6. The use of relatively higher kilovoltage and lower milliampere-second factors.

7. The use of an automatic timer to terminate the exposure at a preset exposure time.

8. The use of shields to the gonads. The amount of radiation received by the gonads from routine radiographic examinations is well brought out in the accompanying table. The gonads, therefore, should be well protected with an appropriate lead shield, provided that the shield does not obscure the area of primary interest when this area is within the bony pelvis.

Appropriate shields containing at least 1 mm. of lead may be obtained commercially or may be made in the department. They may be cut to a specific pattern (see diagrams) as recommended by Ardran and Kemp and by Abram and co-workers. Shields will not protect the gonads from scattered radiation, but they do protect them almost completely from the primary x-ray beam. This results in marked reduction of the gonadal dose.

9. In the childbearing age of the female, the possibility of an early pregnancy that is not yet known to the patient should always be considered. Therefore, radiographic examinations, particularly those which may include the area of the bony pelvis, are best done during the first half of the menstrual cycle. No pregnant woman should be radiographed, especially in the region of the abdomen and pelvis and particularly during the first trimester, unless it is absolutely necessary to do so. Should an examination of the chest, extremities, or skull be necessary, the abdomen and pelvis should be shielded by a lead apron during the radiographic exposures.

REFERENCES

Abram, E., Wilkinson, D. M., and Hodson, C. J.: Gonadal protection from x-radiation for the female, Brit. J. Radiol. **31**:335-336, 1958.

Ardran, G. M.: Dose reduction in diagnostic radiology, Brit. J. Radiol. **30**:436-438, 1957.

Ardran, G. M., and Crooks, H. E.: Gonad radiation dose from diagnostic procedures, Brit. J. Radiol. **30**:295-297, 1957.

Ardran, G. M., and Kemp, F. H.: Protection of the male gonads in diagnostic procedures, Brit. J. Radiol. **30**:280, 1957.

Braestrup, C. B.: Past and present radiation exposure to radiologists from point of view of life expectancy, Amer. J. Roentgen. **78**:988-992, 1957.

Braestrup C. B., and Wyckoff, H. O.: Radiation protection, Springfield, Ill., 1958, Charles C Thomas, Publisher.

International Commission on Radiological Protection: 1954 Recommendations, Brit. J. Radiol., supp. 6, 1955.

International Commission on Radiological Protection, and International Commission on Radiological Units and Measurements: Exposure of man to ionizing radiation arising from medical procedures: an inquiry into methods of evaluation, Phys. Med. Biol. 2:107-151, 1957.

Laughlin, J. S., Meurk, M. L., Pullman, I., and Sherman, R. S.: Bone, skin, and gonadal doses in routine diagnostic procedures, Amer. J. Roentgen. 78:961-982, 1957.

Lincoln, T. A., and Gupton, E. D.: Radiation dose to gonads from diagnostic x-ray exposure, J.A.M.A. 166:233-239, 1958.

Merriam, G. R., Jr., and Focht, E. F.: A clinical study of radiation cataracts and the relationship to dose, Amer. J. Roentgen. 77:759-785, 1957.

Merriam, G. R., Jr., and Focht, E. F.: Radiation dose to the lens and adjacent structures: possibilities of cataract formation, Radiology 71:357-369, 1958.

National Bureau of Standards Handbook 60: X-ray protection, report of NCRP, Washington, D. C., 1955, U. S. Government Printing Office.

Russell, L. B., and Russell, W. R.: Radiation hazards to embryo and fetus, Radiology 58:369-377, 1952.

Stanford, R. W., and Vance, J.: The quantity of radiation received by the reporoductive organs of patients during routine diagnostic x-ray examinations, Brit. J. Radiol. 28:266-273, 1955.

Tievsky, G.: Ionizing radiation and a sense of proportion, J.A.M.A. 166:1667-1672, 1958.

Trout, E. D., Kelley, J. P., and Cathey, G. A.: Use of filters to control radiation exposure to the patient in diagnostic roentgenology, Amer. J. Roentgen. 67:946-962, 1952.

BODY PLANES AND POSITIONS

The *anatomic position* of the body is erect, with the arms at the sides and the palms turned forward. Many of the terms established to describe location or position of parts are based on this body position. Following are the three fundamental planes of the body:

1. The *median sagittal plane* passes vertically through the midline of the body from front to back, dividing it into equal right and left portions. Any plane passing through the body parallel with the median sagittal plane is termed a sagittal plane.

2. The *mid-coronal*, or *mid-frontal*, *plane* passes verti-

cally through the mid-axillary region of the body and through the coronal suture of the cranium at right angles to the median sagittal plane, dividing the body into anterior, or ventral, and posterior, or dorsal, portions. Any plane passing vertically through the body from side to side is called a coronal, or frontal, plane.

3. A *transverse*, or *horizontal*, *plane* passes crosswise through the body at right angles to its longitudinal axis, and to the sagittal and coronal planes, dividing it into superior, or cranial, and inferior, or caudal, portions. Any plane passing through the body at right angles to its longitudinal axis is called a transverse, or horizontal, plane.

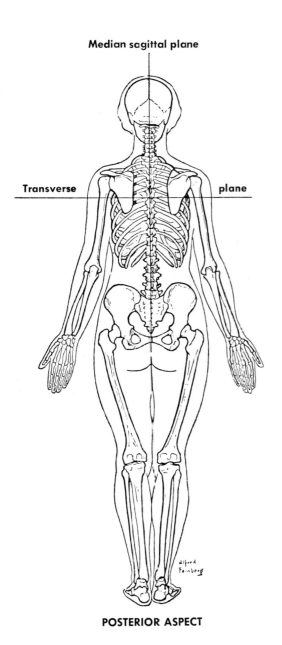

POSTERIOR ASPECT

LATERAL ASPECT

THE JOINTS

The bones of the skeleton are joined together by ligaments, capsules, cartilages, or the dovetailing of bone, as in the sutures of the cranium. The joints, or articulations, are classified according to their movability. The three main classes are as follows:

1. *Synarthrosis* is the term applied to immovable joints. The opposing surfaces of the bones forming these joints are separated only by a thin layer of fibrous tissue or by a layer of cartilage. Epiphyseal articulations are considered synarthrodial joints, and with the exception of the mandible, the articulations of the skull are synarthrodial joints. The latter are called *sutures*.

2. *Amphiarthrosis* is the term applied to joints having limited motion. The articular surfaces of the bones are connected by disks of fibrocartilage, as between the vertebral bodies, the pubes, and the sacroiliac joints, or by fibrous bands, as in the lower tibiofibular articulation.

3. *Diarthrosis* is the term applied to freely movable joints. Here the articular surfaces of the bones are reciprocally shaped for the movement required of the joint, are covered by articular cartilage, and are enclosed in a fibrous envelope called a capsule. The capsule consists of two layers of tissue—an outer fibrous layer and an inner fluid-secreting layer called synovial membrane. In certain joints, an articular disk, or meniscus, is interposed between the articular cartilages to give further protection to the joint. The greatest number of the articulations of the body are diarthrodial joints. The articulations of the extremities, the mandible, and between the vertebral arches are examples of diarthrodial joints.

Depending upon the shape of the articular surfaces of the contiguous bones, four kinds of movement are possible in diarthrodial joints. These movements are circumduction, rotation, angular, and gliding, and they are combined in many of the body actions to produce the great variety of movements.

Where the joint action is such that muscles or tendons slide over underlying parts, fluid-containing sacs called *bursae* are interposed between the sliding surfaces to prevent friction. Bursae are lined with synovial membrane. Important bursae are located at such joints as the shoulder, the elbow, the hip, and the knee, and under such muscles as the deltoid and the trapezius.

ANATOMIC PROJECTIONS AND DEPRESSIONS

Projections are processes that extent beyond or jut out from the main body of a structure, and are designated by the following terms:

Protuberance or **process** general terms for a projection

Tubercle a small, rounded process.

Tuberosity a large, rounded process.

Trochanter either of the two large, rounded processes (greater, or major, and lesser, or minor) located at the junction of the neck and shaft of the femur.

Condyle a rounded projection at an articular extremity.

Epicondyle a projection above a condyle.

Head the expanded end of a long bone.

Coracoid or **coronoid** a beaklike process.

Malleolus a club-shaped process.

Styloid a long, pointed process.

Spine a sharp projection.

Crest a ridgelike projection.

Facet a small, smooth-surfaced process for articulation.

Depressions are hollow, or depressed, areas, and are described by the following terms:

Groove a shallow, linear depression.

Fissure a cleft or groove.

Sulcus a furrow, trench, or fissurelike depression.

Fossa a pit, fovea, or hollow.

Foramen a hole in a bone for the transmission of blood vessels and nerves.

Sinus a recess, groove, cavity, or hollow space:

1. A recess or groove in bone, as used to designate a channel for venous blood on the inner surface of the cranium.

2. An air cavity in bone, or hollow space in other tissue. Used to designate a hollow space within a bone as in the paranasal sinuses.

3. A fistula, or suppurating channel in soft tissues.

PART LOCATION AND POSITION

Following are the standard terms used to describe part location or position:

Anterior and **ventral** refer to the forward part of the body, or to the forward part of an organ. The superior surface of the foot is referred to as the **dorsum** or the **dorsal** surface.

Posterior and **dorsal** refer to the back part of the body, or to the back part of an organ. The inferior surface of the foot is referred to as the **plantar** surface or the **sole**.

Superior, cranial, and **cephalic** are terms used to designate parts toward the head end of the body.

Inferior and **caudal** refer to parts away from the head end of the body.

Medial and **mesial** refer to parts toward the median plane of the body, or toward the middle of a part; opposite of lateral.

Lateral refers to parts away from the median plane of the body, or away from the middle of a part, to the right or the left.

Central refers to the mid-area, or main part, of an organ.

Periphery and **peripheral** refer to parts away from the central mass of an organ and toward its outer limits.

Internal refers to deep structures, those near the center of a part.

External refers to superficial structures, those near the periphery, or outer limits, of a part.

Proximal is the term used to designate nearness to source, or beginning, of a structure, generally used in describing the upper part of an extremity.

Distal is the term used to designate the part away from the source, or beginning, of a structure, generally used in describing the lower part of an extremity.

Parietal refers to the walls of a cavity.

Visceral refers to the organs contained within a cavity.

BODY POSITIONS

The terms used to describe body position are as follows:

Supine lying on the back.

Prone lying face down.

Recumbent or **decubitus** lying down.

Dorsal recumbent supine.

Ventral recumbent prone.

Lateral recumbent lying on the side.

Supinate to turn the arm so that the palm of the hand faces forward.

Pronate to turn the arm so that the palm of the hand faces backward.

Evert or **eversion** to turn outward.

Invert or **inversion** to turn inward.

Flexion a bending movement of a joint whereby the angle between the contiguous bones is diminished; also, a forward bending movement; opposite of extension.

Extension the straightening of a joint; the stretching of a part; also, a backward bending movement; opposite of flexion.

Abduction movement of a part away from the central axis of the body.

Adduction movement of a part toward the central axis of the body.

Decubitus (L *decumbere* to lie down) the act of, and the position assumed in, lying down. The position assumed is described according to the dependent surface: **dorsal decubitus,** lying on the back (supine); **ventral decubitus,** lying face down (prone); **left lateral decubitus,** lying on the left side; **right lateral decubitus,** lying on the right side. These terms are used in radiography to specify the position of the body for *horizontal ray projections*, particularly for those made for the demonstration of air-fluid levels in the chest and abdomen. Thus, a dorsal or ventral decubitus projection denotes a horizontally projected *lateral view* made with the patient lying on the specified posterior or anterior body surface; a left or right lateral decubitus projection denotes a horizontally projected *frontal view* (A.P. or P.A.) made with the patient lying on the specified side

Anatomy and positioning
of the
upper extremity

The upper extremity

For purposes of study anatomists divide the bones of the upper extremities into four main groups: the hand, the forearm, the arm, and the shoulder girdle. The upper end of the arm and the shoulder girdle will be discussed in another section.

THE HAND

The hand consists of twenty-seven bones that are subdivided into three groups: the phalanges, or bones of the fingers; the metacarpus, or bones of the palm; and the carpus, or bones of the wrist.

Fingers. The fingers are both numbered and named; however, the description by number is the more correct terminology. Beginning at the lateral side, the numbers and names are the first finger, or thumb; the second, or index finger; the third, or middle finger; the fourth, or ring finger; and the fifth, or small finger. There are fourteen phalanges in the fingers—two in the thumb and three in each of the other fingers. The phalanges of the first finger are described as first and second, or as proximal and distal. Those of the other fingers are described as first, second, and third, or as proximal, middle, and distal. The phalanges

consist of a cylindrical shaft and two articular ends, and are slightly concave anteriorly. The distal phalanges are small and flattened, and have a roughened rim around their distal anterior end, which gives them a spatular appearance. The interphalangeal articulations are diarthrodial joints of the hinge type, having only forward and backward movement.

Palm. There are five metacarpals, corresponding in position to the palm of the hand. The metacarpals are simply numbered one to five, beginning at the lateral, or thumb, side of the hand. The metacarpals consist of a body, or shaft, and two articular ends. They are cylindrical in shape and are slightly concave anteriorly. They articulate with the phalanges at their distal ends and with the carpus at their proximal ends.

With the exception of the thumb, the metacarpophalangeal articulations are diarthrodial joints of the condyloid type, having the movements of flexion, extension, abduction, adduction, and circumduction. In addition to these movements the thumb has axial rotation, which places it in the saddle joint classification.

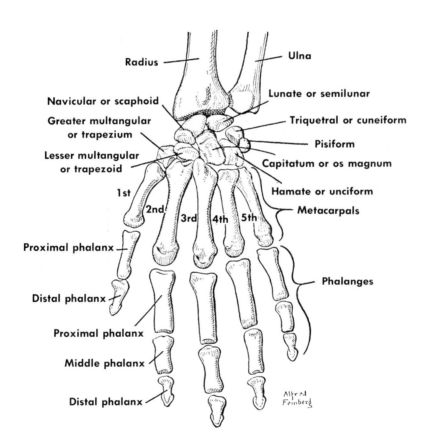

POSTERIOR ASPECT OF HAND AND WRIST

THE WRIST

There are eight carpal bones in the wrist. They are fitted closely together and arranged in two transverse rows. With one exception, each of these bones has two names, both in common usage. The names of those in the proximal row, beginning at the lateral, or thumb, side, are the navicular, or scaphoid; the lunate, or semilunar; the triquetral, or cuneiform (also called the triangular); and the pisiform. In the distal row, beginning at the lateral side, are the greater multangular, or trapezium; the lesser multangular, or trapezoid; the capitatum, or os magnum (also called the capitate); and the hamate, or unciform. The carpals are composed largely of cancellous tissue with an outer layer of compact bony tissue. They are classified as short bones. The carpals articulate with each other, with the metacarpals, and with the radius of the forearm.

In the carpometacarpal articulations, the first metacarpal and the greater multangular form a saddle type of joint, which has great freedom of movement, while the articulations between the second, third, fourth, and fifth metacarpals and the lesser multangular, capitatum, and hamate form gliding joints of limited movement. The midcarpal articulations allow free flexion and extension and slight rotation. The radiocarpal articulation, which is considered the wrist joint proper, is a diarthrodial joint of the condyloid type, which has all movements except rotation.

The dorsal surface of the articulated carpals is convex. The volar surface is concave from side to side, and the groove formed by the concavity is called the carpal sulcus (also carpal canal and carpal tunnel).

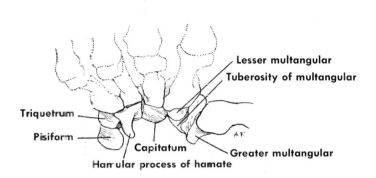

INFEROSUPERIOR ASPECT OF CARPAL CANAL

THE FOREARM

There are two bones in the forearm, the radius and the ulna. Like other long bones, the radius and ulna each consists of a shaft and two articular extremities. The ulna lies on the medial side of the forearm parallel with the radius, which lies on the lateral, or thumb, side.

Ulna. The shaft, or body, of the ulna is long and slender and tapers downward. Its upper extremity is large and presents two beaklike processes and two concave depressions. The upper process, the olecranon, is curved forward and slightly downward, and forms the proximal part of the semilunar notch. The lower, or coronoid, process projects forward from the anterior surface of the shaft to form the lower part of the semilunar notch. The coronoid is triangular in shape and curves slightly upward.

The semilunar notch, which is formed by the smooth, concave surfaces of the olecranon and coronoid processes, articulates with the trochlea of the humerus by a hinge joint. On the lateral side of the coronoid process there is a depression, the radial notch, for articulation with the disklike head of the radius.

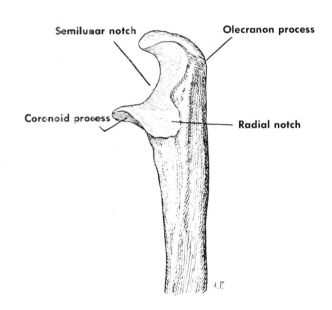

RADIAL ASPECT OF UPPER END OF ULNA

The lower end of the ulna has a rounded process on its lateral side, termed the head of the ulna, which articulates with the lower end of the radius. On its posterior medial side there is a slender conical projection called the styloid process. The head of the ulna is separated from the wrist joint by an articular disk.

Radius. The upper end of the radius is small and presents a flat, disklike head above a constricted area called the neck. Just below the neck, on the medial side of the shaft, is a roughened process called the radial tuberosity. The lower end of the radius is broad and flattened, and has a conical projection on its lateral surface termed the styloid process.

The head of the radius articulates with the capitellum of the humerus above, and with the radial notch of the ulna at the side. The lower end of the radius articulates with the carpus below, and with the head of the ulna at its median side. Both the superior and inferior radioulnar articulations are diarthrodial joints of the pivot type. The movements of supination and pronation of the forearm and hand are largely the result of the combined rotary action of these two joints. In the act of pronation, the radius turns medialward and crosses over the ulna at its upper third, while the ulna makes a slight counterrotation, which obliques the humerus by rotating it medialward.

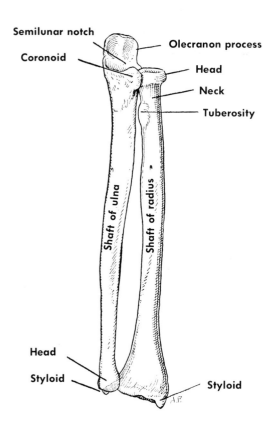

ANTERIOR ASPECT OF RADIUS AND ULNA

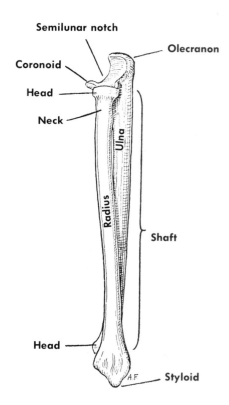

LATERAL ASPECT OF RADIUS AND ULNA

THE ARM

The arm has but one bone, the humerus, which consists of a shaft, or body, and two articular extremities. The shaft is long and cylindrical in shape. The upper extremity of the humerus will be considered with the shoulder girdle. The lower extremity is broad and flattened and presents numerous processes and depressions. It has medial and lateral condyles, and medial and lateral epicondyles. On its inferior surface are two smooth elevations for articulation with the bones of the forearm, the trochlea on the medial side for articulation with the ulna, and the capitellum on the lateral side for articulation with the flattened head of the radius.

On the anterior surface, just above the trochlea, there is a shallow depression called the coronoid fossa for the reception of the coronoid process when the elbow is flexed. Immediately behind the coronoid fossa, on the posterior surface, is the olecranon fossa, which is a deep depression for the accommodation of the olecranon process when the elbow is extended.

The articulation between the humerus and the ulna is a hinge type of joint, allowing forward and backward movement only. The elbow joint proper includes the superior radioulnar articulation as well as the articulations between the humerus and the radius and ulna. The three joints are enclosed in a common capsule.

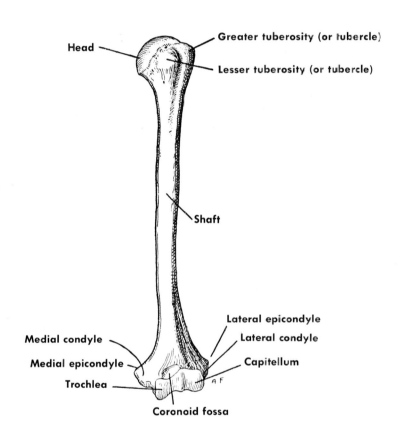

ANTERIOR ASPECT OF HUMERUS

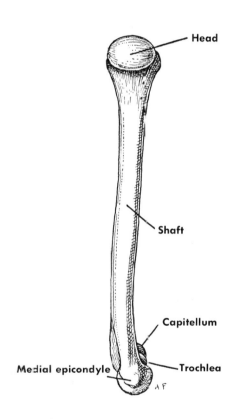

MEDIAL ASPECT OF HUMERUS

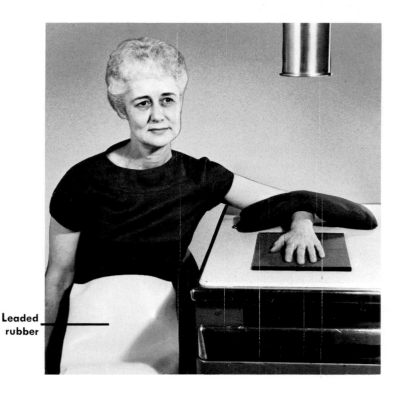

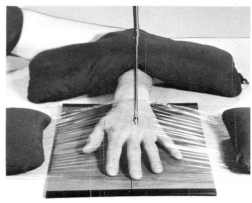

Leaded
rubber

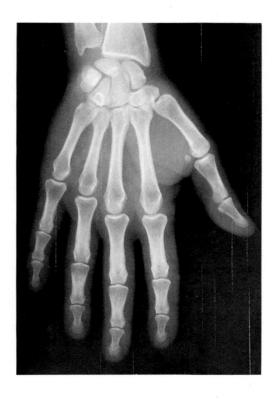

UPPER EXTREMITY

When radiographing the upper extremity, seat the patient at either the side or the end of the table in such a way that it will not be necessary for him to assume a strained or uncomfortable position. Place the film holder at a location and angle that will allow the patient to be positioned most comfortably. Since the degree of immobilization is limited, particularly of the hand and fingers, it is important that the patient be comfortable so that he can relax and cooperate in maintaining the position.

The central ray, unless otherwise specified, is directed at right angles to the midpoint of the film. The joint spaces of the extremities are narrow. Accurate centering is essential in order to avoid obscuring them. When a bilateral examination is requested of the hands and/or wrists, *each side should be correctly, separately positioned.* This is for the purpose of preventing rotation distortion, particularly of the joint spaces, as happens when both sides are placed on the film for simultaneous projection.

The gonadal area should be shielded from scattered radiation with a sheet of lead-impregnated rubber placed as shown in the adjacent photograph.

HAND
Posteroanterior projection
Anteroposterior view
Film: 8″ × 10″ for hand of average size.

Position of part

Have the patient rest his forearm on the table and place his hand on the film holder with the palmar surface down. Center the film to the metacarpophalangeal joints, and adjust it so that the long axis of the film is parallel with the long axis of the hand and forearm. Spread the fingers only slightly.

Ask the patient to relax his hand so as to avoid motion. Place a sandbag across the forearm just above the wrist. Involuntary movement can be prevented by stretching a strip of plastic wrap tautly across the hand and securing it in position with sandbags.

Central ray

Direct the central ray vertically to the third metacarpophalangeal joint.

Structures shown

A posteroanterior projection of the carpals, the metacarpals, and the phalanges (except of the thumb), the interarticulations of the hand, and the lower ends of the radius and ulna. This position demonstrates an oblique view of the first finger.

NOTE: When the metacarpophalangeal joints are the point of interest and the patient cannot extend his hand enough to place its palmar surface in contact with the film holder, reverse the position of the hand for an anteroposterior projection. This position is also used for the metacarpals when, due to injury, pathology, or dressings, the hand cannot be extended.

HAND
Lateral in flexion
Film: 8″ × 10″ lengthwise.

Position of part

Ask the patient to rest his forearm on the table and to place his hand on the film with the ulnar aspect down. Center the film holder to the metacarpophalangeal joints and adjust it so that its midline is parallel with the long axis of the hand and forearm.

With the patient relaxing his fingers so that the natural arch of the hand is maintained, arrange them so they are perfectly superimposed. Support the thumb on a cork or a loofah sponge. Immobilize by placing a sandbag across the lower forearm.

Central ray

Direct the central ray vertically to the metacarpophalangeal joints.

Structures shown

A lateral view of the bony structures and soft tissues of the hand in their normally flexed position.

This view is used to demonstrate forward or backward displacement in fractures of the metacarpals. The exposure should be heavy enough to show the outline of each bone clearly through the superimposed shadows of the other metacarpals. Depending upon the width of the hand, this requires from 12 to 16 kilovolts more than the postero-anterior projection.

Fiolle[1,2] was the first to describe a small bony growth occurring on the dorsal surface of the third metacarpocarpal joint. He termed the condition "carpe bossu," or carpal boss, and found that it could be demonstrated to best advantage in a lateral view with the wrist in palmar flexion.

[1]Fiolle, J.: Le "carpe bossu," Bull. Soc. Chir. Paris **57**:1687, 1931.
[2]Fiolle, J., and Ailland: Nuovelle observation de "carpe bossu," Bull. Soc. Chir. Paris **58**:187-188, 1932.

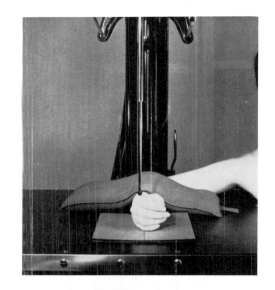

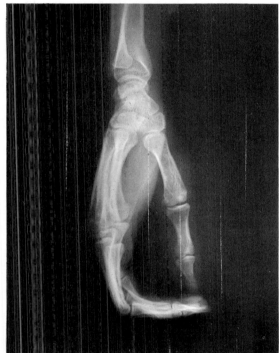

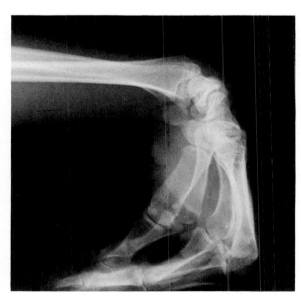

Normal wrist.

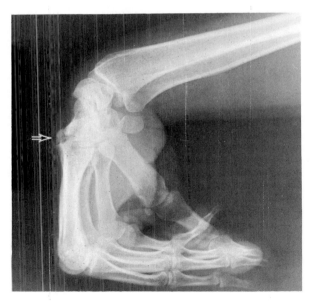

Carpal boss.

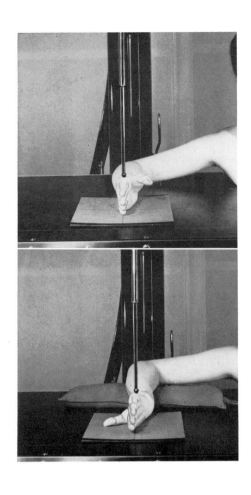

HAND
Lateral in extension

Film: $8'' \times 10''$ for hand of average size.

Position of part

Have the patient completely extend his fingers, with the thumb at right angles to the palm and his hand on the film holder, with either the radial or the ulnar aspect down, as indicated. If the elbow is elevated, support it in position with sandbags.

Center the film holder to the metacarpophalangeal joints and adjust it so that its midline is parallel with the long axis of the hand and forearm. If the hand is resting on the ulnar surface, support the thumb on a cork or loofah sponge. Place a sandbag across the forearm if it is horizontal; against the elbow if the forearm is elevated on sandbags.

Central ray

Direct the central ray vertically to the metacarpophalangeal joints.

Structures shown

A lateral view of the hand in extension. This is the customary position for the localization of foreign bodies. The exposure technique will depend upon the nature of the foreign body. Whereas a heavy exposure can be used for metallic substances, a light exposure should be used for less opaque substances.

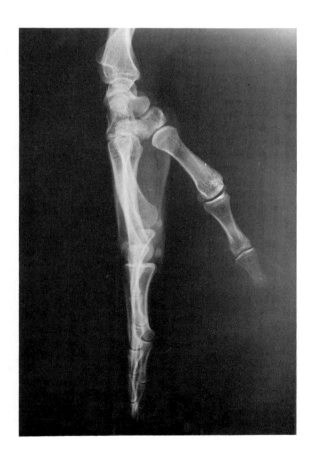

HAND
Posterior oblique projection
Anterior oblique view
Film: 8″ × 10″ lengthwise.

Position of part

Have the patient rest his forearm on the table and place his hand on the film holder in the lateral position, ulnar side down. From the lateral position, rotate the hand medialward with the fingers slightly flexed so that their tips will touch the film holder. Center the film to the metacarpophalangeal joints and adjust it so that its midline is parallel with the long axis of the hand and forearm. Adjust the obliquity of the hand so that the metacarpophalangeal joints form an angle of approximately 45 degrees with the plane of the film.

If it is not possible to obtain the correct position, with all fingertips resting on the film holder, elevate the index finger and thumb on corks, a loofah sponge, or other suitable radiolucent material.

When an oblique view of the interphalangeal joints is desired, a foam wedge should be used to support the fingers in the intended position.

Central ray

Direct the central ray vertically to the third metacarpophalangeal joint.

Structures shown

An oblique projection of the bones and soft tissues of the hand. This position is used largely in pathologic conditions, or as a supplemental view in the investigation of fractures.

NOTE: An excellent device for obtaining oblique views of the hand, and lateral views of the fingers, was developed by Schneider.[1] Referring to the model illustrated, the device can be made up of tongue depressors, corks, and adhesive tape.

[1]Schneider, Cathryn C.: Mechanical devices for immobilizing the head and hand, Xray Techn. **1:**70-71, 1930.

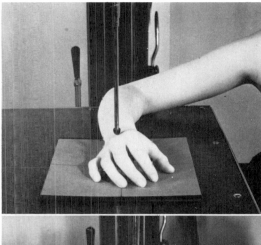

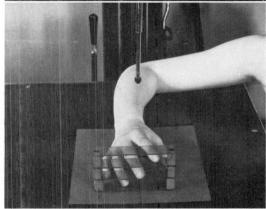

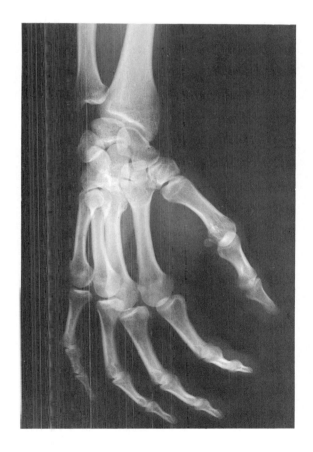

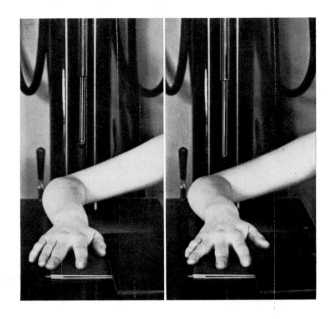

FINGERS (SECOND THROUGH FIFTH)
Posteroanterior projection
Anteroposterior view

Film: 5″ × 7″ crosswise for two views on the one film.

Position of part

When radiographing individual fingers (except the first), place the finger on the unmasked half of the film holder with the palmar surface down.

Separate the fingers slightly and center the finger being examined to the midline of the film, with its proximal interphalangeal joint over the center point of the film. Immobilize by placing a sandbag over the wrist.

Central ray

Direct the central ray vertically to the proximal interphalangeal joint.

NOTE: Fingers that cannot be extended can be examined in small sections with dental films. If a joint is in question, the projection should be from the anteroposterior instead of the posteroanterior position.

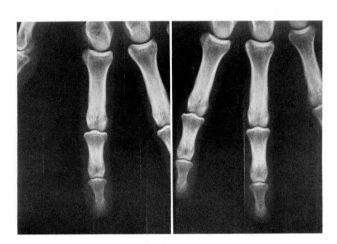

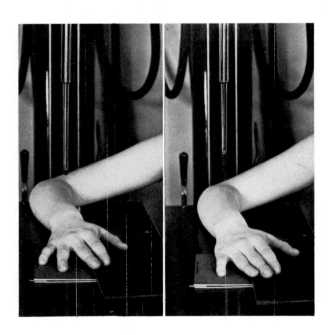

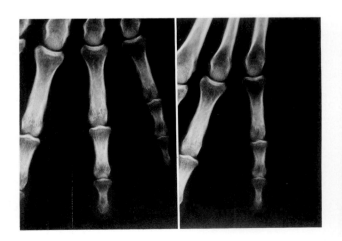

FINGERS (SECOND THROUGH FIFTH)
Lateral projection

Film: 5″ × 7″ crosswise for two views on the one film.

Position of part

Since lateral finger positions are difficult to hold, it is advisable to tell the patient how his finger is to be adjusted on the film holder. Demonstrate with your own finger, and then let him assume the position with his arm in the position that will be most comfortable for him.

Ask the patient to extend the finger to be examined, close the rest of the fingers into a fist, and hold them in complete flexion with his thumb. When it is necessary to elevate the elbow in order to bring the finger into position, support it on sandbags.

With the finger to be examined extended and the other fingers folded into a fist, the patient's hand should rest (1) on the radial surface for the second or third finger, (2) on the ulnar surface for the fourth or fifth finger.

Before the final adjustment of the position of the finger, place the film holder so that the midline of its unmasked half is parallel with the long axis of the finger and center it to the proximal interphalangeal joint.

The second and fifth fingers rest directly on the film holder, but for accurate projection of the bones and joints, the third and fourth fingers must be elevated to place their long axis parallel with the plane of the film.

Immobilize the extended finger by placing a strip of balsa wood, a tongue depressor, or a loofah sponge against its palmar surface. The patient can hold the support with his opposite hand. Finally, adjust the forward or backward rotation of the hand so as to obtain a true lateral position of the finger.

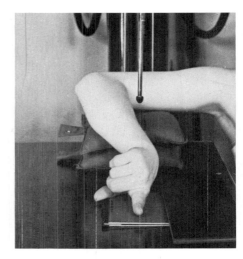

Second finger.

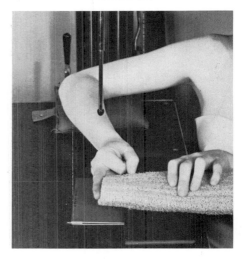

Third finger.

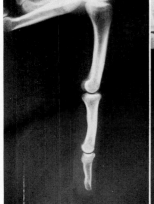
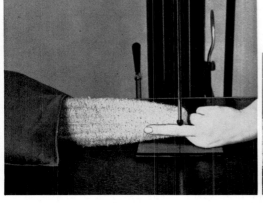

Third finger.

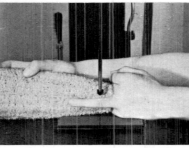

Fourth finger.

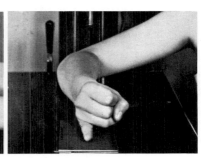

Fifth finger.

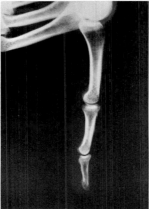

Second finger.   Third finger.

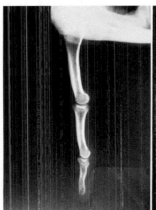
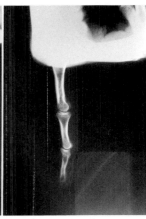

Fourth finger.   Fifth finger.

37

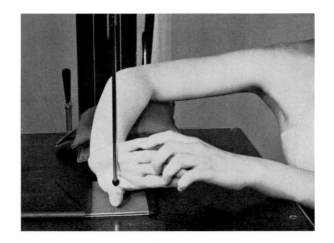

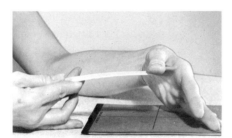

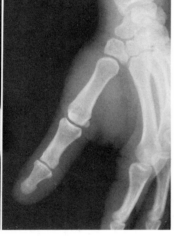

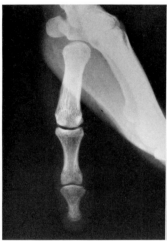

Anteroposterior projection.   Posteroanterior projection.

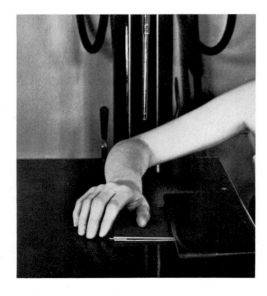

38

FIRST FINGER (THUMB)
Frontal and lateral projections
Film: $5'' \times 7''$ lengthwise, $8'' \times 10''$ crosswise for two views on one film.

Anteroposterior projection, posteroanterior view

In order to avoid motion or rotation, it is advisable for the technologist to demonstrate the desired position with his own hand. The patient can then, by adjusting the position of his body on the chair, place his hand in the correct position with the least amount of strain on his arm. Also, place the film holder under the finger after the hand is in approximately the correct position. The patient will assume a more comfortable position if he is not asked to adjust his hand at a specific point.

Ask the patient to turn his hand to a position of extreme internal rotation and, holding the extended fingers back with his opposite hand, to rest the thumb on the table. If the elbow is elevated, support it with sandbags and have the patient rest the opposite forearm against the table for support.

Place the film holder under the thumb and, with its midline parallel with the long axis of the finger, center to the metacarpophalangeal joint. Adjust the position of the hand so as to secure a true anteroposterior position of the thumb, being careful to have the fifth metacarpal back far enough to avoid superimposition.

Posteroanterior projection, anteroposterior view

It is sometimes necessary to take the frontal view of the first carpometacarpal joint and finger from the dorsal aspect. For this projection, place the hand in the lateral position, rest the elevated and abducted thumb on a radioparent support, and adjust the hand so as to place the dorsal surface of the finger parallel with the film. When the position requires that the wrist be elevated, support it on a small sandbag. An increase of 4 to 6 inches in focal-film distance (with a compensatory increase of 4 to 6 kilovolts) will offset the increase in part-film distance.

Lateral projection

Have the patient place his hand in its natural arched position with the palmar surface down. Place the film holder so that its midline is parallel with the long axis of the finger, and center it to the metacarpophalangeal joint. Adjust the arching of the hand until a true lateral position of the thumb is obtained.

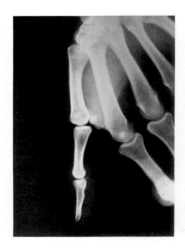

Lateral projection.

FIRST CARPOMETACARPAL JOINT
Anteroposterior projection
Radial shift of the carpal canal position

Burman,[1] who devised this projection, states that it gives a clearer view of the first carpometacarpal joint than does the standard anteroposterior projection, which it may supplement when the wrist can be dorsiflexed.

Film: 5″ × 7″ crosswise.

Position of patient

Seat the patient at the end of the table in such a way that the forearm can be adjusted to lie approximately parallel with the long axis of the table.

Position of part

Hyperextend the hand and have the patient hold it in this position with his opposite hand or with a bandage looped around the fingers, and then rotate the hand so as to place the thumb in the horizontal position. Place the film holder under the wrist and finger and center it about 1 inch proximal to the first carpometacarpal joint; the joint will be projected to the center of the film.

Central ray

Direct the central ray to a point about 1 inch distal to the first carpometacarpal joint at an angle of 45 degrees toward the elbow.

Burman[1] recommends the use of a short focal-film distance (15 to 18 inches) for the purpose of magnifying the projected image.

Structures shown

An anteroposterior projection showing the concavo-convex outline of the first carpometacarpal joint.

[1]Burman, Michael: Anteroposterior projection of the carpometacarpal joint of the thumb by radial shift of the carpal tunnel view, J. Bone Joint Surg. **40-A:** 1156-1157, 1958.

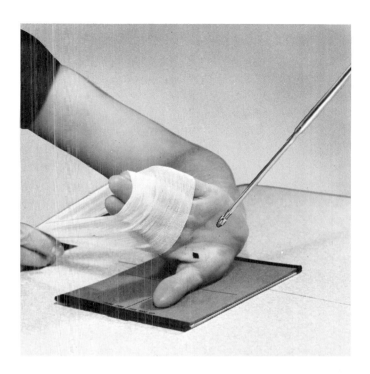

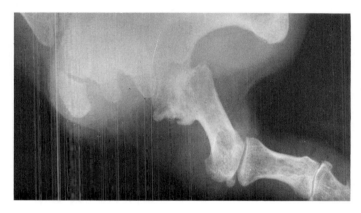

Radial shift projection.

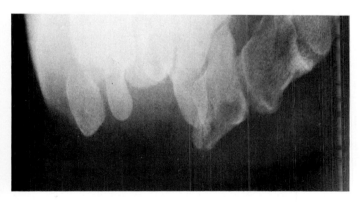

Carpal canal projection showing fracture of greater multangular.

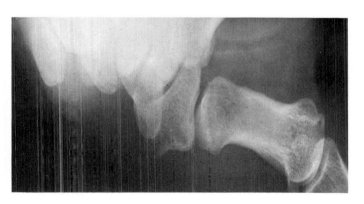

Radial shift projection on opposite patient.

Radiographs courtesy Dr. Michael Burman

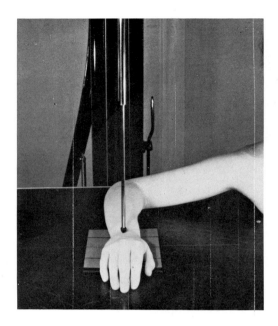

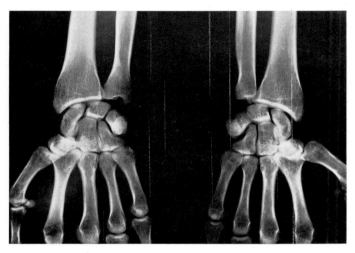

Posteroanterior projection.   Anteroposterior projection.

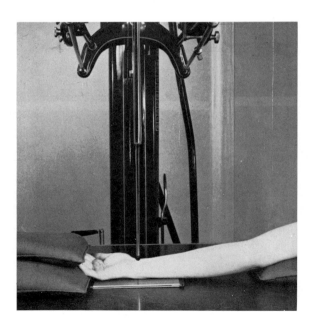

WRIST
Frontal projections

For examinations of the wrist, seat the patient low enough to place the axilla in contact with the table, or elevate the extremity to shoulder level on a suitable support. This is done for the purpose of placing the shoulder, elbow, and wrist joints in the same plane in order to permit right-angle rotation of the ulna as well as of the radius for the lateral view.

Film: $5'' \times 7''$ lengthwise, or $8'' \times 10''$ crosswise for two projections.

When it is difficult to determine the exact location of the carpus due to an obese or swollen wrist, ask the patient to flex the wrist slightly, and then center to the point of flexion. When the wrist is in a cast or a splint, the exact point of centering can be determined by comparison with the opposite side.

Posteroanterior projection, anteroposterior view
Position of part

Have the patient rest his forearm on the table. Place the film holder under the wrist and center to the carpus. Adjust the hand and forearm so that they lie parallel with the long axis of the film. Arch the hand slightly at the metacarpophalangeal joints to place the wrist in close contact with the film.

Place a sandbag across the forearm to immobilize it. When necessary, place one sandbag under the fingers and another on them.

Central ray

Direct the central ray vertically to the midcarpal area.

Structures shown

A posteroanterior projection of the carpals, the lower ends of the radius and ulna, and the upper ends of the metacarpals.

The posteroanterior projection gives a slightly oblique view of the ulna. When this bone is the point of interest, the anteroposterior position should be used.

Anteroposterior projection, posteroanterior view
Position of part

Have the patient rest his forearm on the table in the anteroposterior position. Place the film holder under the wrist and center to the carpals. Elevate the fingers on a sandbag to place the wrist in close contact with the film. Have the patient lean laterally to prevent rotation of the wrist. Place one sandbag over the fingers and another over the forearm.

Central ray

Direct the central ray vertically to the midcarpal area.

Structures shown

The carpal interspaces are better demonstrated in this position since, because of their oblique direction, they are more nearly parallel with the divergence of the beam of roentgen rays.

WRIST
Lateral projection

Film: $8'' \times 10''$ for two projections.

Position of part

Have the patient flex his elbow 90 degrees to rotate the ulna to the lateral position, and have him rest his *arm* and forearm on the table. Center the film to the carpals and adjust the forearm and hand so that the wrist is in a true lateral position.

Immobilize the forearm with a sandbag and, when necessary, place a small sandbag against the palmar surface of the hand and another against the posterior surface.

Central ray

Direct the central ray vertically to the wrist joint.

Structures shown

A lateral view of the carpals, the upper ends of the metacarpals, and the lower ends of the radius and ulna.

NOTE: Stecher[1] recommends that the wrist be adjusted with the radial surface to the film when examining the navicular in order to prevent blurring-out of fracture lines.

Burman and co-workers[2] suggest that the lateral view of the navicular be made with the wrist in palmar flexion because this action rotates the bone anteriorly into a dorsovolar position. They state, however, that this position is of value only when enough flexion is permitted.

[1]Stecher, William R.: Roentgenography of the carpal navicular bone, Amer. J. Roentgen. **37**:704-705, 1937.
[2]Burman, M. S., Sinberg, S. E., Gersh, W., and Schmier, A. A.: Fractures of the radial and ulnar axes, Amer. J. Roentgen. **51**:455-480, 1944.

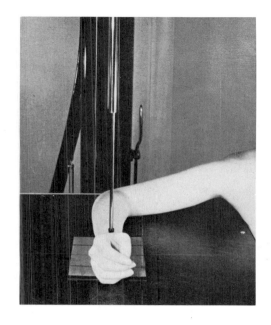

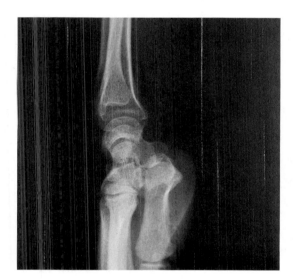

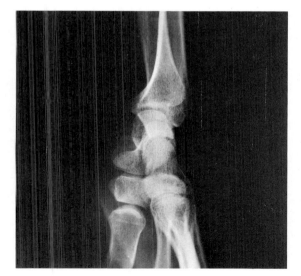

Ulnar surface to film.

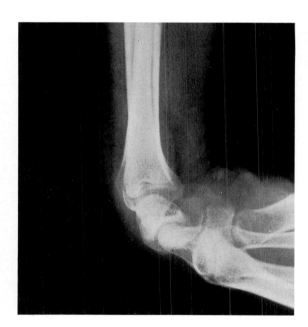

Radial surface to film.

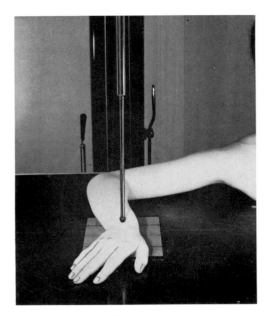

Ulnar flexion.

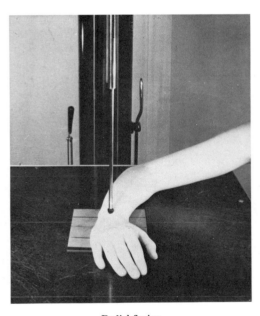

Radial flexion.

WRIST
Bending positions

Film: $8'' \times 10''$ for two projections.

ULNAR FLEXION
Position of part

Position the wrist and center the film holder as for a posteroanterior projection. Next, with one hand cupped over the joint to hold it in position, move the elbow outward, that is, away from the patient's body, and then turn the hand outward until the wrist is in extreme ulnar flexion. Immobilize by placing one sandbag over the forearm and another over the fingers.

Central ray

Direct the central ray vertically to the navicular; according to the direction of the fracture line, its clear delineation sometimes requires a central ray angulation of 10 to 15 degrees either proximally or distally.

Structures shown

This position corrects the foreshortening of the navicular, which is obtained in the direct posteroanterior position, and opens the spaces between the adjacent carpals.

RADIAL FLEXION
Position of part

Position the wrist and center the film holder as for a posteroanterior projection. Cup one hand over the wrist joint to hold it in position and then move the elbow toward the patient's body and the hand medialward until the wrist is in extreme radial flexion. Place one sandbag over the hand and another over the forearm.

Central ray

Direct the central ray vertically to the midcarpal area.

Structures shown

This position opens the interspaces between the carpals on the medial side of the wrist.

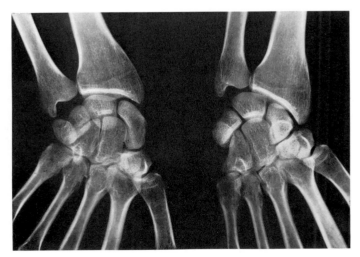

Ulnar flexion.   Radial flexion.

WRIST
Oblique projections
Semisupination and semipronation positions[1]

Film: $8'' \times 10''$ crosswise for two views on one film.

A 45-degree foam wedge placed under the elevated side of the wrist permits exact positioning and ensures duplication in follow-up examinations.

Semisupination oblique projection
Position of part

Have the patient rest his forearm on the table in the lateral position. Place the film holder under the wrist and center it at the dorsal surface of the carpus. Then rotate the wrist lateralward until it forms an angle of approximately 45 degrees to the film. Rest the hand against a small sandbag and put a long sandbag across the forearm.

Central ray

Direct the central ray vertically to the midpoint of the film; it enters the anterior surface of the wrist midway between its medial and lateral borders.

Structures shown

This position separates the pisiform from the adjacent carpal bones. It also gives a more distinct view of the cuneiform (triquetrum) and unciform (hamate).

Semipronation oblique projection
Position of part

Place the wrist, resting on the ulnar surface, on the film holder. Adjust the holder so that its center point is approximately 1½ inches anterior to the carpals; this will place it under the navicular when the wrist is rotated from the lateral position.

From the lateral position, rotate the wrist medialward until it forms an angle of approximately 45 degrees with the plane of the film. Extend the wrist just slightly, and if the fingers do not touch the table, support them on a sandbag. When the navicular is the point of interest, adjust the wrist in ulnar flexion. Place a sandbag across the forearm.

Central ray

Direct the central ray vertically to the navicular; it enters just distal to the radius.

Structures shown

This position demonstrates the carpals on the lateral side of the wrist, particularly the navicular, which is stacked on itself in the direct posteroanterior projection.

[1]McBride, Earl: Wrist joint injuries, a plea for greater accuracy in treatment, J. Okla. Med. Ass. **19**:67-70, 1926.

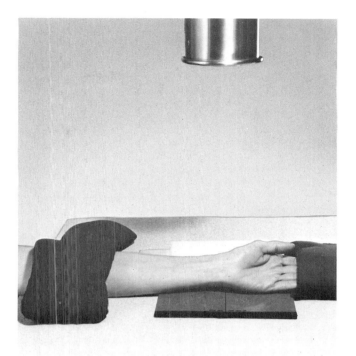

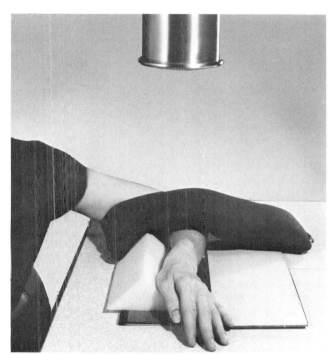

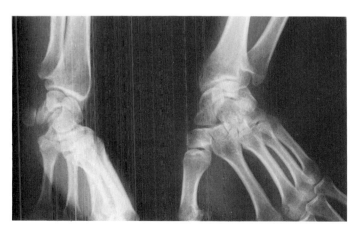

Semisupination.   Semipronation.

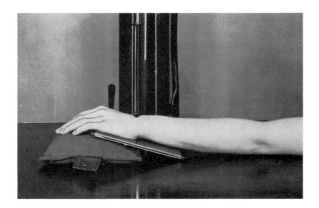

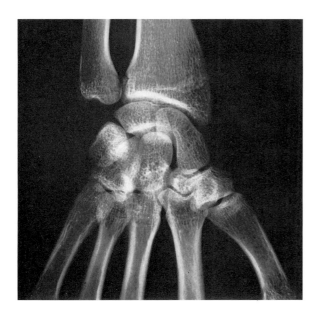

WRIST
Navicular
Stecher position

Film: $5'' \times 7''$ lengthwise.

Position of part

Place one end of the film holder on a sandbag and adjust it so that it forms an angle, inclined toward the elbow, of 20 degrees to the horizontal.

Adjust the wrist on the film holder in the posteroanterior position and center the carpus approximately ½ inch above the midpoint of the film. Bridgman[1] suggests that the wrist be positioned in ulnar flexion for this projection.

Immobilize with a sandbag placed across the forearm.

Central ray

With the central ray perpendicular to the horizontal, direct it to the navicular.

Structures shown

The 20-degree angulation of the wrist places the navicular at right angles to the central ray so that it is projected without self-superimposition.

Variations

1. Stecher[2] recommends the above method as being the preferable one; however, he says that a similar view can be obtained by placing the film and wrist horizontally and directing the central ray 20 degrees toward the elbow.

For the demonstration of a fracture line that angles superoinferiorly, these positions may be reversed; that is, the wrist may be angled downward or, from the horizontal position, the central ray may be angled toward the fingers.

2. A third method recommended by Stecher is to have the patient clench his fist. He says that this tends to elevate the distal end of the navicular so that it will lie parallel with the film, and that it also tends to widen the fracture line. The wrist is positioned as for the posteroanterior projection, and no tilt is used.

[1]Bridgman, C. F.: Radiography of the carpal navicular bone, Med. Radiogr. Photogr. **25**:104-105, 1949.

[2]Stecher, William R.: Roentgenography of the carpal navicular bone, Amer. J. Roentgen. **37**:704-705, 1937.

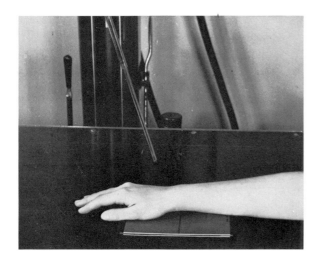

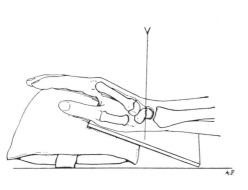

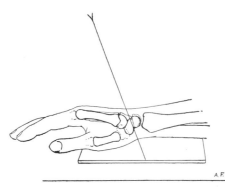

CARPAL CANAL
Inferosuperior projection
Gaynor-Hart position

Film: 5″ × 7″ crosswise.

Position of patient

Seat the patient at the end of the table in such a way that the forearm can be adjusted to lie parallel with the long axis of the table.

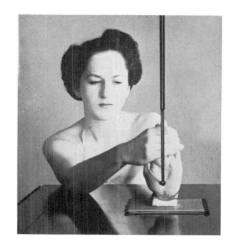

Position of part

Hyperextend the wrist and center the film holder to the joint at the level of the radial styloid. Place a radio-parent pad approximately ¾ inch thick under the lower forearm for support.

Adjust the position of the hand so as to place its long axis, as nearly as possible, vertical. In order to prevent superimposition of the shadows of the hamate and pisiform bones, rotate the hand slightly toward the radial side. Have the patient grasp the fingers with his opposite hand to hold the wrist in the extended position.

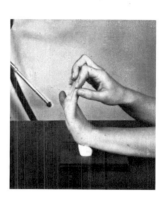

Central ray

Direct the central ray to the palm of the hand, to a point approximately 1 inch distal to the base of the fourth metacarpal, at an angle of 25 to 30 degrees to the long axis of the hand.

Structures shown

An axial projection of the carpal canal (sulcus carpi; carpal tunnel) showing the volar aspect of the greater multangular, the tuberosity of the navicular, the lesser multangular, the capitate, the hamular process of the hamate, the triquetrum, and the entire pisiform.

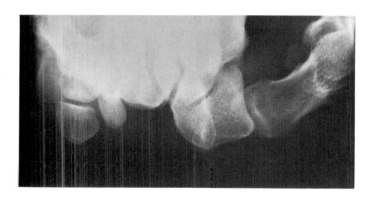

NOTE: When the patient cannot assume or maintain the above position, a similar but not identical view may be obtained by adjusting the wrist as shown in the photograph below. Have the patient dorsiflex his wrist as much as is tolerable and lean forward so as to place the carpal canal tangent to the film. The canal is easily palpable on the volar aspect of the wrist as the concavity between the greater multangular laterally and the hamular hook and pisiform medially.

Templeton and Zim[1] recommend a variation on this position wherein the forearm is placed at right angles to the film. The central ray is then directed through the carpal canal at an angle of 40 degrees toward the fingers.

[1]Templeton, A. W., and Zim, I. D.: The carpal tunnel view, Missouri Med. **61:**443-444, 1964.

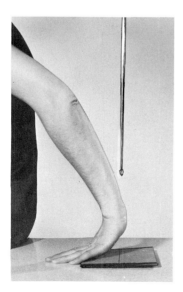

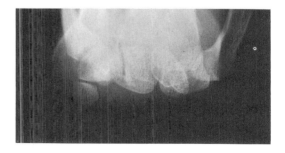

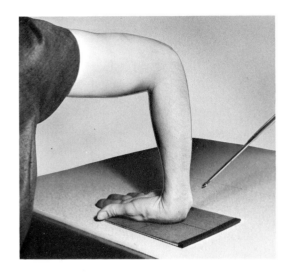

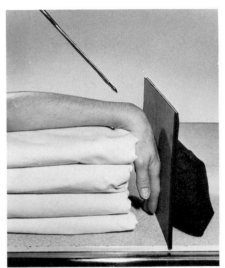

CARPAL BRIDGE
Tangential projection

Film: $5'' \times 7''$ or $8'' \times 10''$ lengthwise.

Position of patient

The patient must be seated at the side of the table to permit the required manipulation of the x-ray tube.

Position of part

The originators[1] of this position recommend that the hand lie palm upward on the film holder, with the arm forming a right angle to the body, the forearm a right angle to the arm, and the hand a right angle to the fore-arm, as shown in the opposite photograph.

When the wrist is too painful to be adjusted in the above position, a similar but not identical view can be obtained by elevating the forearm on sandbags or other suitable support and, with the wrist flexed to a right-angle position, placing the film in the vertical position, as shown in the photograph below.

Central ray

The central ray is directed to a point about $1\frac{1}{2}$ inches proximal to the wrist joint at a superoinferior angle of 45 degrees.

Structures shown

A semiaxial view of the carpus. The originators recommend this projection for the demonstration of (1) fractures of the navicular, (2) lunate dislocations, (3) calcifications and foreign bodies in the dorsum of the wrist, and (4) chip fractures of the dorsal aspect of the carpal bones.

[1]Lentino, W., Lubetsky, H. W., Jacobson, H. G., and Poppel, M. H.: The carpal bridge view, J. Bone Joint Surg. **39-A:**88-90, 1957.

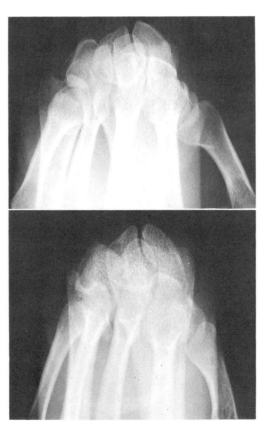

Original method.

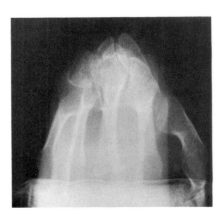

Modified method.

FOREARM
Anteroposterior and lateral projections
Film

Select a film long enough to include the entire forearm from the olecranon process of the ulna to the styloid process of the radius. Take both views of the forearm on one film by alternately covering one-half with a lead mask.

Anteroposterior projection, posteroanterior view
Position of patient

Seat the patient close to the table and low enough to place the entire extremity in the same plane.

Position of part

Supinate the hand, extend the elbow, and center the unmasked half of the film holder to the forearm. Have the patient lean laterally until the forearm is in a true anteroposterior position. Adjust the film holder so that its long axis is parallel with that of the forearm.

The hand *must be supinated*. Pronation of the hand crosses the radius over the ulna at its upper third and rotates the humerus medially, resulting in an oblique view of the forearm.

Immobilize the forearm by placing a sandbag over the palm of the hand and, if necessary, another over the arm just above the elbow.

Lateral projection
Position of patient

The patient must be seated so that the shoulder joint and elbow will lie in the same plane in order to permit the ulna to rotate to the lateral position.

Position of part

Flex the elbow 90 degrees, place the unmasked half of the film holder under the forearm, parallel with its long axis, and center it. Adjust the extremity in a true lateral position. The thumb side of the hand *must be up*.

Immobilize the forearm by placing one sandbag against the palmar surface of the hand and another against the posterior surface.

Structures shown

Anteroposterior and lateral projections of the forearm, the elbow joint, and the proximal row of carpal bones.

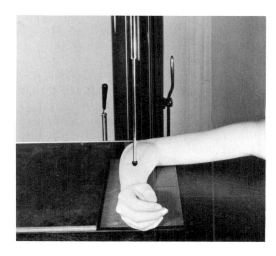

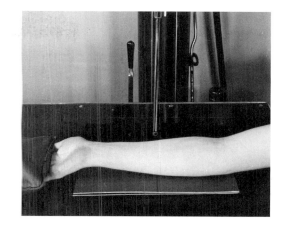

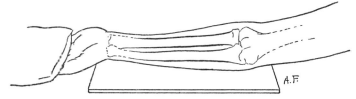

CORRECT POSITION OF HAND

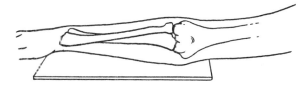

INCORRECT POSITION OF HAND

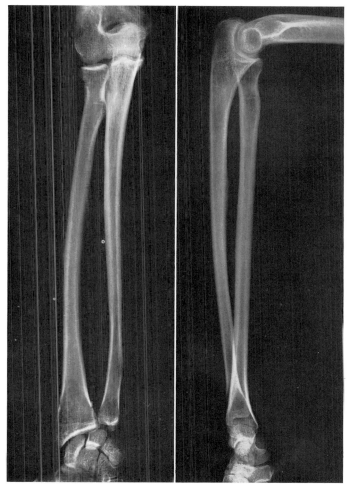

Anteroposterior projection.   Lateral projection.

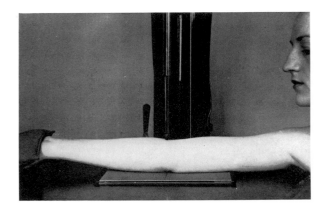

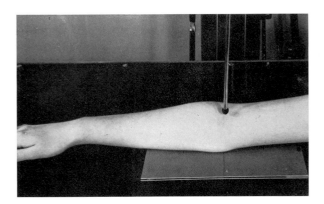

ELBOW
Anteroposterior and oblique projections
Film: 8″ × 10″ lengthwise.

Position of patient
Seat the patient low enough to place the shoulder and elbow joints in the same plane.

Anteroposterior projection, posteroanterior view
Position of part
Extend the elbow, supinate the hand, and center the film holder to the elbow joint. Have the patient lean laterally until the anterior surface of the elbow is parallel with the plane of the film. Adjust the film holder so that it is parallel with the long axis of the part.

The hand *must be supinated* to prevent rotation of the bones of the forearm. Place a sandbag on the upturned palm and, if necessary, another across the mid-arm.

Central ray
Direct the central ray vertically to the elbow joint.

Structures shown
An anteroposterior projection of the elbow joint, the lower end of the arm, and the upper end of the forearm.

Oblique projection
Position of part
Extend the extremity as for the anteroposterior projection and center the midpoint of the film holder to the elbow joint.

Pronate the hand and adjust the elbow so as to place its anterior surface at an angle of 40 to 45 degrees. This degree of obliquity will usually clear the coronoid process of the radial head. Immobilize with a sandbag placed across the hand.

Central ray
Direct the central ray vertically to the midpoint of the film.

Structures shown
An oblique view of the elbow with the coronoid process projected free of superimposition.

Anteroposterior projection.

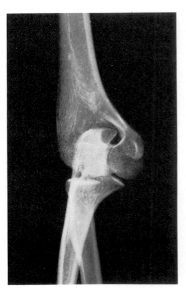

Oblique projection.

ELBOW

Lateral projection

Film: $8'' \times 10''$ lengthwise.

Position of part

From the anteroposterior or oblique position, flex the elbow 90 degrees. Center the film holder to the joint and adjust it so that its long axis is parallel with the long axis of the forearm, as shown in the photograph and the upper radiograph. When it is desired to include more of the arm and forearm, adjust the film holder diagonally, as shown in the lower radiograph.

In order to obtain a lateral view of the elbow (1) the hand must be adjusted in the lateral position, and (2) the humeral epicondyles must be perpendicular to the plane of the film. The latter requirement makes it necessary to place a folded towel or a small pad under the side of the wrist and hand.

Immobilize with a sandbag placed across the wrist, or by having the patient grasp a small sandbag.

Central ray

Direct the central ray vertically to the elbow joint regardless of its location on the film.

Structures shown

A lateral view of the elbow joint, the lower arm, and the upper forearm.

NOTE: When the soft structures about the elbow are in question, the joint should be flexed only 30 or 35 degrees.

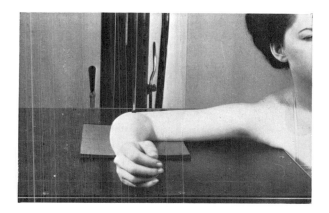

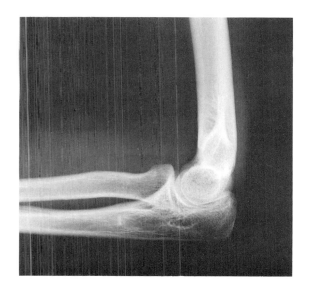

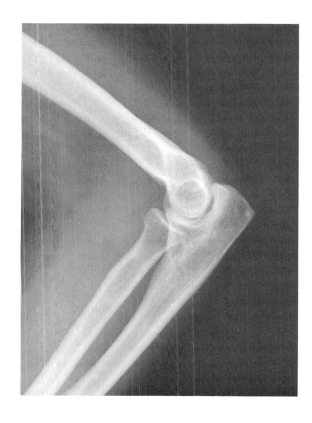

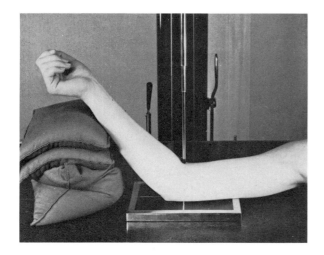

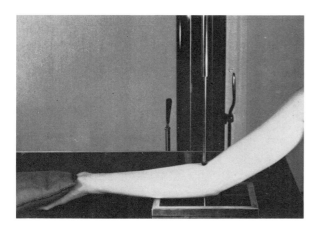

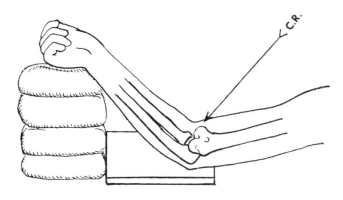

ELBOW
Anteroposterior projection
Partial flexion

When the patient is unable to extend his elbow completely, the lateral position offers little difficulty, but it is necessary to make two anteroposterior exposures in order to avoid distortion. Both exposures can be made on one 8″ × 10″ film placed crosswise by alternately covering one-half of the film with a lead mask. If preferred, use a 5″ × 7″ film placed lengthwise for each exposure.

LOWER HUMERUS

Seat the patient low enough to place the entire humerus in the same plane, and support the elevated forearm on sandbags. If possible, the hand should be supinated. Place the film holder under the elbow and center it to the condyloid area of the humerus.

Central ray

Direct the central ray to the midpoint of the film. Depending upon the degree of flexion, it may be necessary to angle the central ray into the joint.

UPPER FOREARM

Seat the patient high enough to permit him to rest the dorsal surface of the forearm on the table. If this is not possible, elevate the extremity on a suitable support, adjust it in the lateral position, place the film holder in the vertical position behind the upper end of the forearm, and direct the central ray horizontally.

Holly[1] has described an excellent method for obtaining the anteroposterior projection of the radial head. The patient is positioned as described above for the lower end of the humerus. Extend the elbow as much as possible and support the forearm on sandbags. Holly states that the forearm should be supinated enough to place the transverse plane of the wrist at an angle of 30 degrees with the horizontal.

Central ray

The central ray is directed at right angles to the long axis of the forearm and centered to the elbow joint. Adjust the film so that the central ray will pass to its midpoint.

[1]Holly, E. W.: Radiography of the radial head, Med. Radiogr. Photogr. **32**:13-14, 1956.

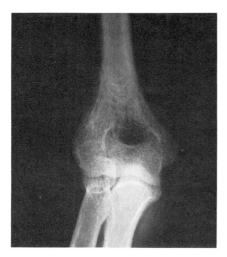

Distal humerus.

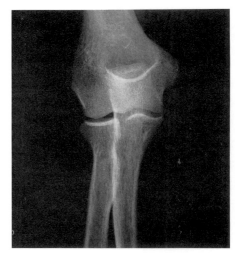

Joint and proximal radius and ulna.

ELBOW
Frontal projection
Acute flexion

Film: 5″ × 7″ lengthwise.

When fractures around the elbow are being treated in the Jones position (complete flexion), the lateral projection offers little difficulty but the frontal view must be made through the superimposed bones of the arm and forearm. The central ray should be directed at right angles either to the humerus or to the radius and ulna, depending upon the location of the fracture.

LOWER HUMERUS

The frontal projection of the lower end of the arm is obtained by centering the film a little above the epicondyloid area of the humerus and directing the central ray at right angles to the film.

Adjust either the arm or the tube and film so that there will be no rotation.

UPPER FOREARM

When the upper end of the forearm is in question, the tube should be tilted so that the central ray will be at right angles to the forearm. The film must be displaced toward the shoulder so that the central ray will pass to its midpoint.

Structures shown

The outlines of the superimposed bones of the arm and forearm in a frontal position. This position gives a very clear view of the olecranon process.

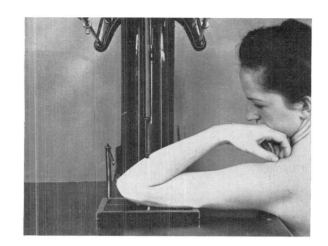

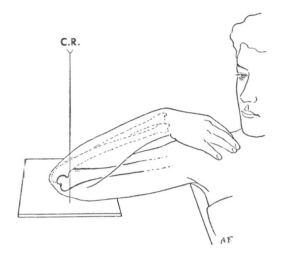

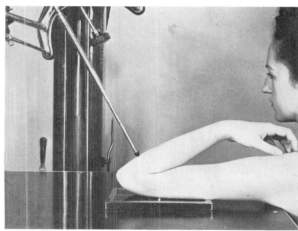

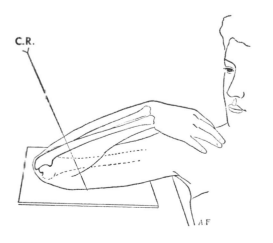

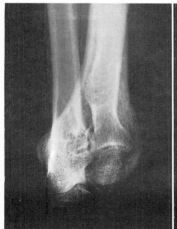

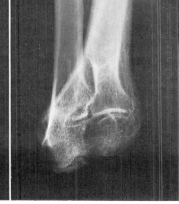

Distal arm.　　　　　Proximal forearm.

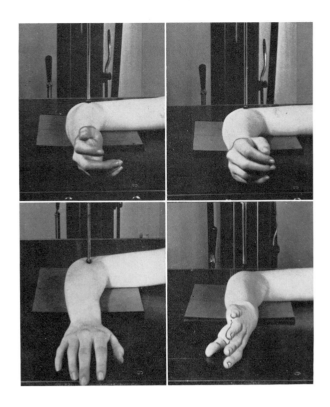

ELBOW
Radial head
Lateromedial rotation

In order to demonstrate the entire circumference of the radial head free of superimposition, it is necessary to make four exposures, varying the position of the hand.

Film: 8″ × 10″ for four exposures on one film.

Place an 8″ × 10″ cassette-changing tunnel in position and cover three-fourths of the film area with sheet lead.

Position of patient

Seat the patient low enough to place the entire extremity in the same plane.

Position of part

Flex the elbow 90 degrees, center the joint to the unmasked fourth of the cassette tunnel, and position it as for a lateral view.

1. Make the first exposure with the hand supinated as much as is possible in this position.

2. Shift the film and make the second exposure with the hand in the lateral position, that is, with the thumb surface up.

3. Shift the film and make the third exposure with the hand pronated.

4. Shift the film and make the fourth exposure with the hand in extreme internal rotation, that is, resting on the thumb surface.

Central ray

Direct the central ray vertically to the elbow joint.

NOTE: When the radial head is in question and it is not possible for the patient to rotate his forearm, the Schmitt[1] method of separating the radial head from the olecranon process can be employed.

The elbow is positioned as for an anteroposterior projection, and one radiograph is made with the central ray directed 45 degrees medially, and one with it directed 45 degrees laterally.

[1]Schmitt, H.: Die röntgenologische Darstellung des Radiusköpfchens, Roentgenpraxis 11:33-36, 1939.

Compare position of radial tuberosity.

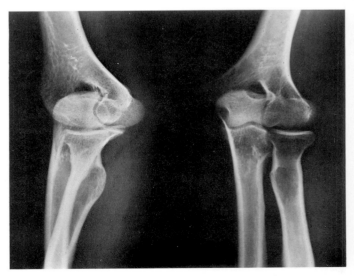

Angled projections.

ELBOW
Radial head
Axial projection

Film: 5″ × 7″ crosswise.

Position of patient

Seat the patient low enough to place the shoulder joint and the elbow in the same plane.

Position of part

Center the humeral epicondyles to the midpoint of the film and flex the elbow so that the forearm forms an angle of 70 degrees to the horizontal (20 degrees to the vertical). Rest the forearm against sandbags or other suitable support.

1. Make the first exposure with the hand supinated.
2. Change the film and make the second exposure with the hand pronated.

Because the thick brachioradialis muscle is drawn over the head of the radius when the hand is pronated, it is necessary to increase 8 or 10 kilovolts for the second view.

Central ray

Direct the central ray perpendicularly to the head of the radius.

Structures shown

These two projections demonstrate the entire articular surface of the radial head free of bony superimposition.

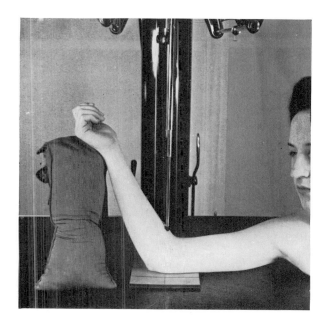

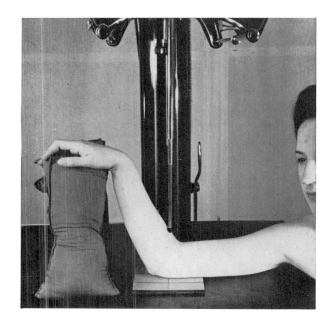

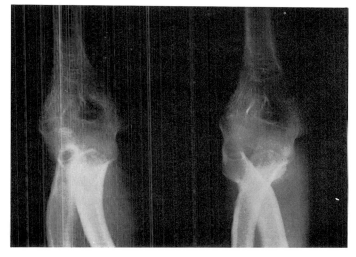

Supination   Pronation

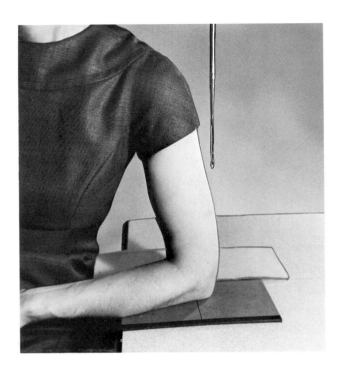

DISTAL HUMERUS AND OLECRANON PROCESS
Axial projections[1,2]

Film: 5″ × 7″ crosswise; 8″ × 10″ for two views on one film.

Position of patient

For an axial projection of the distal end of the humerus, seat the patient high enough to enable him to rest his forearm on the table with the arm in the vertical position. The patient may be seated somewhat lower for an examination of the olecranon process. He must, for either region, be seated so that the forearm can be adjusted to parallel the long axis of the table.

Position of part

Ask the patient to rest his forearm on the table, and then adjust it so that its long axis is parallel with that of the table. Adjust the degree of flexion of the elbow to place the arm at the angle to be used. Center the film holder between the epicondyles, a little anterior to this level when central ray angulation is to be used.

DISTAL HUMERUS
Position of part

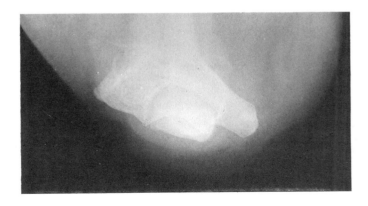

Adjust the patient's arm in a near vertical position (10 to 15 degrees) so that there is no forward or backward leaning. Supinate the hand to prevent rotation of the humerus and ulna, and have the patient immobilize it with his opposite hand.

Central ray

Direct the central ray vertically to the ulnar sulcus, a point just medial to the olecranon process.

Structures shown

This projection demonstrates an axial view of the epicondyles, the trochlea, the ulnar sulcus (the groove between the medial epicondyle and the trochlea), and the olecranon fossa. It is used in cases of radiohumeral bursitis (tennis elbow) for the detection of otherwise obscured calcifications located in the ulnar sulcus.

[1]Laquerrière et Pierquin: De la nécessité d'employer une technique radiographique spéciale pour obtenir certains détails sequelettiques, J. Radiol. Électr. 3:145-148, 1918.
[2]Veihweger, G.: Zum Problem der Deutung der knochernen Gebilde distal des Epikondylus medialis humeri, Fortschr. Roentgenstr. 86:643-652, 1957.

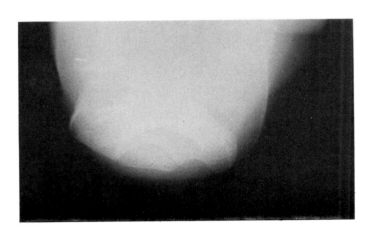

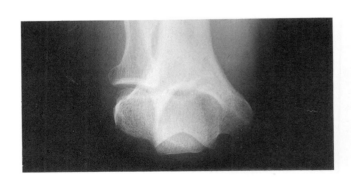

DISTAL HUMERUS AND
OLECRANON PROCESS
Axial projections[1,2]—cont'd

Position of part

For an axial projection of the olecranon process, adjust the arm at an angle of 45 to 50 degrees and so there is no forward or backward leaning. Supinate the hand to place the ulna in the anteroposterior position, and have the patient immobilize it with his opposite hand.

Central ray and structures shown

Direct the centray ray to the olecranon process (1) vertically for the demonstration of the dorsum of the process and (2) at an anterior angle of 20 degrees for the demonstration of the curved extremity and articular margin of the process.

[1]Laquerrière et Pierquin: De la nécessité d'employer une technique radiographique spéciale pour obtenir certains détails sequelettiques, J. Radiol. Electr. 3:145-148, 1918.
[2]Veihweger, G.: Zum Problem der Deutung der knochernen Gebilde distal des Epikondylus medialis humeri, Fortschr. Roentgenstr. 86:643-652, 1957.

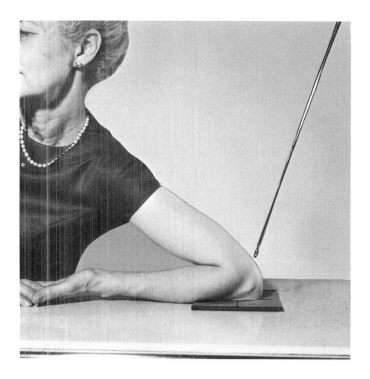

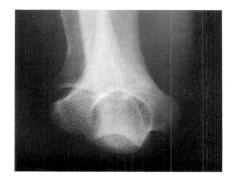

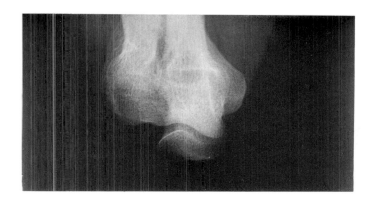

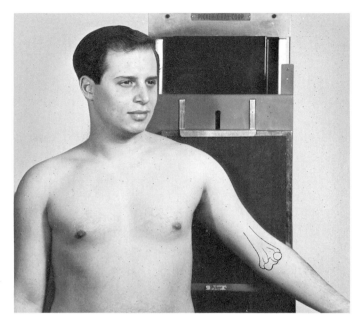

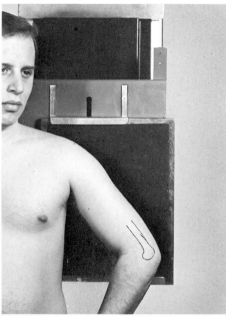

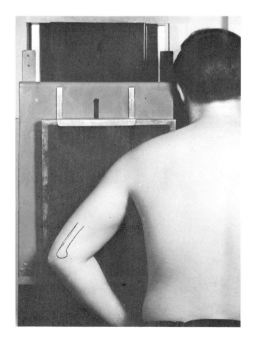

HUMERUS
Frontal and lateral projections
Erect position

Shoulder and arm abnormalities, whether traumatic or pathologic in origin, are extremely painful. For this reason, an erect position, either standing or seated, should be used whenever possible for the examination of these parts. By rotating the patient's body as required, the arm can be positioned quickly and accurately with minimal discomfort to the patient and, in the presence of fracture, with no danger of fragment displacement.

Film

The film selected should be long enough to include the humerus from its head to its condyles inclusively. An 11″ × 14″ film is adequate for adults when the arm can be abducted enough for diagonal placement on the film.

Position of patient

Place the patient in the general position, adjust the height of the cassette to place the upper margin of the film about 1½ inches above the head of the humerus, and then adjust the tube so as to direct the central ray perpendicularly to the midpoint of the film.

The accompanying photographs illustrate the body position used for anteroposterior and lateral projections of the freely movable arm. The body position, whether oblique or facing toward or away from the film, is unimportant, however, so long as true frontal and lateral views of the arm are obtained.

Position of part

Locate the epicondyles, and while holding them between the thumb and index fingers of one hand, adjust the position of the arm or, as indicated, have the patient turn slowly until the desired position is reached. *A coronal plane passing through the epicondyles will be parallel with the plane of the film for the frontal (anteroposterior or posteroanterior) projection, and at right angles to it for the lateral projection.*

Immobilization is usually not necessary because of the short exposure time, the average arm requiring no more than twenty milliampere-seconds at a 6-foot focal-film distance.

Structures shown

Frontal and lateral views of the entire length of the humerus, the accuracy of the positions being shown by the epicondyles.

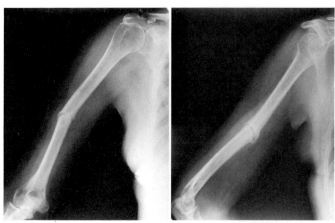

Courtesy Dr. Edward M. Winant.

HUMERUS
Anteroposterior and lateral projections
Recumbent position

Film

The film selected should be long enough to include the bone from its head to its condyles inclusively.

Anteroposterior projection, posteroanterior view

With the patient in the supine position, adjust the cassette so as to include the entire length of the humerus. Elevate the opposite shoulder on a sandbag to place the affected arm in contact with the cassette, or elevate the arm and cassette on sandbags. Supinate the hand and adjust the extremity so as to place the epicondyles parallel with the plane of the film. Immobilize the hand with a sandbag.

Lateral projection

Abduct the arm somewhat and place the cassette under it. Flex the elbow, rotate the forearm medially enough to place the epicondyles at right angles to the plane of the film, and rest the hand against the patient's side. Adjust the position of the cassette so as to include the entire length of the humerus.

Lateral decubitus position

When it is necessary to position the patient in the lateral decubitus position, place the cassette close to the axilla and center the arm to its midline. Flex the elbow, turn the thumb surface of the hand up, and rest it on a suitable support. Adjust the position of the body so as to place the lateral surface of the arm at right angles to the central ray.

Respiration is suspended for these exposures.

Central ray

Direct the central ray perpendicularly to the midpoint of the film.

Structures shown

Anteroposterior and lateral projections of the lower portion or of the entire humerus, depending upon the size of the film.

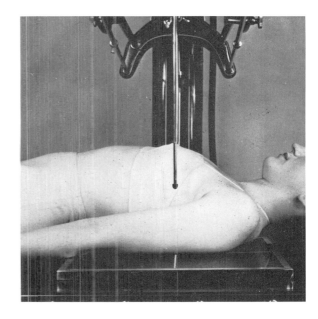

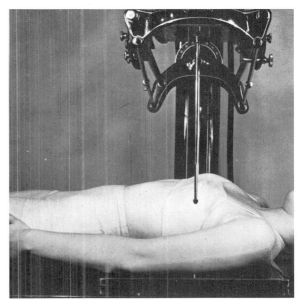

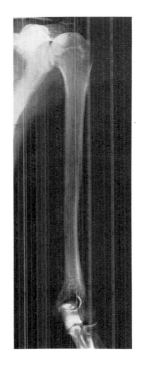
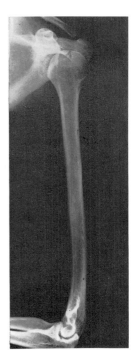

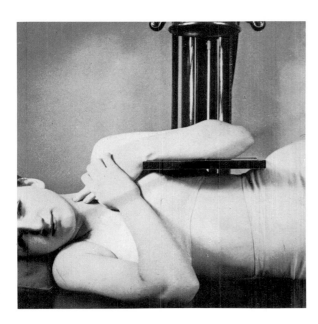

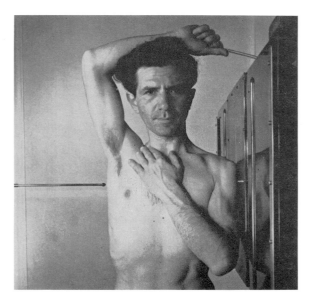

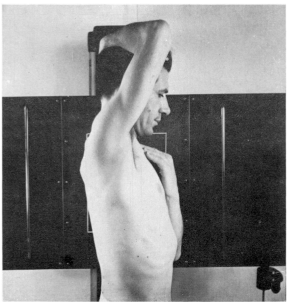

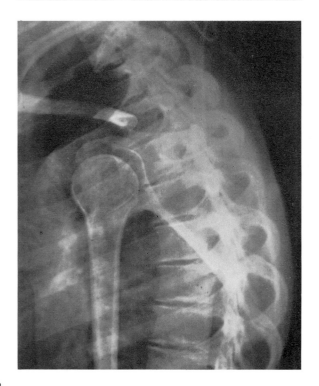

UPPER HUMERUS
Transthoracic lateral projection
Lawrence position

This projection, devised by Lawrence,[1] is used when the arm cannot be abducted for an axial projection.

Film: $8'' \times 10''$ or $10'' \times 12''$ lengthwise.

Position of patient

While this projection can be carried out with the patient in either the supine or the erect position, the latter facilitates accurate adjustment of the shoulder.

Position of part

Seat or stand the patient in the lateral position before a vertical Potter-Bucky stand. Have the patient raise the uninjured arm, rest the forearm on his head, and elevate the shoulder as much as possible. The elevation of the uninjured shoulder will give the desired depression of the injured side, thus separating the shoulders to prevent superimposition. Center the film to the region of the surgical neck of the affected humerus.

While holding the humeral epicondyles between the thumb and forefinger of one hand, adjust the rotation of the patient's body so as to place the lateral aspect of the humeral head parallel with, and *the epicondyles at right angles to*, the plane of the film.

Instruct the patient to hold his breath at full inspiration when ready to make the exposure. Having the lungs full of air improves the contrast and also decreases the exposure necessary to penetrate the body.

When the patient is able to hold his breath for five or six seconds, lung detail may be blurred considerably by the action of the heart. When this is possible, maintain the usual milliampere-second factor but convert to a low current, long exposure time combination.

If the patient can be sufficiently well immobilized to prevent voluntary motion, breathing motion can be utilized. In this case, instruct the patient and have him practice slow, deep breathing. An exposure time of seven to ten seconds will give excellent results.

Central ray

Direct the central ray perpendicularly to the midpoint of the film.

Structures shown

A lateral view of the upper half or two-thirds of the humerus projected through the thorax. While the definition may be poor, the outline of the humerus is clearly shown.

[1]Lawrence, W. S.: A method of obtaining an accurate lateral roentgenogram of the shoulder joint, Amer. J. Roentgen. **5**:193-194, 1918.

Anatomy and positioning of the lower extremity

The lower extremity

The bones of the lower extremities together with their girdle, the pelvis, which will be considered in a later section, are divided into four parts, (1) the foot, (2) the leg, (3) the thigh, and (4) the hip. These bones are so composed, shaped, and placed that they can carry the body in the erect position and transmit its weight to the ground with a minimum amount of stress to the individual parts.

THE FOOT

The foot consists of twenty-six bones, which are subdivided into three parts: (1) the tarsus, or bones of the ankle, (2) the metatarsus, or bones of the instep, and (3) the phalanges, or bones of the toes. For descriptive purposes, the foot is sometimes divided into (1) the forefoot, which includes the metatarsals and toes, (2) the midfoot, which includes the cuneiforms, the navicular, and the cuboid, and (3) the hindfoot, which includes the talus and the calcaneus. The bones of the foot are so shaped and jointed to-

gether that they form a series of longitudinal and transverse arches. This results in a considerable variation in the thickness of the component parts of the foot. In order to overcome the resulting difference in radiopacity, it is necessary to balance the exposure factors in such a way as to obtain the greatest possible range of tissue density. This is best accomplished with nonscreen technique. When screens are used, it is advisable to use a high kilovoltage with a low milliampere-second factor.

Phalanges. There are fourteen phalanges in the toes— two in the great toe and three in each of the other toes. The phalanges of the great toe are termed the first, or proximal, and the second, or distal. The phalanges of the other toes are termed the first, second, and third, or the proximal, middle, and distal. Each phalanx is composed of a shaft and two expanded ends. The distal phalanges are small and flattened and have a roughened rim of cancellous tissue at their distal end for the support of the nail. The interphalangeal articulations are of the hinge type.

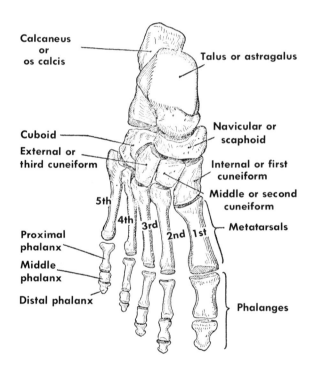

ANTERIOR ASPECT OF FOOT

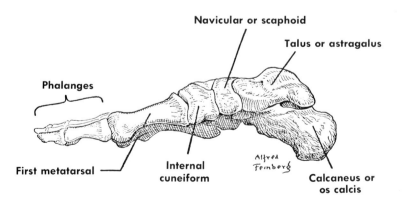

MEDIAL ASPECT OF FOOT

Metatarsus. The five metatarsals are simply numbered beginning at the medial side of the foot. The metatarsals consist of a body, or shaft, and two articular extremities. The distal extremities of the metatarsus, called the heads, form the ball of the foot and articulate with the proximal phalanges to form joints having the movements of flexion, extension, adduction, and abduction. Their proximal extremities articulate with each other and with the tarsals, forming joints that have only slight gliding movements. The first metatarsal is the shortest and thickest of these bones, the second metatarsal is the longest, and the fifth presents a prominent tuberosity at the lateral side on its base. Two sesamoids are always present on the plantar surface of the first metatarsophalangeal joint, and occasionally more. Frequently sesamoids are found on the plantar surface at one or more of the other metatarsophalangeal joints, and at the interphalangeal joints of the first and second toes. These sesamoids begin to appear between the ages of 8 and 12 years.

Tarsus. There are seven tarsals in the ankle—the *calcaneus*, or *os calcis*, the *talus*, or *astragalus*, the *navicular*, or *scaphoid*, the *cuboid*, and three *cuneiforms*. The cuneiform bones are termed, beginning at the medial side of the foot, the first, or internal, the second, or middle, and the third, or external.

The calcaneus is the largest bone of the tarsus, is more or less cuboidal in shape, and projects backward and medialward at the lower posterior part of the foot. It is also directed downward so that its long axis forms an angle of approximately 30 degrees, open forward, with the sole of the foot. The calcaneus supports the talus above, articulating with it by an irregularly shaped, three-faceted joint known as the subtalar joint, and articulates with the

cuboid in front. The talus is the second largest of the tarsus, is irregular in form, and occupies the highest position. It rests on the calcaneus, articulates with the navicular anteriorly, supports the tibia above, and articulates with the malleoli of the tibia and fibula at its sides.

The cuboid lies on the lateral side of the foot between the calcaneus and the fourth and fifth metatarsals. The navicular lies on the medial side of the foot between the talus and the three cuneiforms. The cuneiforms lie at the central and medial side of the foot between the navicular and the first, second, and third metatarsals. The first cuneiform is the largest, and the second is the smallest of the three cuneiforms.

The intertarsal and tarsometatarsal articulations allow only slight gliding movements between the bones. The joint spaces are narrow and are obliquely situated. Those lying in the transverse plane slant downward and backward at an angle of approximately 15 degrees to the vertical. The joints lying in the longitudinal plane slant downward and medialward at an angle of approximately 15 degrees to the vertical. When the joint surfaces of these bones are in question, it is necessary to angle the tube or adjust the foot, so as to place the joint spaces parallel with the central ray. Several positions with varying central ray angulations are required for the demonstration of the subtalar joint. Each of the three parts of the joint is formed by reciprocally shaped facets situated on the inferior surface of the talus and the superior surface of the calcaneus. Study of the superior and medial aspects of the calcaneus (left illustrated below) will aid the student technologist to better understand the problems involved in radiography of this joint.

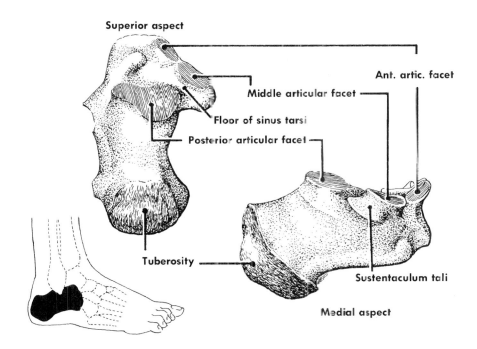

Superior aspect

Middle articular facet

Ant. artic. facet

Floor of sinus tarsi

Posterior articular facet

Tuberosity

Sustentaculum tali

Medial aspect

THE LEG

There are two bones in the leg—the tibia, or shin bone, and the fibula, or calf bone. The tibia is the second longest bone in the body and is situated on the medial side of the leg slightly anterior in position to the fibula, which is placed on the lateral side of the leg.

Tibia. The tibia is the larger of the two bones of the leg. It consists of a shaft and two expanded extremities. The upper end of the tibia is called the head of the bone and presents two prominent processes, which are termed the medial and lateral condyles. The upper surfaces of the condyles form smooth facets for articulation with the condyles of the femur. Between the two articular surfaces is a sharp projection, the intercondyloid eminence, or tibial spine, which terminates in two peaklike processes called tubercles. The lateral condyle has a facet at its lower posterior surface for articulation with the head of the fibula. On the anterior surface of the tibia, just below the condyles, is a prominent process that is called the tuberosity. Extending along the anterior surface of the shaft from the tuberosity to the medial malleolus is a sharp ridge called the anterior crest, or border. The lower end of the tibia is broad, and its medial surface is prolonged into a large process called the medial malleolus. Its lateral surface is flattened and presents a triangular depression for the inferior tibiofibular articulation. Its undersurface is smooth and shaped for articulation with the talus.

Fibula. The fibula is slender in comparison to its length. It consists of a shaft and two articular extremities. The upper end of the fibula is expanded into a head, which articulates with the posteroinferior surface of the lateral condyle of the tibia. At the lateral and posterior part of the head is a conical projection called the apex or styloid process. The enlarged distal end of the fibula is termed the lateral malleolus. The lateral malleolus is pyramidal in shape, articulates with the talus at its medial surface, and is marked by several depressions at its inferior and posterior surfaces.

Ankle joint. The ankle joint is formed by the articulation of the talus with the tibia and the fibula. It is a diarthrosis of the hinge type, which permits the movements of flexion and extension only. Other movements at the ankle are largely dependent upon the gliding movements of the intertarsal joints, particularly that between the talus and calcaneus.

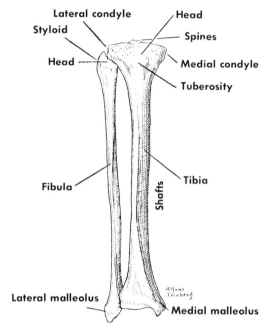

ANTERIOR ASPECT OF TIBIA AND FIBULA

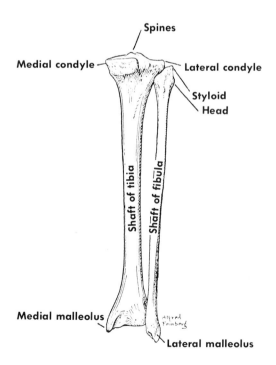

POSTERIOR ASPECT OF TIBIA AND FIBULA

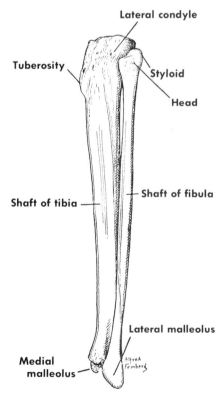

LATERAL ASPECT OF TIBIA AND FIBULA

62

THE THIGH

The femur, or thigh bone, is the longest, strongest, and heaviest bone in the body. It consists of a shaft and two articular extremities. The shaft is cylindrical in form and slightly convex forward. The shaft slants obliquely downward and medialward, the degree of the medial inclination depending upon the breadth of the pelvic girdle. The upper extremity of the femur will be considered with the hip.

The lower end of the femur is broadened and presents two large eminences—the larger medial condyle and the smaller lateral condyle. Anteriorly the condyles are separated by a shallow, triangular depression, the patellar surface, which articulates with the patella. Posteriorly, the condyles are separated by a deep depression called the intercondyloid fossa, or notch. The inferior surfaces of the condyles articulate with the tibia. A slight prominence, the medial and lateral epicondyles, is above each condyle.

The patella, or kneecap, is the largest and most constant sesamoid bone in the body. It is a flat, triangular bone situated at the lower anterior surface of the femur with its apex directed downward. The patella develops in the tendon of the quadriceps femoris muscle between the ages of 3 and 5 years. The tip of the apex lies slightly above the joint space of the knee and is attached to the tuberosity of the tibia by the patellar ligament. The patella articulates with the patellar surface of the femur and functions to protect the front of the knee joint. When the knee is extended in a relaxed state, the patella is freely movable over the patellar surface of the femur. When the knee is flexed, the patella is locked in position in front of the intercondyloid fossa.

Knee joint. The knee joint, a diarthrosis of the hinge type, is the largest joint in the body. Two menisci, one medial and one lateral, are interposed between the articular surfaces of the tibia and the condyles of the femur. The joint is enclosed in an articular capsule and held together by numerous ligaments. There are many bursae around the anterior, lateral, and medial surfaces of the joint.

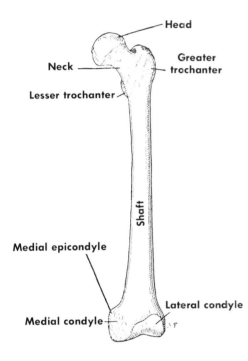

ANTERIOR ASPECT OF FEMUR

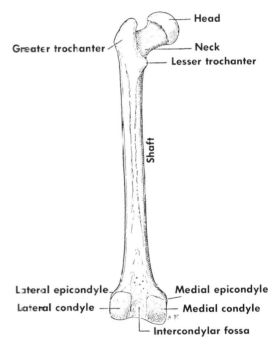

POSTERIOR ASPECT OF FEMUR

PATELLA

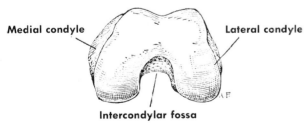

INFERIOR ASPECT OF FEMUR

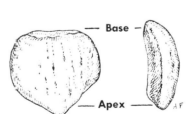

ANTERIOR ASPECT   LATERAL ASPECT

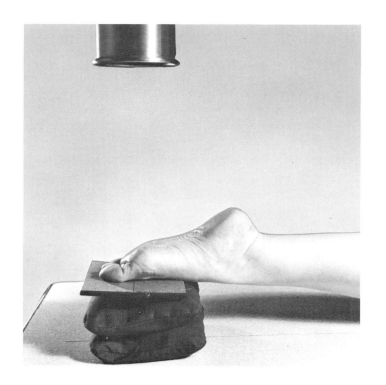

TOES
Frontal projections

Gonadal shielding should be applied for examinations of the lower extremities, most particularly where cranial angulation of the beam of radiation is required, and when the extremity must be adjusted in an acutely flexed position.

Film: 5″ × 7″ crosswise; 8″ × 10″ for two views on one film.

Position of patient

Because of the natural curve of the toes, demonstration of the interphalangeal joint spaces, and of the phalanges without foreshortening, requires that the foot be adjusted in the plantodorsal position or, from the dorsoplantar position, that the toes be elevated on a 15-degree foam wedge. The patient may therefore be placed in either the prone or the supine position.

Position of part

Plantodorsal projection. With the patient in the prone position, elevate the toes on one or two small sandbags and adjust the support so as to place the toes in the horizontal position.

Place the film holder under the toes with its midline parallel with the long axis of the foot and center it to the second metatarsophalangeal joint.

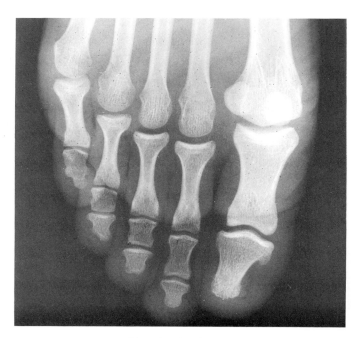

Plantodorsal projection.

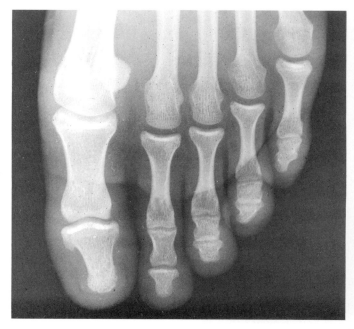

Dorsoplantar projection on opposite patient.

TOES

Frontal projections

Position of part—cont'd

Dorsoplantar projection. With the patient in the supine position, have him flex his knees, separate his feet about 6 inches, and rest his knees together for immobilization.

Place a 15-degree foam wedge well back under the foot so as to rest the toes near the base of the wedge. Adjust the film holder under the wedge with its midline parallel with the long axis of the foot and center it to the second metatarsophalangeal joint.

The toes may be immobilized with plastic wrap, as shown in the second photograph.

Central ray

Direct the central ray vertically to the midpoint of the film.

Structures shown

A frontal view (plantodorsal or dorsoplantar) of the fourteen phalanges of the toes, the interphalangeal joints, and the lower ends of the metatarsals. The metatarsophalangeal joints are not always shown as well in these projections as in the direct dorsoplantar projection.

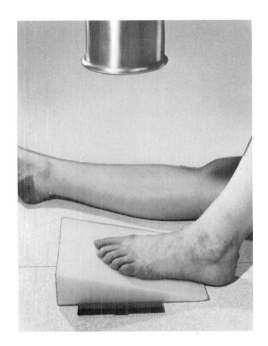

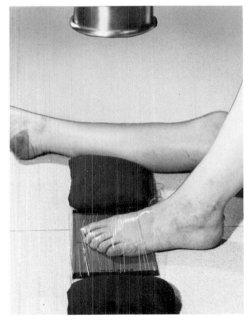

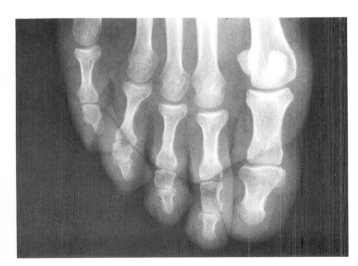

Toes on 15-degree wedge.

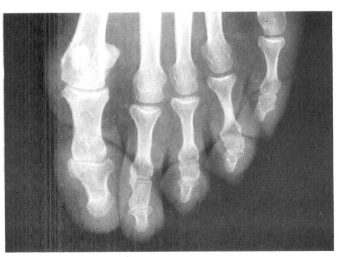

Toes horizontal, opposite patient.

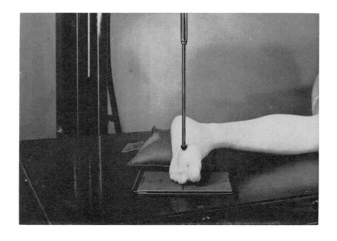

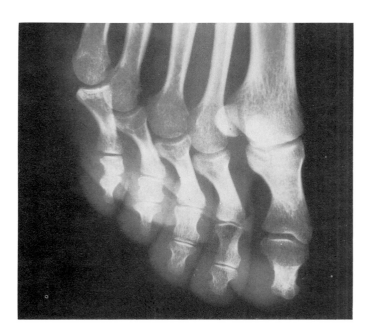

TOES
Oblique projection
Film: $5'' \times 7''$ crosswise.

Position of patient
Have the patient lie in the lateral recumbent position on his affected side.

Position of part
Adjust the affected extremity in a partially extended position. Have the patient turn toward the prone position until the ball of the foot forms an angle of approximately 30 degrees with the horizontal, or have him rest his foot against a 30-degree foam wedge.

Center the film holder to the second metatarsophalangeal joint and adjust it so that its central line is parallel with the long axis of the foot. Support the elevated heel on a small sandbag. Immobilize by placing a sandbag across the ankle.

Central ray
Direct the central ray vertically to the second metatarsophalangeal joint.

Structures shown
An oblique view of the phalanges of the toes and the lower ends of the metatarsals.

Lateral projection
Film: $5'' \times 7''$, occlusal or dental, depending upon the size of the toe.

Position of patient
Have the patient lie in the lateral recumbent position on his unaffected side. Support the affected extremity on sandbags and adjust it in a comfortable position.

To prevent superimposition, tape the toe or toes, above the one being examined, into a flexed position.

Position of part
Great toe. Place a $5'' \times 7''$ film holder under the toe and center to the proximal phalanx. Grasp the extremity by the heel and knee and adjust its position so as to place the great toe in a true lateral position. Adjust the film holder so that its center line is parallel with the long axis of the great toe. Immobilize with a sandbag across the ankle.

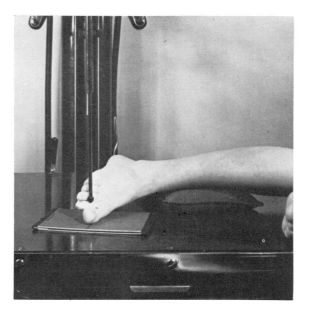

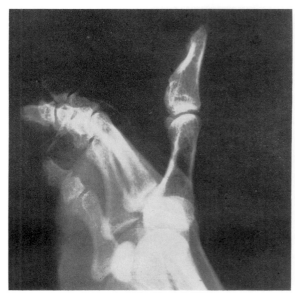

TOES

Lateral projection

Position of part—cont'd

Lesser toes. Depending upon the size of the toe, select either a dental or an occlusal film. Place the film packet, pebbled surface up, between the toe being examined and the subadjacent toe. Adjust the position of the extremity so as to place the toe and film in a horizontal position. Support the elevated heel on a sandbag and place another across the ankle.

Central ray

With the central ray at right angles to the plane of the film, direct it to the proximal interphalangeal joint.

Structures shown

A lateral view of the phalanges of the toe and the interphalangeal articulations, projected free of the other toes.

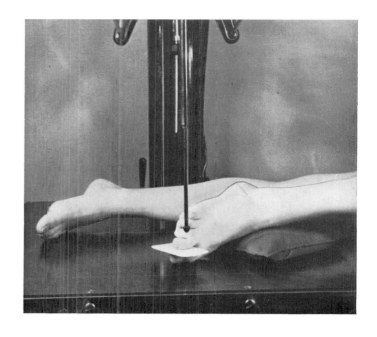

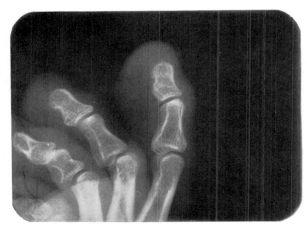

Second toe.

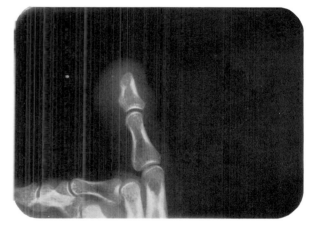

Third toe.

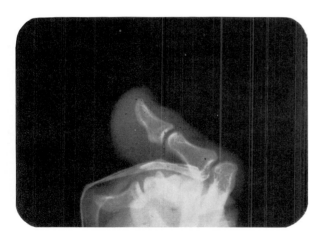

Fourth toe.

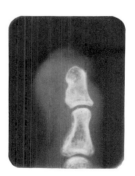

Fifth toe.

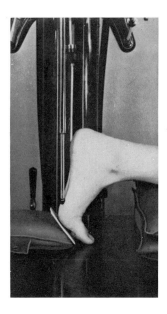
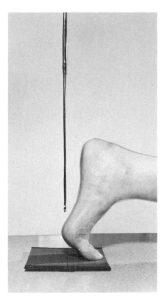

SESAMOIDS (Metatarsophalangeal)
Axial projection
Lewis position[1]

Film: Occlusal lengthwise.

Position of patient

Place the patient in the prone position. Elevate the ankle of the affected side on sandbags and put a folded towel under the knee.

Position of part

Rest the great toe on the table in a position of dorsiflexion and adjust it so as to place the ball of the foot perpendicular to the horizontal.

1. Place an occlusal film packet in close contact with the undersurface of the ball of the foot, center it to the first metatarsal, and support it in position with a sandbag.

2. If the plantar surfaces of the heads of the metatarsals are in question, use a $5'' \times 7''$ film placed crosswise and centered to the second metatarsal.

Central ray

Direct the central ray vertically to the first metatarsophalangeal joint.

Structures shown

An axial projection of the sesamoids of the first metatarsophalangeal joint, and of the plantar surface of the metatarsal head. All the metatarsal heads, and other sesamoids when present, are shown when a $5'' \times 7''$ film is used.

Holly[2] has described the reverse of this position, which he believes to be more comfortable for the patient. With the patient seated on the table, the foot is adjusted so that the medial border is vertical and the plantar surface is at an angle of 75 degrees with the plane of the film. The patient holds the toes in a flexed position with a strip of gauze bandage. The central ray is directed vertically to the head of the first metatarsal bone.

[1]Lewis, Raymond W.: Non-routine views in roentgen examination of the extremities, Surg. Gynec. Obstet. **69**:38-45, 1938.
[2]Holly, E. W.: Radiography of the tarsal sesamoid bones, Med. Radiogr. Photogr. **31**:73, 1955.

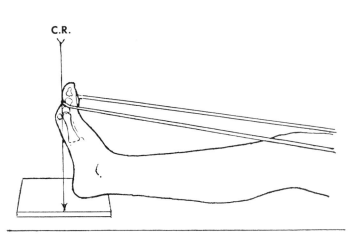

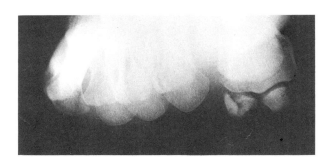

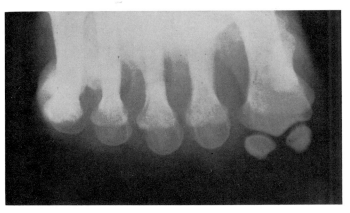

Courtesy Dr. Hudson J. Wilson, Jr.

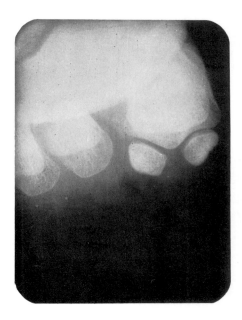

SESAMOIDS (Metatarsophalangeal)
Lateromedial projection
Causton position[1]

Film: Occlusal lengthwise.

Position of patient

Place the patient in the lateral recumbent position on his unaffected side, and flex the knees.

Position of part

Partially extend the extremity being examined and put sandbags under the knee and foot. Adjust the height of the sandbag under the knee so as to place the foot in the *lateral position* with the first metatarsophalangeal joint perpendicular to the horizontal.

Place an occlusal film under the lower metatarsal region and adjust it so that its midpoint will coincide with the central ray.

Immobilize the foot with a sandbag placed across the ankle.

Central ray

Direct the central ray to the prominence of the first metatarsophalangeal joint at an angle of 40 degrees toward the head.

Structures shown

This projection separates the shadows of the first metatarsophalangeal sesamoids and gives an oblique view of them.

[1]Causton, J.: Projection of sesamoid bones in the region of the first metatarsophalangeal joint, Radiology **9:**39, 1943.

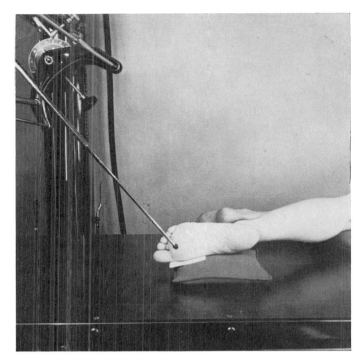

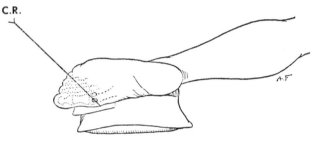

C.R.

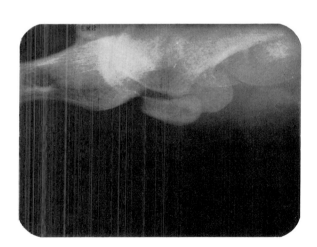

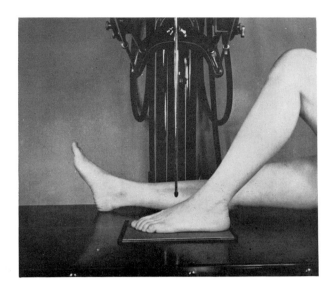

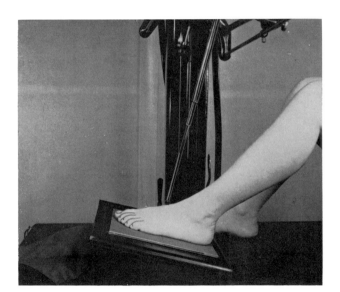

FOOT
Dorsoplantar projection
Plantodorsal view

Film: $8'' \times 10''$ or $10'' \times 12''$, depending upon the length of the foot.

Position of patient

Place the patient in the supine position. Flex the knee of the affected side enough to have the sole of the foot rest firmly on the table.

Position of part

Position the film holder under the foot, center to the base of the third metatarsal, and adjust the holder so that its midline is parallel with the long axis of the foot. The leg can be held in the vertical position by having the patient flex his opposite knee and lean it against the knee of the affected side.

In this position of the foot the entire plantar surface rests on the film holder, so that it is necessary to take precaution against slipping. A nonskid rubber mat may be placed under the film holder, or a bandage may be looped around the knee for the patient to hold. If necessary, the foot can be positioned on an angle block that is held in place with sandbags. In this case, the tube is tilted so as to direct the central ray at right angles to the plane of the film.

Central ray

Direct the central ray vertically to the base of the third metatarsal.

Structures shown

A dorsoplantar projection of the tarsals anterior to the talus, the metatarsals, and the phalanges. This projection is used for foreign body localization, for determining the position of fragments in fractures of the metatarsals and anterior tarsals, and as a general survey of the bones of the foot.

Dorsoplantar projection.

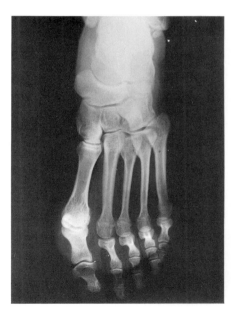

Plantodorsal projection.

FOOT
Oblique plantodorsal projections
Grashey positions

Film: $8'' \times 10''$ or $10'' \times 12''$, depending upon the length of the foot.

Position of patient

Place the patient in the prone position. Elevate the affected foot on sandbags and put a folded towel under the knee.

Position of part

Adjust the elevation of the foot so as to place its dorsal surface in contact with the film. Position the film holder under the foot, parallel with its long axis, and center to the base of the third metatarsal.

1. To demonstrate the interspace between the first and second metatarsals, rotate the heel medially approximately 30 degrees.

2. To demonstrate the interspaces between the second and third, the third and fourth, and the fourth and fifth metatarsals, adjust the foot so that the heel is rotated laterally approximately 20 degrees.

Central ray

Direct the central ray vertically to the midpoint of the film.

Structures shown

Oblique plantodorsal projections of the bones of the foot, and the interspaces of the proximal ends of the metatarsals.

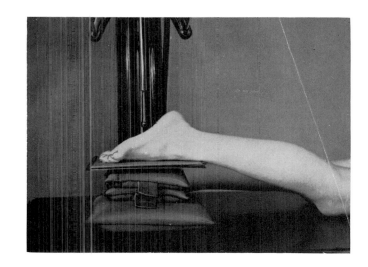

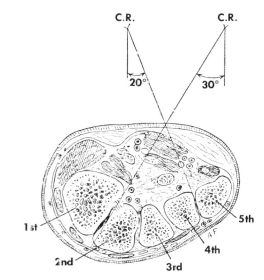

CORONAL SECTION NEAR BASE OF METATARSALS OF RIGHT FOOT

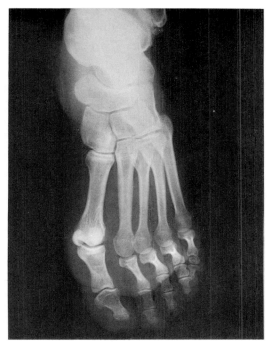

Medial rotation.

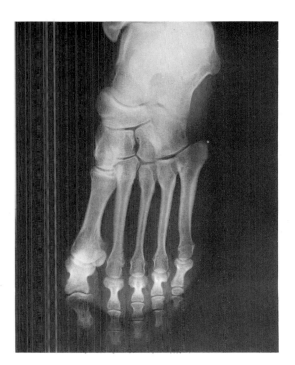

Lateral rotation.

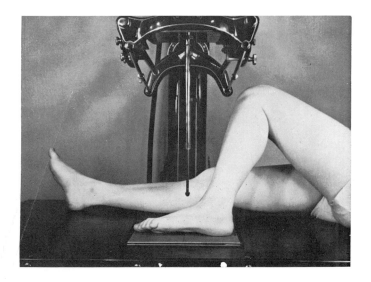

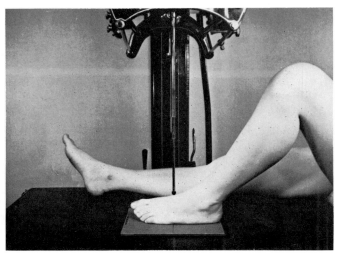

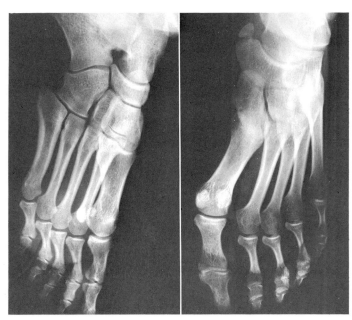

Medial oblique projection. Lateral oblique projection.

FOOT
Medial and lateral oblique projections

Film: $8'' \times 10''$ or $10'' \times 12''$, depending upon the length of the foot.

Position of patient

With the patient in the supine position, flex the knee of the affected side enough to have the sole of the foot rest firmly on the table.

Position of part

Place the film holder under the foot, parallel with its long axis, and center to the midline of the foot at the level of the base of the fifth metatarsal.

Medial oblique projection. Rotate the leg medially until the sole of the foot forms an angle of 30 degrees to the plane of the film.

Lateral oblique projection. Rotate the leg laterally until the sole of the foot forms an angle of 30 degrees to the film.

The elevated side of the foot should be supported on a 30-degree foam wedge to ensure consistent results.

Central ray

Direct the central ray vertically to the midpoint of the film.

Structures shown

Medial oblique projection. The interspaces between the cuboid and calcaneus, between the cuboid and the fourth and fifth metatarsals, between the cuboid and the third cuneiform, and between the talus and the navicular. The sinus tarsi is also well shown in this projection.

Lateral oblique projection. The interspaces between the first and second metatarsals, and between the first and second cuneiforms.

Badgley[1] and Doub[2] recommended the 30-degree medial oblique position for the demonstration of calcaneonavicular coalition.

[1]Badgley, C. E.: Coalition of the calcaneus and the navicular, Arch. Surg. **15:**75, 1927.
[2]Doub, Howard P.: A useful position for examining the foot, Radiology **16:**764-766, 1931.

FOOT

Oblique plantodorsal projection

Film: $8'' \times 10''$ or $10'' \times 12''$, depending upon the length of the foot.

Position of patient

Place the patient in the lateral recumbent position on the affected side, and have him flex his knees.

Position of part

Fully extend the leg of the side being examined. Have the patient turn toward the prone position until the sole of the foot forms an angle of about 45 degrees to the plane of the film. Center the film opposite the base of the fifth metatarsal and adjust it so that its midline is parallel with the long axis of the foot. In order to obtain uniform results, rest the dorsum of the foot against a foam wedge of the desired angle. The general survey study is usually made with the foot at an angle of 45 degrees.

Immobilize the foot by placing a sandbag across the lower leg.

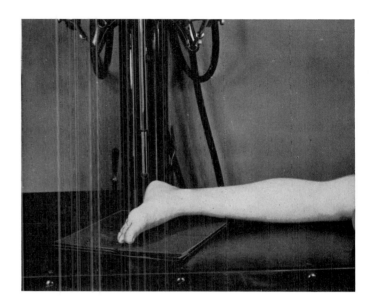

Central ray

Direct the central ray vertically to the midpoint of the film.

Structures shown

An oblique view of the bones of the foot. The articulations between the cuboid and the adjacent bones—the calcaneus, the third cuneiform, and the fourth and fifth metatarsals—are clearly shown. The articulations between the talus and the navicular, between the navicular and the cuneiforms, and between the sustentaculum tali and the talus, are usually shown.

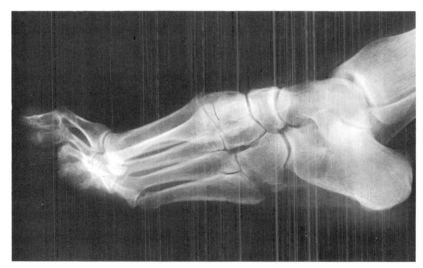

Foot obliqued 45 degrees.

FOOT

Lateral projections

Film: Approximately 2 inches longer than foot.

Position of patient

Whenever possible, lateral views of the foot should be made with its medial side in contact with the film holder. In the absence of an unusually prominent medial malleolus, hallux valgus, or other deformity, the foot assumes an exact or nearly exact lateral position when resting on its medial side. True lateral projections are therefore more easily and consistently obtained with the foot in this position.

Lateromedial projection

Position of part

Have the supine patient turn away from the affected side until the leg and foot are laterally placed. Elevate the knee enough to place the patella perpendicular to the horizontal, and support the knee on a sandbag.

Center the film holder to the mid-area of the foot and adjust it so that its midline is parallel with the long axis of the foot. Adjust the foot so that its plantar surface is perpendicular to the film.

Central ray

Direct the central ray vertically to the midpoint of the film.

Structures shown

A true lateral projection of the foot, the ankle joint, and the distal ends of the tibia and fibula.

Lateromedial position.

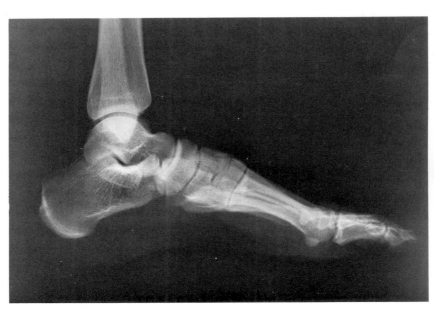

Lateromedial projection.

FOOT
Lateral projections—cont'd
Mediolateral projection

Position of part

Place the patient on the table and have him turn toward the affected side until the leg and foot are placed approximately laterally. Elevate the knee enough to place the patella perpendicular to the horizontal and to adjust a sandbag support under the knee.

Center the film holder to the mid-area of the foot and adjust the holder so that its midline is parallel with the long axis of the foot.

Dorsiflex the foot enough to rest it on its lateral surface, and adjust it so that the plantar surface is perpendicular to the film.

Central ray

The central ray is directed vertically to the midpoint of the film.

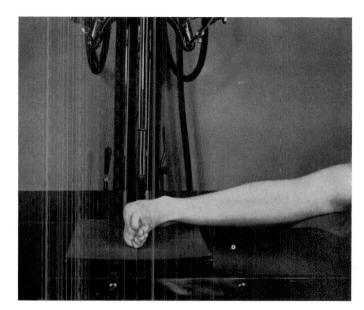

Mediolateral position.

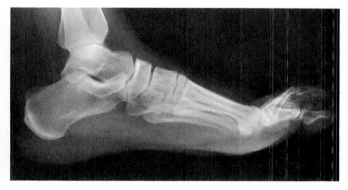

Lateromedial projection.

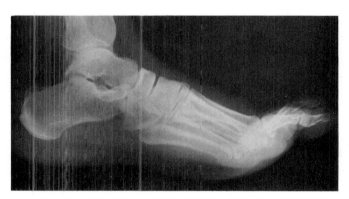

Mediolateral projection on opposite patient.

CALCANEUS

Use a 5″ × 7″ film, or the unmasked half of an 8″ × 10″ film, for a lateral view of the calcaneus, and center to the midportion of the heel, about 1 to 1½ inches distal to the medial malleolus. Adjust the film holder so that its long axis is parallel with the plantar surface of the heel.

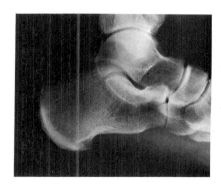

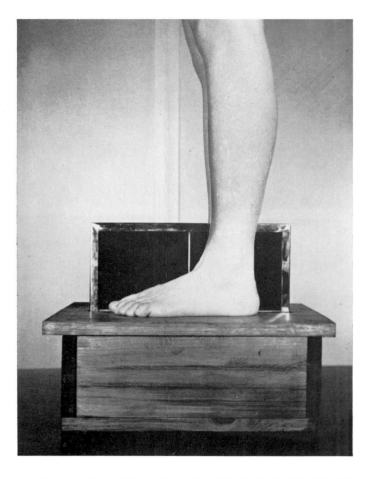

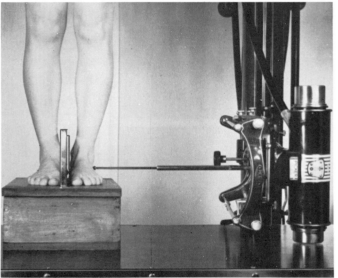

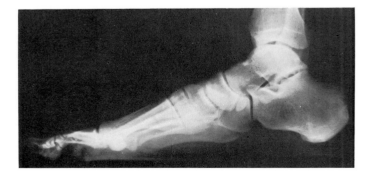

FOOT
Longitudinal arch
Lateral projection
Weight-bearing position

If the radiology department is not equipped with a mobile unit, or if the tube stand does not permit the tube to be lowered enough to allow the patient to stand on a low stool, this examination should not be undertaken unless the equipment is completely shock-proof. The patient must not be placed in the erect position on the radiographic table if the overhead system is not shock-proof.

Film

Select an $8'' \times 10''$ or a $10'' \times 12''$ film, depending upon the length of the foot and whether a unilateral or a bilateral examination is being done.

Position of patient

The patient is placed in the erect position, preferably on a low bench that has a film well such as that described by Gamble.[1] If such a bench is not available, blocks can be used to elevate the feet to tube level and to support the lead mat for the protection of the lower half of the film.

Position of part

Place the film holder in the film well of the bench, or between blocks, with a lead mat to protect its lower half.

Have the patient stand in a natural position, one foot on each side of the projecting film holder, with the weight of the body equally distributed on the feet. Adjust the film holder so that it is centered to the base of the fifth metatarsal.

After the first exposure has been made, lift the film holder out of the film well, turn it over to face the opposite foot, and place it back into the film well, being careful to center to the same point. Swing the tube around to the opposite side and make the second exposure.

Central ray

Direct the central ray perpendicularly to a point just above the base of the fifth metatarsal.

Structures shown

A lateral view of the bones of the foot in their weight-bearing position. This position is used to demonstrate the structural status of the longitudinal arch. Both sides are examined for comparison.

[1]Gamble, Felton O.: A special approach to foot radiography, Radiogr. Clin. Photogr. **19:**78-80, 1943.

FOOT

Composite dorsoplantar projection
Weight-bearing, axial view of entire foot

Film: $8'' \times 10''$ or $10'' \times 12''$, depending upon the length of the foot.

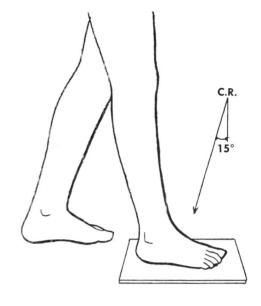

Position of patient

The patient is placed in the standing-erect position. Because the x-ray tube must be placed at a short distance from the patient, *this projection must never be used with equipment that is not shock-proof.* A unit of the mobile type is best suited for the examination because it allows the patient to stand at a comfortable height on a low bench, or on the floor. *The patient must never be placed in a standing position on the radiographic table where the overhead system is not shock-proof.*

Position of part

With the patient standing erect, adjust the film holder under the foot so as to center its midline to the long axis of the foot.

In order to prevent superimposition of the leg shadow on that of the ankle joint, have the patient place the opposite foot one step backward for the exposure of the forefoot, and one step forward for the exposure of the calcaneus.

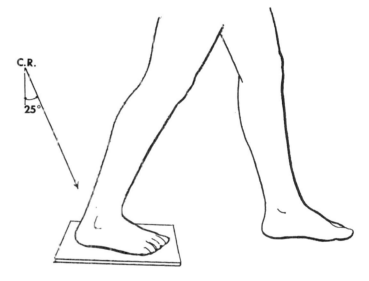

Central ray

In order to utilize the masking effect of the leg, the central ray must be directed along the plane of alignment of the foot in both exposures.

1. With the tube in front of the patient and adjusted for a posterior angulation of 15 degrees, center to the scaphoid for the first exposure.

Caution the patient to carefully maintain the position of the affected foot, and then have him place the opposite foot one step forward in preparation for the second exposure.

2. Place the tube behind the patient, adjust it for an anterior angulation of 25 degrees, and direct the central ray to the posterior surface of the ankle. It emerges on the plantar surface at the level of the lateral malleolus.

Structures shown

A weight-bearing, axial view of all the bones and the full outline of the foot projected free of the shadow of the leg.

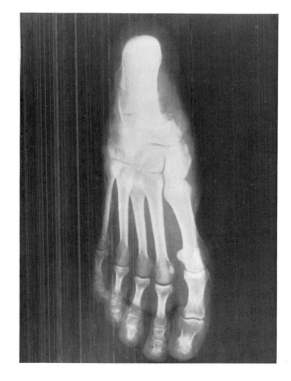

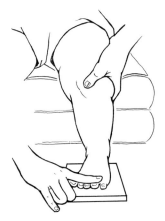

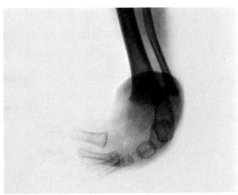

Dorsoplantar projection showing near 90-degree adduction of forefoot.

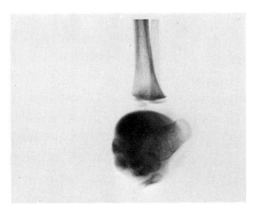

Lateral projection showing pitch of calcaneus, but other tarsals are obscured by adducted forefoot.

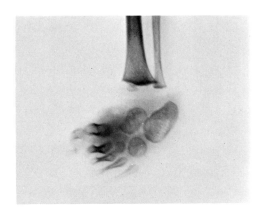

Oblique projection.

Above pretreatment studies and posttreatment studies on opposite page courtesy Dr. J. Hiram Kite.

CONGENITAL CLUBFOOT

The typical clubfoot, called talipes equinovarus, shows three deviations from the normal alignment of the foot in relation to the weight-bearing axis of the leg. These deviations are plantar flexion and inversion of the calcaneus (equinus), medial displacement of the forefoot (adduction), and elevation of the medial border of the foot (supination). There are numerous variations of the typical clubfoot and varying degrees of deformity in each of the typical abnormalities described above.

Kite positions

The classic Kite[1,2] positions—exactly placed dorsoplantar and lateral projections—for radiography of the clubfoot are employed to demonstrate the anatomy of the foot, and the bones and/or ossification centers of the tarsus and their relation to each other. *This objective makes it essential that no attempt be made to change the abnormal alignment of the foot when placing it on the cassette.* Kite[3] and Davis and Hatt[4] stated that even slight rotation of the foot can show marked alteration in the radiographically projected relation of the ossification centers. When special views are required, the physician either positions the foot or gives specific directions for its placement.

Dorsoplantar projection

This view demonstrates the degree of adduction of the forefoot and the degree of inversion of the calcaneus.

Position of patient

The infant is placed in the supine position, with the hips and knees flexed to permit the foot to rest flat on the cassette. Elevation of the body to knee height on firm pillows simplifies both gonadal shielding and leg adjustment.

Position of part

The feet are rested flat on the cassette, with the ankles extended slightly to prevent superimposition of the leg shadow. One parent is instructed to hold the infant's knees either together or in such a way that the legs are exactly vertical; that is, so that they do not lean medially or laterally. The other parent is instructed to hold the baby's toes. When the adduction deformity is too marked to permit correct placement of the legs and feet for bilateral projection without overlap of the feet, they must be separately examined.

Central ray

The central ray is directed *vertically* to the tarsus, midway between the tarsal areas for a bilateral projection. Kite stressed the importance of directing the central ray vertically for the purpose of projecting the true relationship of the bones and ossification centers.

[1]Kite, J. Hiram: Principles involved in the treatment of congenital clubfoot, J. Bone Joint Surg. 21:595-606, 1939.
[2]Kite, J. Hiram: The clubfoot, New York, 1964, Grune & Stratton, Inc.
[3]Kite, J. Hiram: Personal communication.
[4]Davis, L. A., and Hatt, W. S.: Congenital abnormalities of the feet, Radiology 64:818-825, 1955.

CONGENITAL CLUBFOOT
Kite positions—cont'd
Lateral projection

This view demonstrates the anterior talar subluxaticn and the degree of plantar flexion (equinus).

Position of patient

The infant is placed on his side in as near the lateral position as possible. The uppermost extremity is flexed, drawn forward, and so held by one parent.

Position of part

After adjusting the cassette under the foot, place a support having the same thickness as the cassette under the knee to prevent angulation of the foot. Instruct the other parent to hold the baby's toes.

Central ray

The central ray is directed vertically to the midtarsal area.

NOTE: For the demonstration of the degree of equinus deformity and of the relationship and concentricity of the opposing surfaces of the tibia and the talus, Marique[1] recommends that lateral studies of the ankle joint be made both before and after treatment. For these studies the foot should be dorsiflexed as much as possible without causing discomfort to the infant.

Kandel position

Suroplantar (dorsoplantar) projection

Kandel[2] recommends the inclusion of a suroplantar (dorsoplantar) projection in the examination of clubfeet.

For this view the infant is held in a vertical or a bending-forward position. The sole of the foot should rest on the cassette, although a moderate elevation of the heel is acceptable when the equinus is well marked. The central ray, at an anterior angulation of 40 degrees, is directed through the lower leg, as for the usual dorsoplantar projection of the calcaneus.

[1]Marique, Pierre: La réintégration non saglante de l'astragale, Rev. d'Orthop. 28:37-50, 1942.
[2]Kandel, B.: The suroplantar projection in the congenital clubfoot of the infant, Acta Orthop. Scand. 22:161-173, 1952.

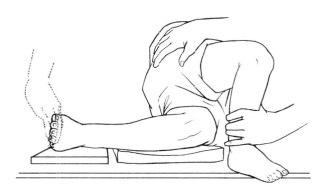

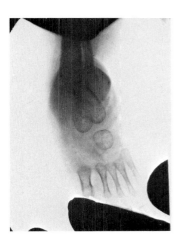

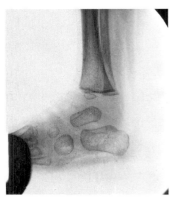

Dorsoplantar and lateral studies after correction of clubfoot deformity shown on the facing page.

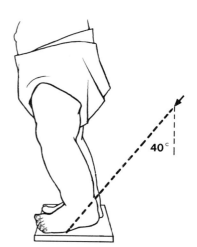

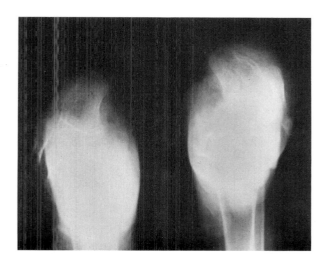

Dorsoplantar projection.

Courtesy Dr. Alex Norman.

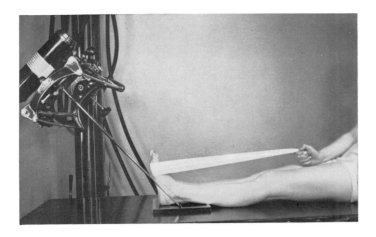

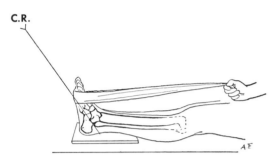

C.R.

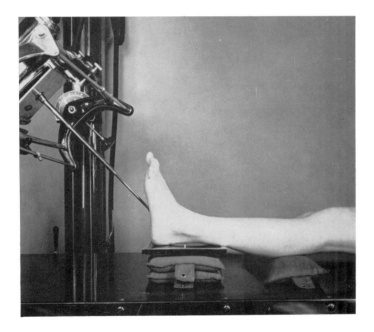

TARSUS
Calcaneus
Plantodorsal projection
Film: $8'' \times 10''$ for a bilateral examination.

Position of patient

Place the patient in either the supine position or in a seated position with the legs fully extended.

Position of part

Place the film holder under the ankles and center it midway between the ankle joints.

Put a long strip of gauze bandage around the balls of the feet and have the patient grasp it to hold the ankles in right-angle dorsiflexion. If the ankles cannot be flexed enough to place the plantar surfaces of the feet at right angles to the horizontal, elevate the extremities on sandbags to obtain the correct position.

Central ray

Direct the central ray to the midpoint of the film at a cranial angle of 40 degrees to the long axis of the feet. The central beam of rays will enter the plantar surfaces of the feet at the level of the bases of the fifth metatarsals and emerge just proximal to the ankle joints.

Structures shown

A semiaxial projection of the calcanei from the tuberosity to the sustentaculum tali and trochlear processes.

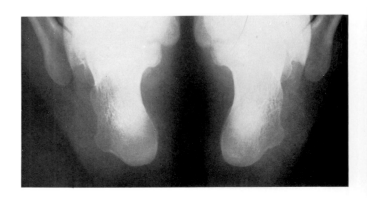

TARSUS
Calcaneus
Dorsoplantar projection

Film: $8'' \times 10''$ for a bilateral examination.

Position of patient

Place the patient in the prone position.

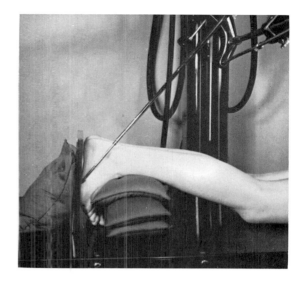

Position of part

Elevate the ankles on sandbags. Adjust the height and position of the sandbags under the ankles in such a way that the patient can dorsiflex his ankles enough to place the long axes of the feet at right angles to the horizontal.

Place the film holder against the plantar surfaces of the feet, center it midway between them, and support it in position with sandbags.

Central ray

Direct the central ray to the midpoint of the film at a caudal angle of 40 degrees to the long axes of the feet. The central beam of rays will enter the dorsal surfaces of the ankle joints and emerge on the plantar surfaces at the level of the bases of the fifth metatarsals.

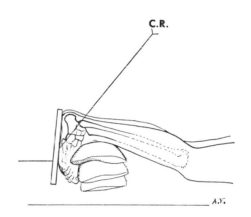

Structures shown

A semiaxial projection of the body of the calcanei from the tuberosity to the sustentaculum tali and trochlear processes.

Weight-bearing "coalition view"

This position, described by Lilienfeld[1] (cit. Holz-knecht), has come into use for the demonstration of cal-caneotalar coalition.[2,3,4] For this reason, it has been called the "coalition view."[2]

Place the patient in the standing-erect position. Center the film to the long axis of the calcaneus with the posterior surface of the heel at the edge of the film. To prevent superimposition of the leg shadow, ask the patient to place the opposite foot one step forward.

With the central ray at an anterior angle of exactly 45 degrees, direct it through the posterior surface of the flexed ankle to a point on the plantar surface at the level of the base of the fifth metatarsal.

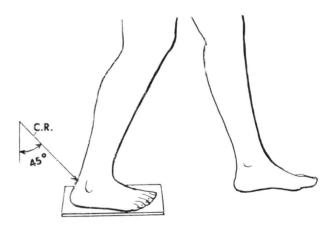

[1]Lilienfeld, Leon: Anordnung der normalisierten Röntgenaufnahmen des menschlichen Körpers, ed. 4, Urban & Schwarzenberg, p. 36, 1927.
[2]Harris, R. I., and Beath, T.: Etiology of peroneal spastic flat foot, J. Bone Joint Surg. **30-B:**624-634, 1948.
[3]Coventry, M. B.: Flatfoot with special consideration of tarsal coalition, Minnesota Med. **33:**1091-1097, 1950.
[4]Vaughan, W. H., and Segal, G.: Tarsal coalition, with special reference to roentgenographic interpretation, Radiology **60:**855-863, 1953.

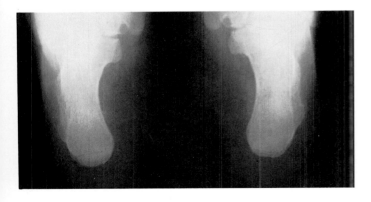

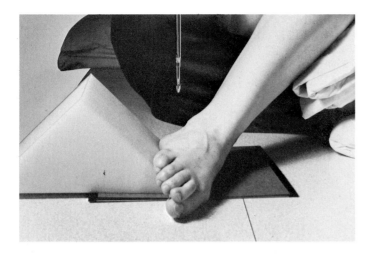

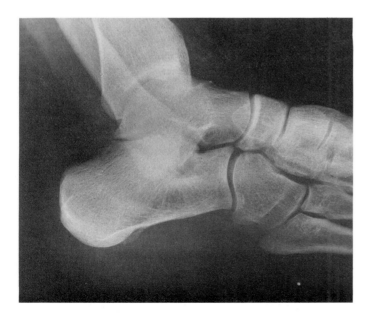

TARSUS AND SUBTALAR JOINT
Lateromedial oblique projection
Feist-Mankin position

Film: $8'' \times 10''$ crosswise.

Position of patient

Have the patient turn toward the unaffected side into a comfortable oblique position. Place a support under the hips. The patient is sometimes more comfortable when he turns from a seated position and supports himself on the outstretched hand.

Position of part

Ask the patient to flex his knee enough to place the ankle in near right-angle flexion and then to lean the leg and foot medialward.

With the medial border of the patient's foot in contact with the film holder, place a 45-degree foam wedge under the elevated lateral side of the foot. Adjust the leg so as to place its long axis coextensive with that of the foot, and adjust a support under the knee. The foot and leg can be easily adjusted at the required 45-degree angle by placing the foam wedge on the medial side, as shown in the lower photograph. A second 45-degree foam wedge may be placed under the lateral side of the foot when necessary.

Central ray

Direct the central ray vertically to a point just distal to the lateral malleolus.

Structures shown

A 45-degree, oblique projection of the tarsus. The cuboid and navicular bones and the subtalar joint are well shown.

The originators[1] state that the basic position can be modified, as indicated for individual patients, by increasing or decreasing the obliquity of the foot or, keeping the foot in contact with the foam wedge, by inversion or eversion of the foot.

[1]Feist, J. H., and Mankin, H. J.: The tarsus: basic relationships and motions in the adult and definition of optimal recumbent oblique projection, Radiology **79:**250-263, 1962.

SUBTALAR JOINT
Middle and posterior articulations
Superoinferior oblique lateral projection
Film: $8'' \times 10''$ lengthwise.

Position of patient

Have the patient lie on the affected side in the lateral position. Flex the uppermost knee to a comfortable position and support it on sandbags to prevent too much forward rotation of the body.

Position of part

Ask the patient to extend the affected extremity. Let it roll slightly forward from the lateral position. Center the film holder 1 to 1½ inches distal to the ankle joint, and adjust it so that its midline is parallel with the long axis of the leg.

Adjust the obliquity of the foot so that the heel is elevated about 1½ inches from the exact lateral position. The ball of the foot (the metatarsophalangeal area) will be angled forward some 25 degrees. Immobilize the foot with a sandbag placed across the leg.

Central ray

Direct the central ray to the ankle joint at an eccentric angle of 5 degrees anteriorly and 23 degrees distally.

Structures shown

This projection demonstrates the middle and posterior articulations of the subtalar joint, and gives an "end-on" view of the sinus tarsi and an unobstructed view of the lateral malleolus.

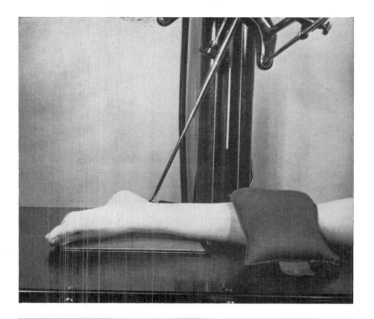

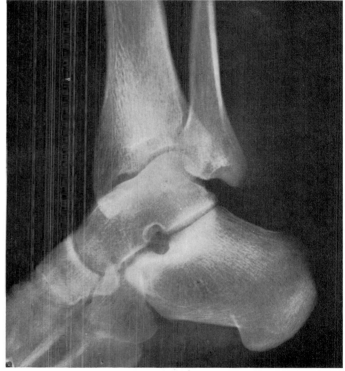

83

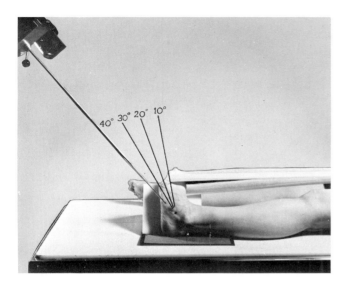

SUBTALAR JOINT
Posterior articulation
Broden positions

Broden[1] recommends these right-angle oblique projections for the demonstration of the posterior articular facet of the calcaneus to determine the presence of joint involvement in cases of comminuted fracture.

Film

Use an $8'' \times 10''$ film for each projection. Because several projections are made at different central ray angulations in each position, a film tunnel should be used to obviate the need to reposition the foot for each projection.

Position of patient

Place the patient in the supine position. Adjust a small sandbag under each knee and under the unaffected ankle. Have a sandbag ready for placement under the elevated hip when the extremity is rotated medially.

Position of part

Place the film tunnel under the lower leg and heel, and with its midline parallel with, and centered to, the leg, adjust its position so that the lower edge of the film will be about 1 inch distal to the plantar surface of the heel.

Loop a strip of 2- or 3-inch bandage around the ball of the foot. Ask the patient to grasp the ends of the bandage, dorsiflex his foot enough to obtain right-angle flexion at the ankle joint, and then maintain the flexion with pull on the bandage.

Medial oblique projections
Position of part

With the patient's ankle joint maintained in right-angle flexion, rotate the leg and foot 45 degrees medially and rest the foot against a 45-degree foam wedge.

[1]Broden, Bror: Roentgen examination of the subtaloid joint in fractures of the calcaneus, Acta Radiol. **31**:85-91, 1949.

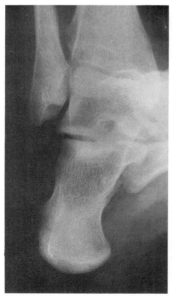

40-degree projection.

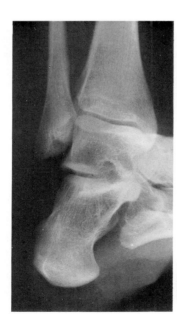

30-degree projection.

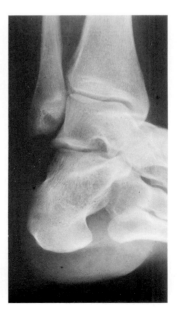

20-degree projection.

10-degree projection.

SUBTALAR JOINT
Posterior articulation
Broden positions
Medial oblique projection—cont'd

Central ray

Four projections are taken with the central ray angled toward the head at 40, 30, 20, and 10 degrees, respectively. For each of the projections, the central ray is directed to a point 2 or 3 cm. caudoanteriorly to the lateral malleolus, to about the midpoint of an imaginary line extending between the most prominent point of the lateral malleolus and the base of the fifth metatarsal.

Structures shown

The 40-degree projection shows the anterior portion of the posterior facet to best advantage. The 10-degree projection shows the posterior portion. The articulation between the talus and the sustentaculum tali is usually shown best in one of the intermediate projections.

Lateral oblique projections

Position of part

With the ankle joint held in right-angle flexion, rotate the leg and foot 45 degrees laterally and rest the foot against a 45-degree foam wedge.

Central ray

Two or three studies may be made with a 3- or 4-degree difference in central ray angulation. The central ray is directed to a point 2 cm. distal and 2 cm. anterior to the medial malleolus, at a cranial angulation of 15 degrees for the first exposure.

Structures shown

The posterior facet of the calcaneous in profile. The articulation between the talus and the sustentaculum tali is usually shown.

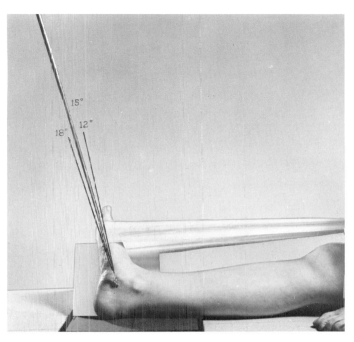

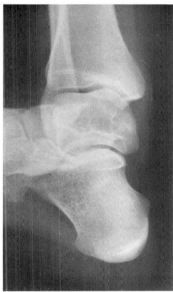

15-degree projection.

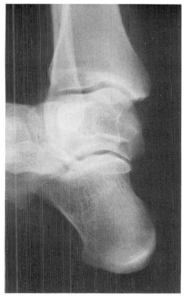

18-degree projection.

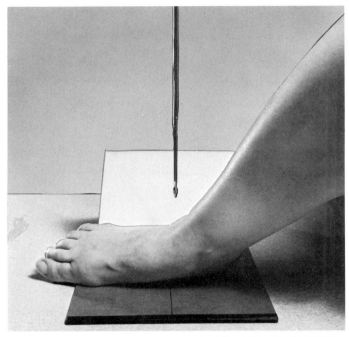

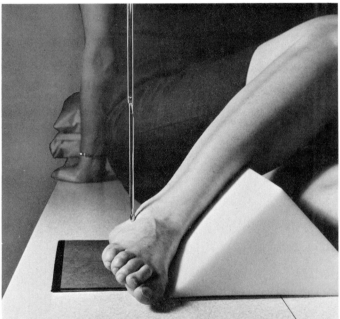

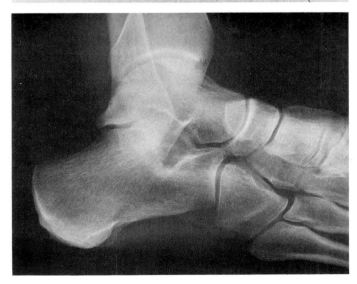

Anterior articulation.

SUBTALAR JOINT
Isherwood positions

Isherwood[1] devised a position for each of the three separate articulations of the subtalar joint—an *oblique lateral* projection for the demonstration of the anterior articulation, a *medial oblique axial* projection for the middle articulation, and a *lateral oblique axial* projection for the posterior articulation.

Film: $8'' \times 10''$ for each projection.

Oblique lateral projection

Position of patient

Place the patient in a semisupine or seated position, and have him turn away from the side being examined. Ask him to flex his knee enough to place the ankle joint in near right-angle flexion and then to lean the leg and foot medially.

Position of part

With the medial border of the foot resting on the film holder, place a 45-degree foam wedge under the elevated lateral side. Adjust the leg so that its long axis is coextensive with that of the foot. Place a support under the knee. Accurate adjustment of the leg is ensured by placing the foam wedge under the medial side of the foot and ankle, as shown in the second photograph. A second 45-degree foam wedge may be placed under the lateral side of the foot.

Central ray

Direct the central ray vertically to a point 1 inch distal and 1 inch anterior to the lateral malleolus.

Structures shown

The anterior subtalar articulation and an oblique view of the tarsus. The Feist-Mankin position produces a similar view (page 82).

[1]Isherwood, Ian: A radiological approach to the subtalar joint, J. Bone Joint Surg. **43-B:**566-574, 1961.

SUBTALAR JOINT
Isherwood positions—cont'd
Medial oblique axial projection

Position of patient

Have the patient assume a seated position on the table and turn with his weight resting on the flexed hip and thigh of the unaffected side. The patient may be adjusted in a semilateral recumbent position if it is more comfortable.

Position of part

Ask the patient to rotate the leg and foot medially, enough to rest the side of the foot and ankle against a 30-degree foam wedge. Place a support under the knee, and if the patient is recumbent, place another under the greater trochanter. Dorsiflex the foot, invert it when possible, and have the patient maintain the position by pulling on a strip of 2- or 3-inch bandage looped around the ball of the foot.

Central ray

Direct the central ray to a point 1 inch distal and 1 inch anterior to the lateral malleolus at an angle of 10 degrees toward the head.

Structures shown

The middle articulation of the subtalar joint and an "end-on" view of the sinus tarsi.

Lateral oblique axial projection
Position of patient

The patient may be placed in either the supine or the seated position.

Position of part

Ask the patient to rotate the leg and foot laterally until the side of the foot and ankle rests against a 30-degree foam wedge. Dorsiflex the foot, evert it when possible, and have the patient maintain the position by pulling on a broad bandage looped around the ball of the foot.

Central ray

Direct the central ray to a point 1 inch distal to the medial malleolus at an angle of 10 degrees toward the head.

Structures shown

The posterior articulation of the subtalar joint in profile.

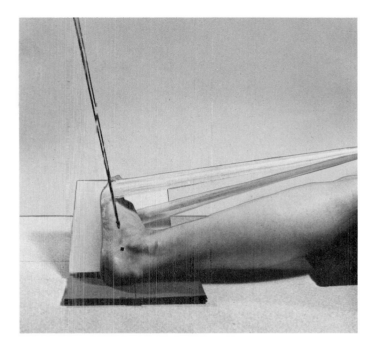

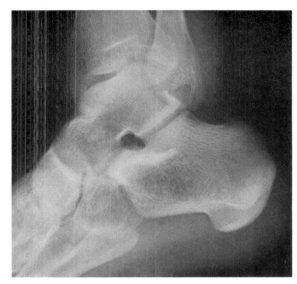

Middle articulation.

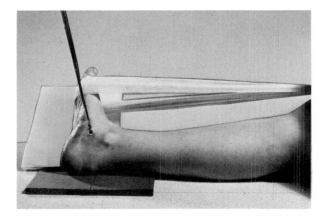

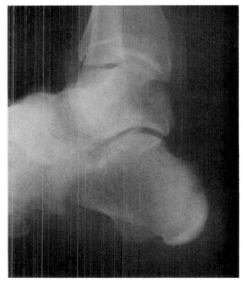

Posterior articulation.

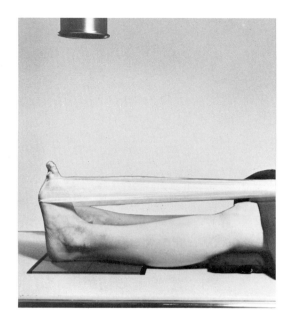

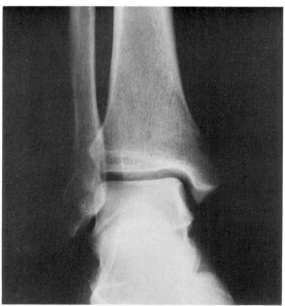

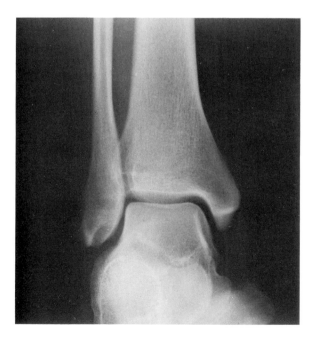

ANKLE
Anteroposterior projection
Posteroanterior view

Film: 8″ × 10″ lengthwise, 10″ × 12″ crosswise for two views on one film.

Position of patient

Place the patient in the supine position and place a small sandbag under each knee to relieve strain.

Position of part

Adjust the ankle joint in the anteroposterior position by flexing the ankle and pronating the foot enough to place its long axis in the vertical position. Slight inversion of the foot, using care not to rotate the leg, will open up the talofibular articulation, as shown in the lower radiograph. Immobilize with sandbags adjusted against the plantar surface of the foot or, preferably, by having the patient support the position with a strip of bandage looped around the ball of the foot.

Ball and Egbert[1] state that the appearance of the ankle mortise will not be appreciably altered by moderate plantar flexion or dorsiflexion as long as the leg is rotated neither laterally nor medially. Lauge-Hansen[2] recommends that the foot be elevated 5 cm., pronated to the greatest possible extent, and dorsiflexed.

If a larger area of the leg is desired, use a longer film, and position the plantar surface of the heel to the lower edge of the film. However, if the joint is involved, always direct the central ray to the joint.

Central ray

Direct the central ray vertically to the ankle joint at a point midway between the malleoli.

Structures shown

An anteroposterior projection of the ankle joint, the lower ends of the tibia and fibula, and the upper portion of the astragalus. Neither the inferior tibiofibular articulation nor the inferior portion of the lateral malleolus is well demonstrated in this projection.

[1]Ball, R. P., and Egbert, E. W.: Ruptured ligaments of the ankle, Amer. J. Roentgen. **50**:770-771, 1943.
[2]Lauge-Hansen, N.: Fractures of the ankle, Amer. J. Roentgen. **71**:456-471, 1954.

ANKLE

Lateral projection

Film: 8" × 10" lengthwise.

When possible, lateral views of the ankle joint should be made with the medial side of the ankle in contact with the film holder. This position places the joint closer to the film and thus provides considerable improvement in its projected image. A further advantage is that exact positioning of the ankle is more easily and more consistently obtained when the extremity is rested on its comparatively flat medial surface.

Lateromedial projection

Have the supine patient turn away from the affected side until the leg is approximately laterally placed.

Position of part

Center the film holder to the ankle joint and adjust it so that its midline is parallel with the long axis of the leg. Adjust the foot in the lateral position. Have the patient turn forward or backward, as required, to place the patella perpendicular to the horizontal. If necessary, place a support under the knee.

Mediolateral projection

Have the supine patient turn toward the affected side until the leg is approximately laterally placed.

Position of part

With the midline of the film holder parallel with the long axis of the leg, center it to the ankle joint. Have the patient turn forward or backward, as required, to place the patella perpendicular to the horizontal, and place a support under the knee. Dorsiflex the foot somewhat and adjust it in the lateral position; dorsiflexion is required here to prevent lateral rotation of the ankle.

Central ray

Direct the central ray vertically through the ankle joint.

Structures shown

A true lateral view of the lower third of the tibia and fibula, of the ankle joint, and of the tarsus.

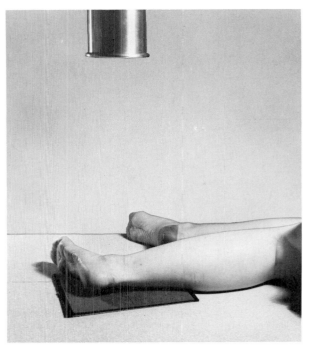

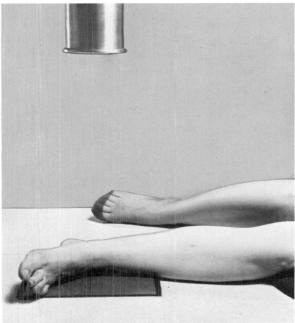

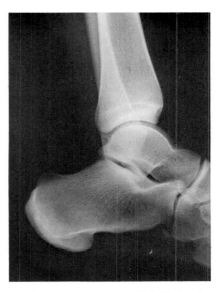

Lateromedial projection (medial side down).

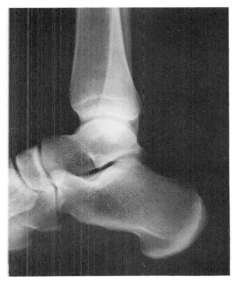

Mediolateral projection (lateral side down).

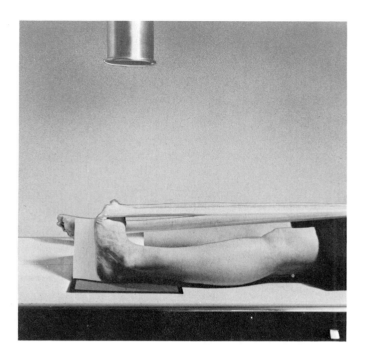

ANKLE
Oblique projections
Film: $8'' \times 10''$ lengthwise; $10'' \times 12''$ crosswise for two views on one film.

Position of patient

The patient is examined in the recumbent position. Because the anteroposterior and lateral projections are usually made on one film, either the lateral view or the oblique view or views should be made first in order to spare the patient unnecessary movement.

Position of part

The leg as well as the foot must be rotated for oblique projections of the ankle, and since the knee is a hinge joint, rotation of the extremity can come only from the hip joint.

An increase in the normal anteversion of the femoral neck rolls the extremity laterally when the body is supine. Positioning for a lateral oblique requires only that the side of the ankle and foot be rested against a 45-degree foam wedge and that the foot be adjusted in dorsiflexion.

In order to rotate the extremity medially, the femoral neck must be rotated forward. This is done by elevating the hip on a suitable support placed under the greater trochanter.

Center the film holder to the ankle joint midway between the malleoli and adjust it so that its midline is parallel with the long axis of the leg. Adjust the support under the hip so that the medial side of the ankle and foot rests against a 45-degree foam wedge. Place a sandbag support under the knee.

Dorsiflex the foot enough to prevent superimposition of the lateral malleolus and the calcaneus, and enough to place the ankle at near right-angle flexion when possible. Immobilize the ankle with sandbags placed against the sole of the foot or by having the patient hold the ends of a strip of bandage looped around the ball of the foot.

Central ray

Direct the central ray vertically to the ankle joint.

Structures shown

An oblique view of the distal ends of the tibia and fibula, the lateral malleolus being particularly well shown in the medial oblique view. The view obtained of the talus and the talocalcaneal articulation depends upon the degree of dorsiflexion of the foot.

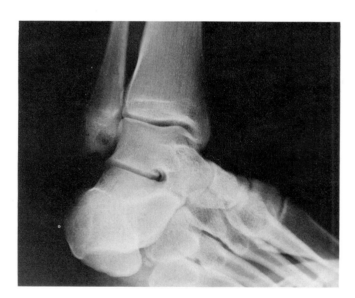

Medial oblique projection, 45 degrees.

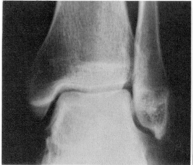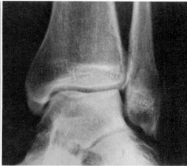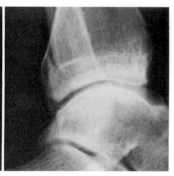

Fracture films courtesy Dr. Hudson J. Wilson, Jr.

ANKLE

Anteroposterior stress studies

Stress studies of the ankle joint are made, usually following an inversion or supination injury, to verify the presence of a ligamentous tear. Rupture of a ligament is demonstrated by widening of the joint space on the side of the injury when, with the ankle kept in the anteroposterior position, the foot is forcibly turned toward the opposite side.

When the injury is recent and the ankle is acutely sensitive to movement, the orthopedic surgeon may inject a local anesthetic into the sinus tarsi preceding the examination. The physician adjusts the foot when it must be turned into extreme stress, and he either holds or straps it in position for the exposure. Under local anesthesia or when the ankle is not too painful, the patient can usually hold the foot in the stress position by asymmetrical pull on a strip of bandage looped around the ball of the foot.

A short exposure-time screen technique is used in all stress studies.

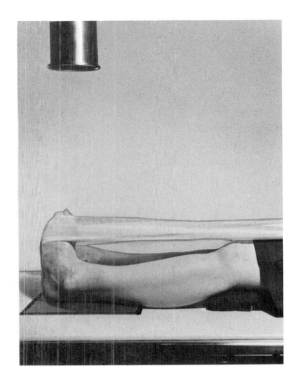

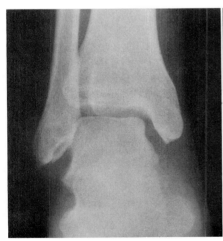 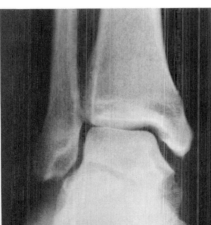 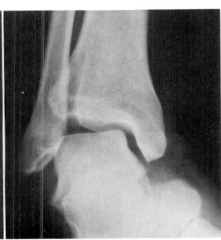

Neutral position.

Eversion stress. No damage to medial ligament indicated.

Inversion stress. Note change in joint. Rupture of lateral ligament.

Stress studies and diagnostic information courtesy Dr. William H. Shehadi.

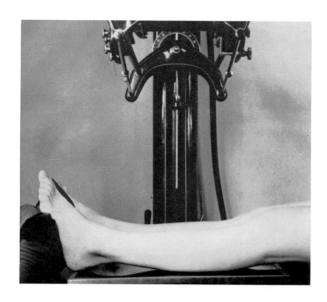

LEG
Anteroposterior, lateral, and oblique projections

Film: $7'' \times 17''$, or $14'' \times 17''$ for two views on one film.

For each of these projections, the cassette is placed parallel with the long axis of the leg and centered to the mid-shaft. Unless the leg is unusually long, the film will extend beyond the knee and ankle joints enough to prevent their being projected off the film by the divergency of the beam of roentgen rays. The film should, depending upon the focal-film distance, extend from 1 to 1½ inches beyond the joints. When the leg is too long for these allowances and the site of the lesion is not known, two films must be used. Place the longer film high enough to include the knee joint, and use a small film for the distal end of the leg. If the site of the lesion has been localized, adjust the film to include the nearer joint.

Position of patient

The patient is placed in the supine position. Less movement of the patient is involved by taking the oblique views first, then the anteroposterior, followed by the lateral, or by reversing this order.

Position of part

Anteroposterior projection. With the patient supine, adjust the body so that there is no rotation of the pelvis. Adjust the leg in the anteroposterior position; invert the foot slightly, but do not rotate the leg. Place a sandbag against the sole of the foot to immobilize it in the correct position.

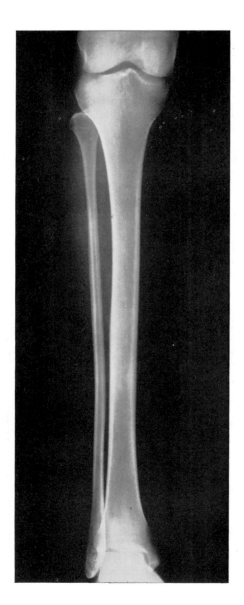

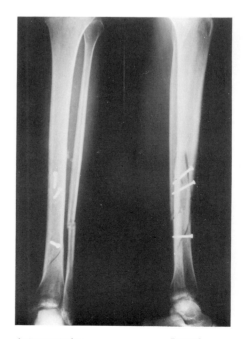

Anteroposterior.   Lateral.

Courtesy Dr. Hudson J. Wilson, Jr.

LEG

Anteroposterior, lateral, and oblique projections

Position of part—cont'd

Lateral projection. From the supine position, the patient may be turned either toward or away from the affected side. Adjust the rotation of the body in order to place the patella perpendicular to the horizontal, and place sandbag supports where needed for the patient's comfort and to stabilize the body position.

After the placement of the cassette, readjust the leg to place the patella perpendicular to the plane of the film. Place a sandbag against the sole of the foot.

When the patient cannot be turned from the supine position, the lateral view must be made by cross-table projection. Lift the leg just enough for an assistant to slide a strip of bakelite, or other rigid support, under it, and then place a small sandbag under each end of the support in order to center the leg to a vertically placed cassette.

Oblique projections. Oblique projections of the leg are taken by alternately rotating the extremity 45 degrees laterally and medially. Because of the increased anteversion of the femoral neck in the supine position, the adjustment of the leg for the lateral oblique projection usually requires only that the lateral side of the foot and ankle be rested against a 45-degree foam wedge. For the medial oblique projection, abduct the extremity somewhat, or shift the pelvis away from the affected extremity when it cannot be moved. Then elevate the hip enough to rest the medial side of the foot and ankle against a 45-degree foam wedge, and place a support under the greater trochanter.

Central ray

The central ray is directed vertically to the midpoint of the film.

Structures shown

Anteroposterior, lateral, and 45-degree oblique projections of the bones and soft tissues of the leg, and one or both of the adjacent joints.

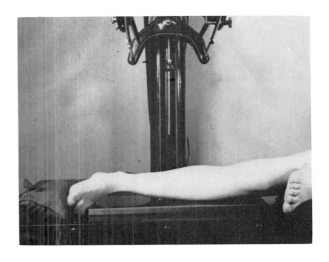

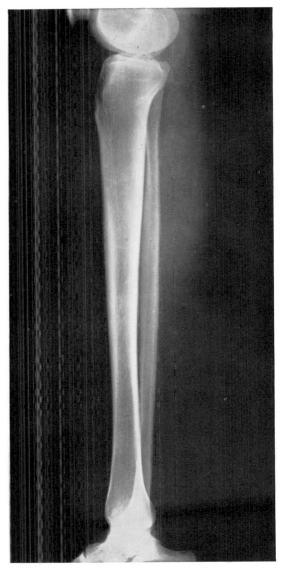

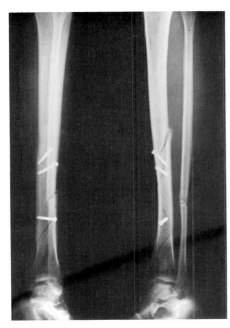

45-degree oblique projections.
Courtesy Dr. Hudson J. Wilson, Jr.

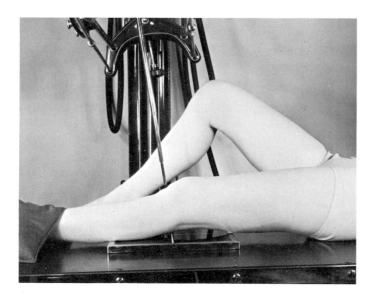

KNEE
Anteroposterior projection
Posteroanterior view

Attention is again called to the need for gonadal shielding in examinations of the lower extremities A sheet of lead rubber is easy to use.

Film: $8'' \times 10''$ lengthwise.

Position of patient

Place the patient in the supine position and adjust the body so that there is no rotation of the pelvis. Place a sandbag under the ankle of the affected side.

Position of part

With the cassette under the patient's knee, flex the joint slightly, locate the apex of the patella and, as the patient extends the knee, center the cassette about ½ inch below the patellar apex. This will center the film to the knee joint.

Adjust the leg in a true anteroposterior position; the patella will lie slightly off center to the medial side. Place a sandbag across the ankle to immobilize it.

If the knee cannot be fully extended, elevate the cassette on sandbags to bring it in contact with the part; if the degree of flexion is fairly great, use a curved cassette or a flexible film holder.

Central ray

When radiographing the joint space, tilt the tube so that the central ray will be directed to the joint at an angle of 5 to 7 degrees toward the head.

When radiographing the distal end of the femur or the proximal ends of the tibia and fibula, the central ray may be directed at right angles to the joint.

Structures shown

An anteroposterior projection of the knee structures. If the position is correct and the knee is normal, the interspace between the medial femoral condyle and the medial tibial plateau and the interspace between the lateral femoral condyle and the lateral tibial plateau will be equal in width.

NOTE: Some radiologists prefer that the frontal view of the knee joint be taken from the posteroanterior direction. The patient is adjusted in the prone position with the ankles and feet extended over sandbag supports. Because the knee is balanced on the medial side of the obliquely placed patella, care must be used in adjusting and immobilizing the extremity in a direct posteroanterior position.

The central ray is directed to the popliteal depression, usually vertically.

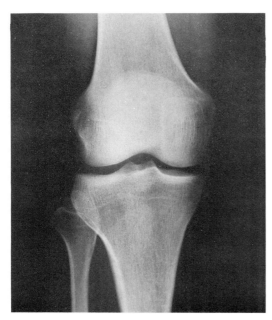

5-degree central ray angulation.

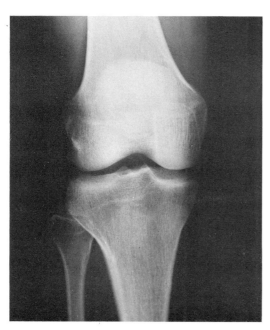

0-degree central ray angulation.

KNEE
Lateral projection

Film: $8'' \times 10''$ lengthwise.

Position of patient

Ask the patient to turn onto his affected side. When the knee is to be adjusted in right-angle flexion, have the patient bring it forward and extend the other extremity behind it, as shown in the opposite photograph. When the knee is to be examined in extension or partial flexion, the opposite extremity is brought forward and the flexed knee is then supported on sandbags to prevent forward rotation of the pelvis.

A flexion of 20 to 30 degrees is usually preferred for survey studies because, as pointed out by Scheller[1], this position relaxes the muscles and shows the maximal volume of the joint cavity.

In order to prevent fragment separation in new or unhealed patellar fractures, the knee should not be flexed more than 10 degrees, if at all; in any case, it should be flexed just enough to relax the muscles.

Position of part

Flex the knee to the desired angle. Center the film to the knee joint; the joint can be easily located by palpating the depression between the femoral and tibial condyles on the medial side of the knee just below the level of the patellar apex.

Place a sandbag under the ankle, grasp the medial and lateral borders of the patella between the thumb and index finger of one hand, and adjust the sandbag so as to place the long axis of the leg in a horizontal position; the patella will be perpendicular to the plane of the film.

Central ray

Direct the central ray to the knee joint at an angle of 5 degrees toward the head. This slight angulation of the central ray will prevent the joint space from being obscured by the magnified shadow of the medial femoral condyle.

Structures shown

A lateral view of the lower end of the femur, the patella, the knee joint, the upper ends of the tibia and fibula, and the adjacent soft parts. If the position is correct and there is no rotation, the interspace between the patella and the femoral condyles will be well demonstrated.

[1]Scheller, Sven: Roentgenographic studies on epiphyseal growth and ossification in the knee, Acta Radiol. **195**:12-16, 1960.

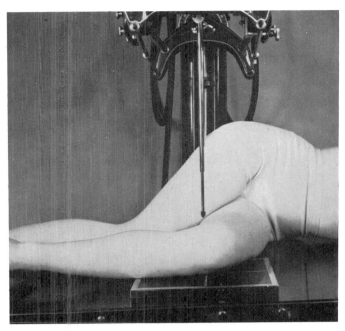

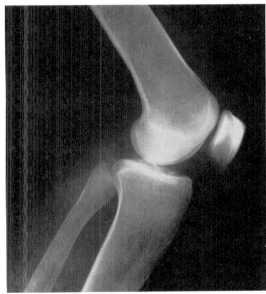

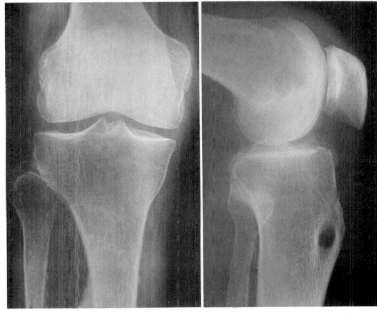

Courtesy Dr. Henry K. Taylor.

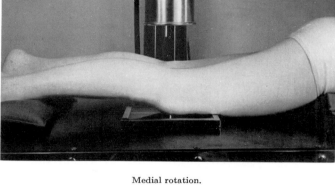

Medial rotation.

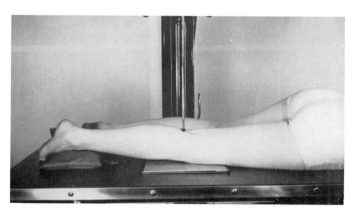

Lateral rotation.

KNEE
Posterior oblique projections
Anterior oblique views

Film: $8'' \times 10''$ lengthwise, or $10'' \times 12''$ crosswise for two views on one film.

Position of patient

Place the patient on the table in the prone position and support the ankles on small sandbags.

Position of part

Posteromedial oblique projection. Elevate the hip of the affected side enough to rotate the extremity medially 45 degrees, and support the hip on sandbags. Place the cassette under the knee, parallel with its long axis, and center to the joint.

Posterolateral oblique projection. Reverse the above position by elevating the opposite hip enough to rotate the affected extremity laterally about 45 degrees. Support the elevated hip on sandbags.

Holmblad[1] recommended that the knee be flexed about 10 degrees on both of these views.

Central ray

Direct the central ray vertically through the knee joint.

Structures shown

Posterior oblique projections of the femoral condyles, the patella, the tibial condyles, and the fibular head. The head of the fibula and the proximal tibiofibular articulation are particularly well shown with the posterolateral oblique projection.

[1]Holmblad, Edward C.: Improved x-ray technic in studying knee joints, Southern Med. J. **32**:240-243, 1939.

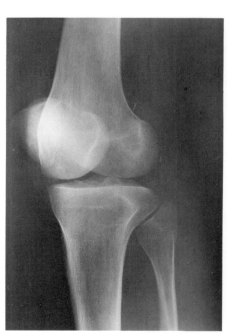

Posteromedial oblique projection.

Posterolateral oblique projection.

KNEE
Anterior oblique projections
Posterior oblique views

Film: 8″ × 10″ lengthwise, or 10″ × 12″ crosswise for two views on one film.

Position of patient

Place the patient on the table in the supine position, and support the ankles on small sandbags.

Position of part

Anterolateral oblique projection. Elevate the hip of the unaffected side enough to rotate the affected extremity 45 degrees laterally. Support the elevated hip and knee of the unaffected side on sandbags and adjust the sandbag under the ankle of the affected side to prevent flexion of the knee.

With the cassette parallel with the long axis of the knee, center approximately ½ inch below the apex of the patella. Immobilize the knee with sandbags placed across the ankle.

Anteromedial oblique projection. Reverse the above position by elevating the hip of the affected side enough to rotate the extremity 45 degrees medially; place a support under the hip. Adjust a sandbag under the film holder to place it in contact with the knee, which is elevated several inches in this position.

Central ray

Direct the central ray vertically to the knee joint.

Structures shown

Anterior oblique projections of the femoral condyles, the patella, the tibial condyles, and the head of the fibula. The proximal tibiofibular articulation is well demonstrated in the anteromedial oblique projection.

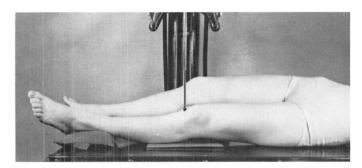

Lateral rotation.

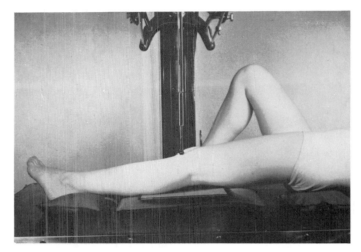

Medial rotation.

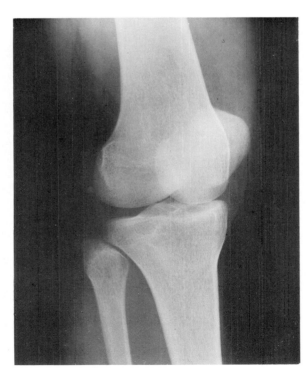

Anteromedial oblique projection.

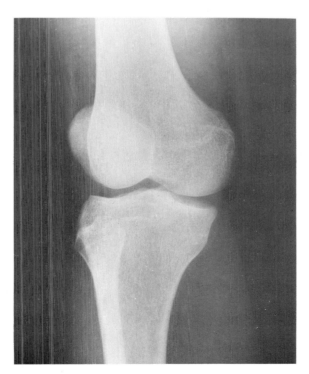

Anterolateral oblique projection.

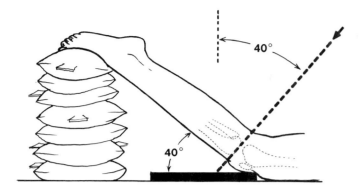

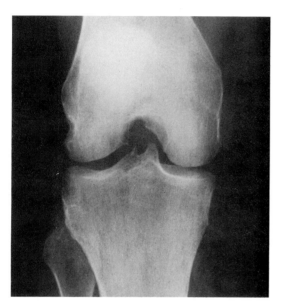

40-degree flexion of knee.

INTERCONDYLOID FOSSA
Semiaxial posteroanterior projection
Camp-Coventry position[1]
Film: $8'' \times 10''$ lengthwise.

Position of patient

Ask the patient to turn to the prone position, and then adjust the body so that there is no rotation. Place a sandbag under the ankle and foot of the unaffected side for the patient's comfort.

Position of part

Because of the high elevation of the foot and the number of sandbags required to support it in position, it is expedient to use a firm, hair-filled cushion or a light-weight, wooden box for this purpose. By moving the support closer to, or farther away from, the knee, the correct angulation of the leg can be easily obtained.

Flex the knee to the approximate angle to be used and rest the foot on a suitable support. Center the proximal half of the cassette to the knee joint; the central ray angulation projects the joint to the center of the film.

According to the preference of the radiologist, set the protractor arm at an angle of either 40 or 50 degrees from the horizontal and place it beside the leg. Adjust the position of the foot support so as to place the anterior surface of the leg parallel with the arm of the protractor. Adjust the leg so that there is no medial or lateral rotation of the knee.

[1]Camp, John D., and Coventry, M. B.: Use of special views in roentgenography of the knee joint, U. S. Naval Med. Bull. **42:**56-58, 1944.

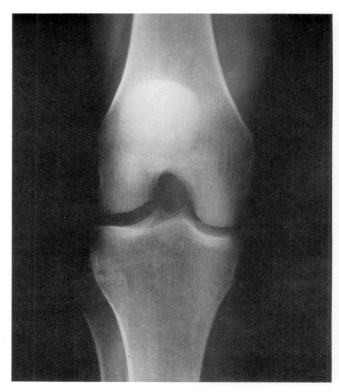

40-degree flexion of knee on opposite patient.

INTERCONDYLOID FOSSA
Semiaxial posteroanterior projection
Camp-Coventry position—cont'd

Central ray

Tilt the tube to direct the central ray at right angles to the long axis of the leg and center to the popliteal depression; the central ray will be angled 40 degrees when the knee is flexed 40 degrees, and 50 degrees when the knee is flexed 50 degrees.

Structures shown

A superoinferior projection giving a somewhat more "open" view of the intercondyloid fossa than is obtained with the positions described on the two following pages.

NOTE: An intercondyloid fossa projection is usually included in routine examinations of the knee joint for the detection of loose bodies (joint mice). The projection is also used in evaluating split and displaced cartilage in cases of osteochondritis dissecans, and flattening or underdevelopment of the lateral femoral condyle in cases of congenital slipped patella.

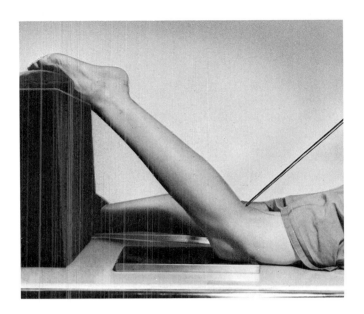

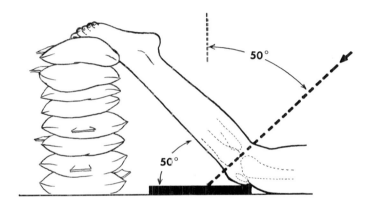

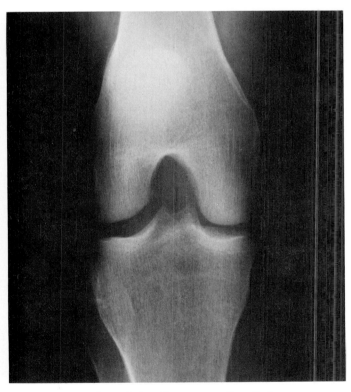

50-degree flexion of knee on opposite patient.

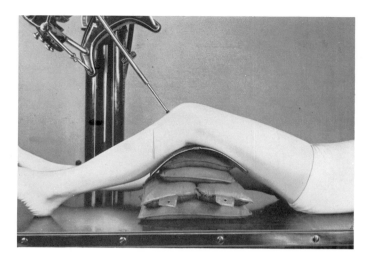

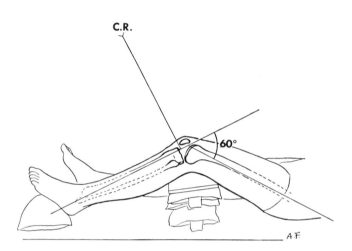

INTERCONDYLOID FOSSA
Semiaxial anteroposterior projection
Béclère position
Film

A 5″ × 7″ film placed crosswise is satisfactory, but it is preferable to use a curved cassette or a flexible film holder in order to obtain better part-film contact.

Position of patient

Place the patient in the supine position and adjust the body so that there is no rotation.

Position of part

Flex the affected knee enough to place the long axis of the femur at an angle, open upward, of 60 degrees to the long axis of the tibia. Support the knee on sandbags.

Place the cassette under the knee and position it so that its center point will coincide with the central ray. Adjust the leg in the anteroposterior position and immobilize the foot with sandbags.

Central ray

Direct the central ray at right angles to the long axis of the tibia and center to the knee joint.

Structures shown

An inferosuperior projection giving a profile view of the intercondyloid fossa, the tibial spine, and the knee joint.

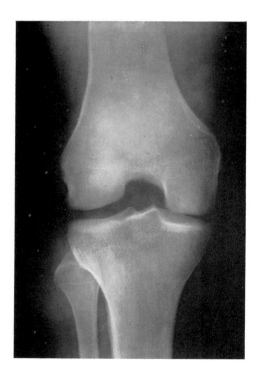

INTERCONDYLOID FOSSA
Semiaxial posteroanterior projection
Holmblad position[1]

Film: 8″ × 10″ lengthwise for a unilateral examination, 10″ × 12″ crosswise for a bilateral examination.

Position of patient

Place the patient on the table in a kneeling position with the feet extended over the end of the table so that the long axes of the legs will be parallel with the table. Have the patient lean forward on his hands.

Position of part

Place the film holder under the knee, parallel with the long axis of the tibia, and center to the apex of the patella. When performing a bilateral examination, center the film midway between the patellar apices.

Adjust the position of the body, that is, the degree of leaning, so that the long axes of the femora form an angle of 70 degrees to the horizontal (20 degrees to the vertical). Adjust the legs in a true posteroanterior position and immobilize them with sandbags.

Central ray

Direct the central ray vertically to the midpoint of the film.

Structures shown

The intercondyloid fossa of the femur and the tibial spines in profile. Holmblad[1] says that the degree of flexion used in this projection widens the joint space between the femur and tibia and gives a better view of the joint and of the surfaces of the tibia and femur.

[1]Holmblad, Edward C.: Postero-anterior x-ray view of the knee in flexion, J.A.M.A. **109**:1196-1197, 1937.

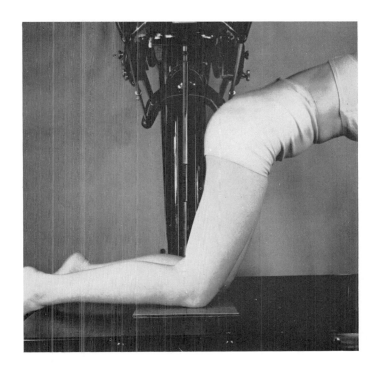

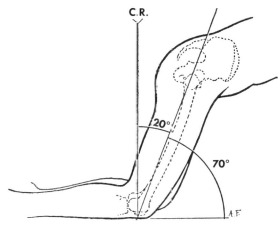

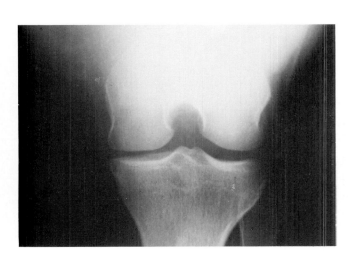

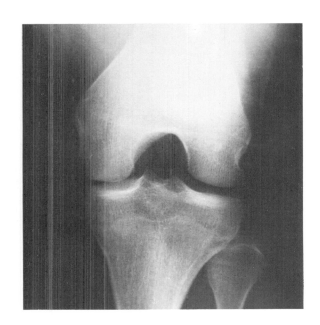

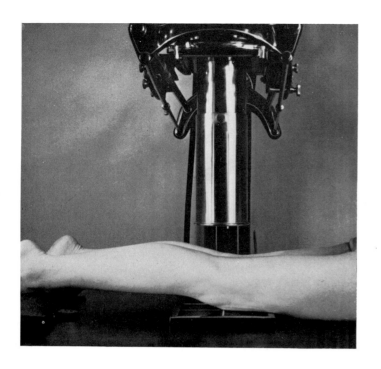

PATELLA
Posteroanterior projection
Anteroposterior view
Film: $8'' \times 10''$ lengthwise.

Position of patient

Place the patient in the prone position with the ankles and feet extended over sandbags. If the knee is painful, place one sandbag under the thigh and another under the leg to relieve pressure on the patella.

Position of part

With the cassette parallel to the long axis of the knee, center to the patella.

Adjust the position of the leg so as to place the patella parallel with the plane of the film; this usually requires that the heel be rotated 5 to 10 degrees outward. Immobilize with a sandbag across the ankle.

In order to demonstrate the patella through the superimposed femoral condyles, it is necessary to increase the exposure approximately 10 kilovolts; use a small cone to reduce secondary radiation.

Central ray

Direct the central ray vertically to the midpoint of the film.

Structures shown

A posteroanterior projection of the patella giving sharper detail than can be obtained in the anteroposterior position.

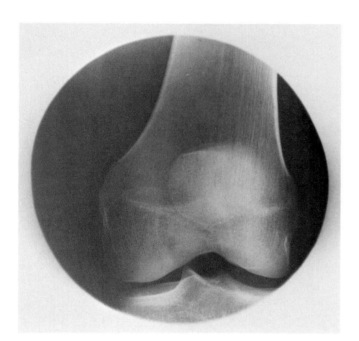

PATELLA
Superoinferior projection
Kuchendorf position
Film: 8″ × 10″ lengthwise.

Position of patient

Place the patient in the prone position. Elevate the hip of the affected side 2 or 3 inches and support it on sandbags. Place a sandbag under the ankle and foot and adjust it so that the knee will be slightly flexed, approximately 10 degrees, to relax the muscles.

Position of part

Center the film holder to the patella. With the knee turned slightly away from the posteroanterior position, place the index finger against the medial border of the patella, press it lateralward, and rest the knee on its anteromedial side to hold the patella in a position of lateral displacement. Immobilize with a sandbag placed across the ankle.

Central ray

Direct the central ray to the joint space between the patella and the femoral condyles at an angle of 25 to 30 degrees toward the feet; it enters the posterior surface of the patella.

Structures shown

A slightly oblique posteroanterior projection of the patella showing three- or four-fifths of the bone free of superimposed structures.

This position is more comfortable for the patient than the direct posteroanterior position since no pressure is placed on the injured kneecap. The slight pressure required to displace the patella laterally is rarely objectionable to the patient even in painful injuries.

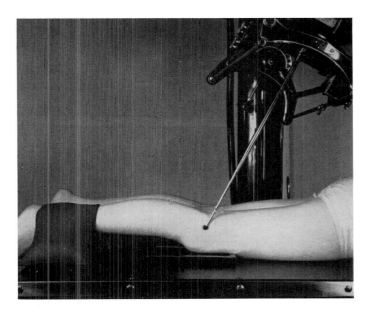

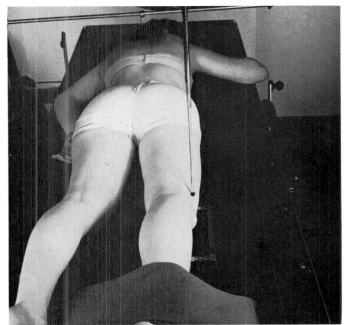

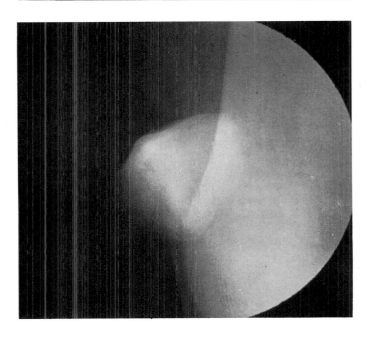

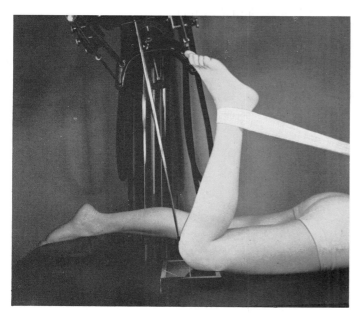

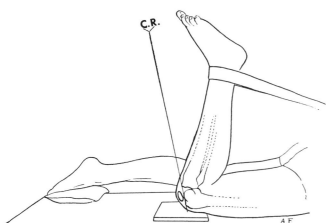

PATELLA
Axial projection
Settegast position

Because of the danger of fragment displacement by the acute flexion of the knee required for this view, it should not be attempted until a transverse fracture of the patella has been ruled out with a lateral view.

Film: 5″ × 7″ crosswise for unilateral examination, 8″ × 10″ or 10″ × 12″ crosswise for bilateral examination.

Position of patient

The patient may be placed in either the supine or the prone position. The latter is preferable because the knee can usually be flexed to a greater degree, and immobilization is easier. When the supine position is used, the film holder must be either held or strapped in position.

Position of part

With the patient in the prone position, flex the knee *slowly* as much as possible, or until the patella is standing at right angles to the film. *By slow, even flexion, the patient will be able to tolerate the position, whereas quick, uneven flexion will cause too much pain.*

Loop a long strip of bandage around the ankle or foot, and have the patient grasp the ends over his shoulder to hold the leg in position. Adjust the leg so that its long axis is vertical, that is, so that there is no sideways leaning.

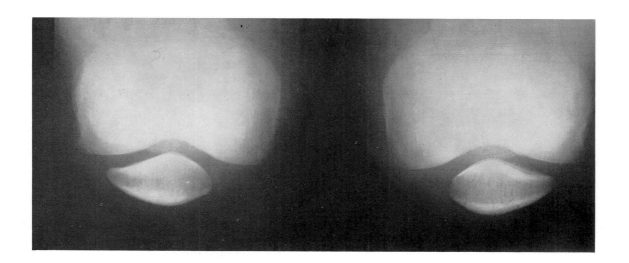

PATELLA
Axial projection
Settegast position
Position of part—cont'd

Place the film holder transversely under the knee and center to the joint space between the patella and the femoral condyles.

When performing a bilateral examination, place the knees in contact with each other and flex them as far as the injured side allows. Have the patient hold one end of the strip of bandage over each shoulder to hold the legs in the vertical position. Center the film holder midway between the knees parallel to the femoropatellar joint spaces.

By maintaining the part-film and tube-film relationships, this view can be obtained with the patient in the lateral position or in a seated position, as circumstances require.

Central ray

Direct the central ray at right angles to the joint space between the patella and the femoral condyles; the degree of central ray angulation, if any, will depend upon the degree of flexion of the knee.

Structures shown

An axial view of the patella used to demonstrate vertical fractures of this bone, and to investigate the articulating surfaces of the femoropatellar articulation.

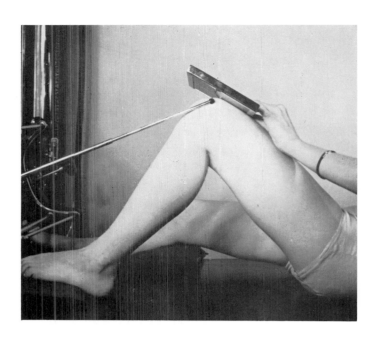

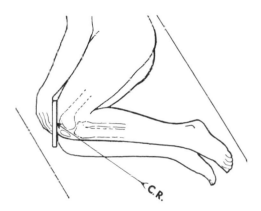

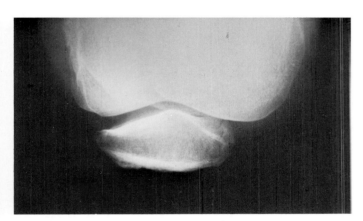

Courtesy Dr. Edward M. Winant.

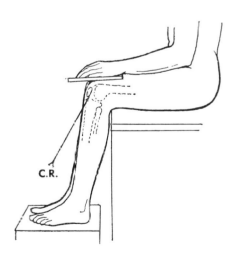

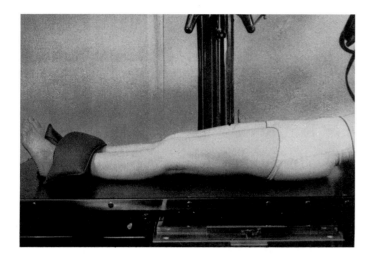

FEMUR
Anteroposterior projection
Posteroanterior view

Film: $7'' \times 17''$ for a unilateral examination; $14'' \times 17''$ for a bilateral examination.

If the femoral heads are separated by an unusually broad pelvis, the shafts will be strongly angled toward the midline and will require a $14'' \times 17''$ film for a unilateral examination. A bilateral examination will require two exposures: one on a $14'' \times 17''$ film placed crosswise for the upper portions of the femora, and one on a smaller film for the lower portions of the femora and the knee joints. This same procedure must be followed where pathology has caused abnormal bowing of the femora.

Position of patient

Place the patient in the supine position and adjust the body in a true anteroposterior position.

Position of part

For a bilateral examination, center the median sagittal plane of the body to the midline of the table. For a unilateral examination, center the affected thigh to the midline of the table.

Place a long sandbag under the ankles, invert the feet approximately 15 degrees to overcome the anteversion of the femoral necks, and place a sandbag across the ankles.

Apply a gonadal shield.

Central ray

Direct the central ray vertically to the midpoint of the film.

Structures shown

An anteroposterior projection of the femur, and of the hip and/or the knee joint.

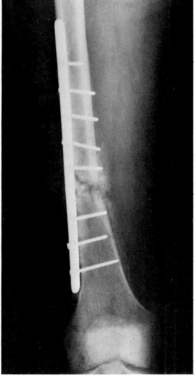

Radiographs courtesy Dr. Edward M. Winant.

FEMUR

Lateral projection

Film: $7'' \times 17''$ lengthwise.

Position of patient

Ask the patient to turn onto his affected side. Adjust the body position so as to center the dependent thigh to the midline of the table. Have the patient grasp the side of the table with the upper hand to aid in maintaining the position.

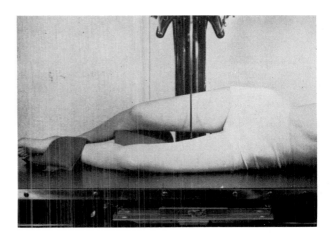

Position of part

1. If the hip joint is to be included, draw the upper extremity backward and support it on sandbags. Adjust the pelvis so that it is rolled backward just enough to prevent superimposition; 10 to 15 degrees from the lateral position is sufficient.

2. If only the knee joint is to be included, draw the uppermost extremity forward and support it at hip level on sandbags. Adjust the pelvis in a true lateral position.

Flex the dependent knee somewhat, place a sandbag under the ankle, and adjust it and the body rotation so as to place the patella perpendicular to the horizontal. Immobilize the leg with a sandbag across the ankle.

Adjust the position of the Potter-Bucky tray so that the film will project approximately 2 inches beyond the joint to be included.

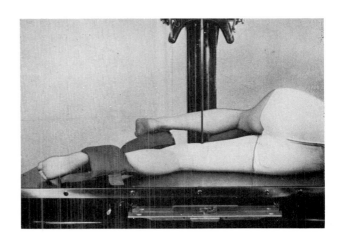

Central ray

Direct the central ray vertically to the midpoint of the film.

Structures shown

A lateral view of about three-fourths of the femur and of the adjacent joint. Two films must usually be taken for the demonstration of the entire length of the adult femur.

NOTE: Because of the danger of fragment displacement, the above position is not recommended for fracture cases, nor should it be used if there is a question of destructive disease. These subjects should be examined in the supine position by placing the cassette vertically along either the medial or the lateral aspect of the thigh and knee, and directing the central ray horizontally. A wafer grid or a grid-front cassette should be used to minimize secondary radiation.

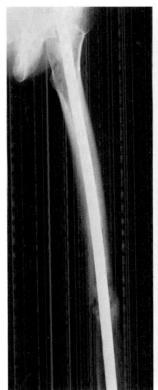
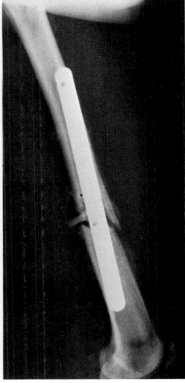

Radiographs courtesy Dr. Edward M. Winant.

LONG BONE MEASUREMENT

Radiography provides the most reliable means of obtaining accurate measurements of the length of long bones, specifically of length differences between the two sides. Measurement studies are made of the upper extremities, but the procedure is most frequently applied to the lower extremities. Various radiographic methods have been devised for long bone measurement, only a few of which will be considered here. For a detailed description of the different procedures and their modifications, the reader is referred to the bibliography for a listing of original papers.

RADIATION PROTECTION

Extremity length differences, which are more common in children, result from any one of a variety of disorders. Patients usually require yearly examinations for evaluation of any inequality in growth. More frequent examinations may follow surgical intervention to equalize length by controlling the growth of the normal side. This is usually done by means of a diaphysial-epiphysial fusion at the distal femoral or proximal tibial level. Patients have interval checkups extending over a period of years. It is therefore necessary to guard their well-being by the application of local gonadal shielding and by avoiding repeated exposures through careful positioning, secure immobilization, and accurate centering of a closely coned beam of radiation.

POSITION OF PATIENT

The patient is placed in the supine position for all methods, and both sides are examined for comparison. When a soft tissue abnormality (swelling or atrophy) is causing rotation of the pelvis, the low side must be elevated on a radioparent support to overcome the rotation and thereby place the upper femora equidistant from the film for comparable sized projection.

POSITION OF PART

The upper extremities are alternately adjusted and immobilized in the anteroposterior position for unilateral projection.

The lower extremities are extended and immobilized in the anteroposterior position with the ankles separated 5 or 6 inches. When the knee of the abnormal side cannot be fully extended, the normal knee must be flexed to the same degree and each knee supported on one of a pair of *identical-sized* supports to ensure that the joints are flexed to the same degree and are equidistant from the film.

Sandbags or other suitable supports should be placed against the sole of the feet to immobilize them and to dorsiflex them enough to place the ankles in near right-angle flexion. When possible, the extremities can be immobilized and the ankles correctly adjusted by having the feet firmly pressed against the footboard. The form of immobilization does, however, depend upon the age of the patient and his ability to cooperate.

LOCALIZATION OF JOINTS

For the methods that require centering over the joints, each joint must be accurately localized and marked to indicate the centering point. Both sides are examined for comparison, and since there is usually a bone-length discrepancy, the joints of each side must be marked. This is done with a skin-marking pencil after the patient is placed in the supine position.

For the upper extremity, the mark for the shoulder joint is placed over the head of the humerus near its upper border; that for the elbow joint, midway between the epicondyles of the humerus; and that for the wrist, midway between the styloid processes of the radius and ulna.

For the lower extremity, the *hip joint* is localized by placing a mark ½ to 1 inch, according to the age and size of the patient, laterodistally at exact right angles to the midpoint of an imaginary line extending from the anterior superior iliac spine to the pubic symphysis. The *knee joint* is located just below the apex of the patella at the level of the depression between the femoral and tibial condyles. The *ankle joint* is located directly under the depression midway between the malleoli.

LOADING OF LONG CASSETTES

When placing two or more films in a long cassette, it is important that the films be exactly abutted and then taped together to prevent displacement that might cause a discrepancy in measurement.

LONG BONE MEASUREMENT
Orthoroentgenographic method

Orthoroentgenography was introduced by Hickey[1] in 1924. He used a cassette long enough for the inclusion of the entire length of the extremities and made a single exposure at a focal-film distance of 7 feet. This method, now with the use of a long, finely graduated metal ruler and, usually, a 6-foot focal-film distance, is still in wide use.

Modifications of the orthoroentgenographic method vary. In one method, a long cassette tunnel—the Potter-Bucky diaphragm, when indicated—is used. A metal ruler is taped to the top of the tunnel or table so that the part of it included in the exposure fields records the position of each joint, and measurements can then be quickly determined. The cassette is placed in the tunnel or grid tray which permits it to be shifted for centering at the three joint levels without moving the patient. By alternately masking two-thirds of the film, three exposures are made on one 14″ × 17″ film.

The median sagittal plane of the patient's body is centered to the midline of the tunnel or table. The unmasked third of the film and the tube are successively centered at the previously marked level of the hip joints, the knee joints, and the ankle joints for simultaneous bilateral projections. When there is a difference in level between contralateral joints, the film and the tube are centered midway between the two levels.

[1]Hickey, Preston M.: Teleoroentgenography as an aid in orthopedic measurements, Amer. J. Roentgen. 11:232-233, 1924.

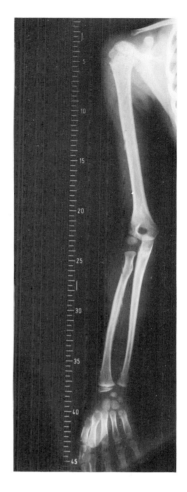

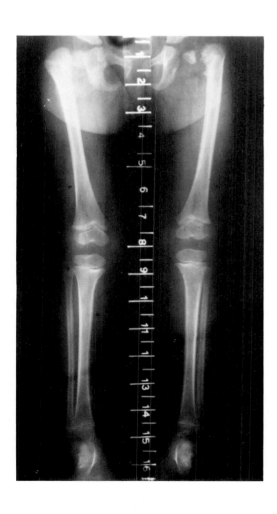

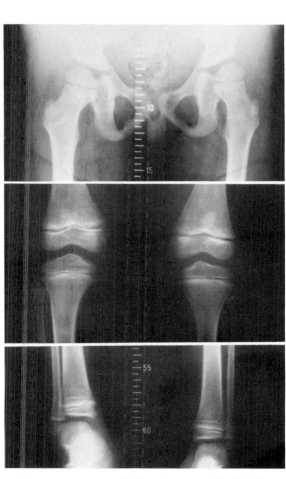

Radiographs courtesy Dr. Alex Norman.

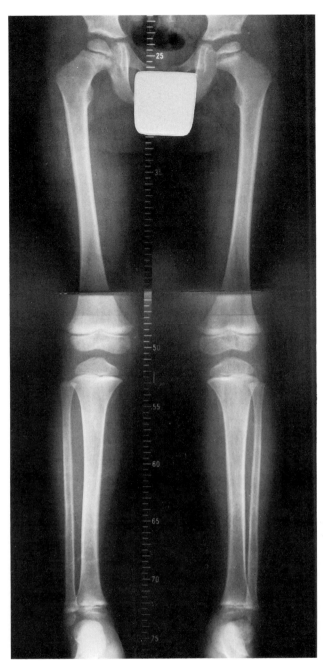

Slit scanogram.

Courtesy Dr. Alex Norman.

LONG BONE MEASUREMENT
Slit scanography

Slit scanography was introduced by Millwee[1] in 1937. This method utilizes a slitlike beam of radiation to scan a part as the narrow beam is moved over it, in the direction of its long axis for length measurement. Slit scanography requires the use of a lead filter measuring *exactly* 1/8 inch in thickness to fit the filter slot and having, centered under the focal-spot of the x-ray tube, a transverse slit measuring *exactly* 1/16 inch in width and, according to the focal-film distance used, 3½ to 4 inches in length. The lead blocks the passage of all but a narrow beam of the central, perpendicular radiation. The length of the slit permits the passage of laterally divergent rays, with resultant distortion in this direction, but blockage of the longitudinally divergent rays results in no distortion in this direction.

As the slit scanograph is moved along the part during the exposure, the instantaneous projection of the longitudinal dimension of each point of the part is recorded by perpendicular, nondistorting radiation. As can be demonstrated by scanning a rod, the *exact length* of the part is projected onto the film irrespective of the part-film distance and of the focal-film distance used.

The patient is placed on a cassette long enough to include the entire length of the extremities. A mark should be placed 1 to 1½ inches above the level of the hip joints to indicate the starting point of the tube movement; the tube should travel the same distance beyond the ankle joints. After placing the metal ruler and positioning and immobilizing the patient, apply local gonadal shielding.

The duration of the exposure depends on the length of the extremities, usually ranging from five to ten seconds. The tube travel time required for each subject should be determined before the actual exposure is made.

The tube movement must be smooth in order to prevent a stroboscopic effect, but the speed of its movement may be varied with the variation in the thickness of the part, the movement being slower over the hips and upper thighs, where greater exposure is required. When the tube movement cannot be varied, the milliamperage can be gradually reduced, or the distal half of the back screen can be blocked out with a sheet of paper. The need for these compensatory measures can be eliminated by having the cassette lined with three pairs of screens of varying speed—high for the hips and upper thighs, medium for the knees, and low for the ankles.

With practice, the technologist can move the tube by hand for an occasional patient, but a motor-driven arrangement is a necessity where such examinations are performed frequently. The motor of a standard tomographic unit can be used for this purpose by disconnecting the Potter-Bucky attachment.

[1]Millwee, Robert H.: Slit scanography, Radiology **28**:483-486, 1937.

LONG BONE MEASUREMENT
Spot scanography

Spot scanography was introduced by Gill[1] in 1944. This is the procedure wherein a closely coned exposure is made over each joint, a restriction of the exposure field that considerably reduces radiation to the patient's body.

All three joints of both extremities of the infant can be made on one film of standard length, but two films, sometimes three or four placed diagonally, are required for children. For the examination of adults and teen-age children by this method, a long grid-front cassette is a necessity. The long cassette obviates exposing the knee joints twice, as must be done with the use of shorter cassettes. It also eliminates the need to use separate, diagonally placed films for long extremities.

After the localization marks are made, the patient is positioned and immobilized, and local gonadal shielding is applied. The extension cone, or collimator, is adjusted to delimit the exposure field as much as possible, according to the age and size of the patient. Alternately and successively centering to the localization marks, the right and left sides are exposed without moving the patient.

A practical modification of the spot method of long bone measurement utilizes a long cassette tunnel or, when indicated, the Potter-Bucky diaphragm. A finely graduated metal ruler is taped to the top of the tunnel or table, where it will be included in the exposure fields to record the location of the joints. When both sides are projected onto the same film, one ruler serves for the measurement of both. By suitable masking, a 14″ × 17″ cassette can be shifted in the tunnel or grid tray for the projection of three unilateral joints on large patients, and for the projection of all six joints on small patients.

[1]Gill, Gerald G.: A simple roentgenographic method for the measurement of bone length; modification of Millwee's method of slit scanography, J. Bone Joint Surg. 26:767-769, 1944.

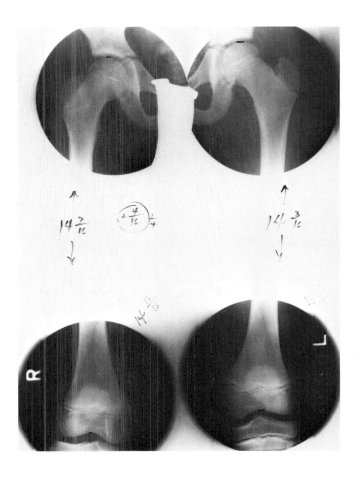

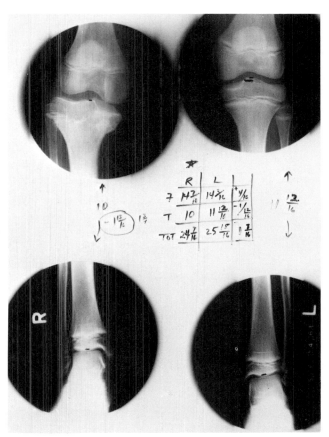

Radiographs courtesy Dr. Hudson J. Wilson, Jr.

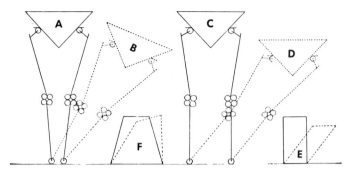

Diagrams showing why it is necessary to have the patient's feet at the same distance apart as the femoral heads during measurements of differences of leg length. *A, B,* If feet are too close together, any sway of the body to the left will make it appear that the left leg is shorter, and vice versa. *C, D, E,* If feet are at correct distance apart, swaying does not affect measurements. *F,* If feet are too far apart, the effect of swaying will be to make the right leg appear too short upon swaying to the left, and vice versa. The significant centers of the ball and socket surfaces of the femoral heads are usually about 7 inches apart. If the feet are placed parallel with each other, and 7 inches apart between centers, no difficulty will be experienced in obtaining accurate measurements.

Courtesy Dr. W. Edward Chamberlain.

MEASUREMENT OF DIFFERENCES OF LEG LENGTH
Chamberlain method

When a patient has low back pain, it is necessary to determine whether the causative factor may be faulty statics resulting from a difference of leg length, and to determine the thickness of the corrective lift required to equalize the leg length. Chamberlain[1] believes that the radiographic method is neither so accurate nor so foolproof as the radioscopic method, but that with reasonable care it is possible to use the radiographic method successfully.

Film: $14'' \times 17''$ lengthwise.
Position of patient

Have the patient stand erect, barefooted, before a vertical Potter-Bucky diaphragm. Adjust the height of the diaphragm to center the film midway between the anterior superior iliac spines and the iliac crests.

Position of part

With the patient standing in the anteroposterior position, center the median sagittal plane of the body to the midline of the Potter-Bucky diaphragm. *Place the feet parallel with each other and 7 inches apart between centers,* that is, between the midline of each foot. The weight of the body must be equally distributed on the feet.

Chamberlain[2] specifies that the feet must be placed the same distance apart as the centers of curvature of the femoral heads in order to obtain accurate measurements of differences of leg length. Chamberlain states that the distance between the significant centers of the surfaces of the femoral heads is usually about 7 inches, so that this spacing of the feet is satisfactory in a majority of cases. When the feet are placed farther apart or nearer together than the distance between the femoral heads, any lateral tilting of the body results in false measurements.

Apply a compression band across the pelvis, being careful not to rotate the body. Respiration is suspended for the exposure.

[1]Chamberlain, W. Edward: Personal communication.
[2]Chamberlain, W. Edward: Reprint from Proceedings of the California Academy of Medicine, 1937-1938.

MEASUREMENT OF DIFFERENCES OF LEG LENGTH
Chamberlain method—cont'd
Central ray

Special precautions are necessary: the focal spot of the tube must be the same distance from the floor as the hip joints. With a yardstick or tape measure, determine the distance from the patient's hip joints to the floor, adjust the tube so that the focal spot is at this distance above the floor, and then direct the central ray obliquely upward to the center of the film. Place a lead marker on the cassette front at the same distance above the floor as the hip joints, and close enough to the edge of the film to avoid superimposition upon important structures. Note that the center of the film is several inches higher than the focal spot of the tube (see instructions for centering of film under *Position of patient*).

The purpose of the above special arrangement of the central ray and focal spot level is to avoid misinformation concerning the relative lengths of the two legs while at the same time utilizing the full length of the 14″ × 17″ film for delineation of the lumbar column.

Structures shown

An anteroposterior projection of the pelvis, hip joints, and lumbar vertebrae, with the lead marker indicating the exact level of the focal spot during the exposure. If the image of the lead marker is more than 1 inch higher or lower than those of the hip joints, the possibility of significant error in the determination of the relative leg lengths, through distortion, must be admitted. (If one could assume that the hip joints were exactly the same distance from the film at the moment of exposure, the requirements concerning the level of the focal spot with relation to the hip joints would not be so exacting.) From this roentgenogram the radiologist can determine the thickness of the corrective lift that must be placed under the foot of the shorter leg in order to bring the hip joints level with each other.

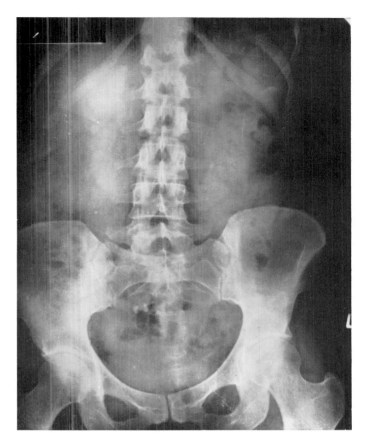

This anteroposterior projection was made with the patient standing barefooted, with the feet parallel and 7 inches apart, weight borne equally on the two legs, focal spot at approximately the same distance above the floor as the patient's hip joints. The actual level of the focal spot is shown by the lower edge of the image of the letter L near one edge of the film. Since the centering indicator (lower edge of the lead letter) is very nearly at the level of the hip joints, we know that the portion of the x-ray beam that projected the images of the hip joints was composed of almost exactly horizontal rays. (The "central ray" was not horizontal but was inclined upward toward the midpoint of the film, which was at a higher level than the hip joints.)

Courtesy Dr. W. Edward Chamberlain.

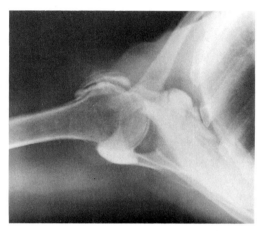

Frontal view with arm in external rotation, showing normal filling of subscapular bursa. Note extension of contrast material into bicipital groove.

Axial view of above patient.

CONTRAST ARTHROGRAPHY

Arthrography (Gr. *arthron*, joint) indicates radiography of a joint or joints. *Pneumoarthrography, opaque arthrography, and double-contrast arthrography* are terms used to denote radiologic examinations of the soft tissue structures of joints (menisci, ligaments, articular cartilage, bursae) following the injection of a contrast agent or of two contrast agents into the capsular space. A gaseous medium is employed in pneumoarthrography, a water-soluble iodinated medium in opaque arthrography, and a combination of both in double-contrast arthrography. While contrast studies may be made on any encapsuled joint, the knee is the most frequent site of investigation. Other joints sometimes examined by contrast arthrography are the shoulder, the hip, the elbow, the wrist, and the temporomandibular joints.

These examinations are usually performed with local anesthesia only. The injection is made under careful aseptic conditions, usually in a combination radioscopic-radiographic examining room, which should be carefully prepared in advance. The sterile items required, particularly the length and gauge of the needles, varies according to the part being examined. The sterile tray and the nonsterile items should be set up on a conveniently placed instrument cart or a small two-shelf table.

After aspirating any effusion, the doctor injects the contrast agent or agents and manipulates the joint to ensure proper distribution of the contrast material. Where an image intensifier is available, the examination may be carried out by radioscopy and spot films. Conventional studies are then made when special views, such as an axial projection of the shoulder or an intercondyloid fossa projection of the knee, are desired.

Bilateral opaque arthrogram of hip joints in patient with bilateral congenital dislocations.

Above radiographs and diagnostic information courtesy Dr. William B. Seaman.

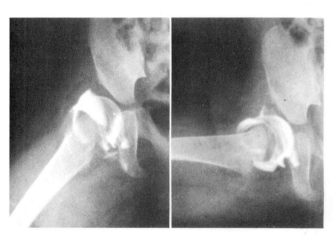

Frontal and "frog" views following contrast injection of a treated congenitally dislocated right hip.

Radiographs and diagnostic information courtesy Dr. Robert H. Freiberger.

CONTRAST ARTHROGRAPHY OF KNEE

Vertical ray method

Contrast arthrography of the knee by the vertical ray method requires the use of a special frame. The extremity is adjusted and strapped into the frame to widen or "open up" the side of the joint space under investigation. This widening, or spreading, of the intrastructural spaces permits better distribution of the contrast material around the meniscus.

After the contrast material is injected, the extremity is placed in the frame, and the thigh band is snugly applied. For the delineation of the medial side of the joint, the curved wooden block is placed in the frame against the lateral femoral condyle. The leg is then fully abducted on the femur and secured in this position with the ankle strap. This positioning of the wooden block and the leg is reversed for the demonstration of the lateral side of the joint.

When contrast arthrograms are to be made by conventional radiography, the radiologist turns the patient to the prone position and radioscopically localizes and marks the centering point for each side of the joint. The mark ensures accurate centering for closely coned studies of each side of the joint and permits multiple exposures to be made on one film. The views taken of each side of the joint usually consist of a direct frontal projection and 20-degree right and left oblique projections. The oblique projections may be obtained by rotation of the leg or by central ray angulation. Following completion of these studies, the frame is removed for a lateral and an intercondyloid fossa projection.

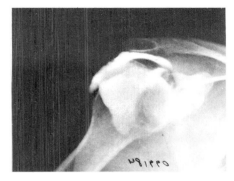

Opaque arthrogram of shoulder. Posterior dislocation with cuff tear. Subacromial bursa opacified.

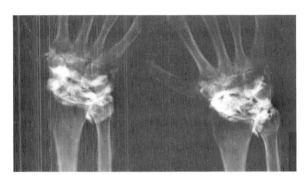

Opaque arthrogram of wrist. Rheumatoid arthritis.

Above radiographs and diagnostic information courtesy Dr. Robert H. Freiberger.

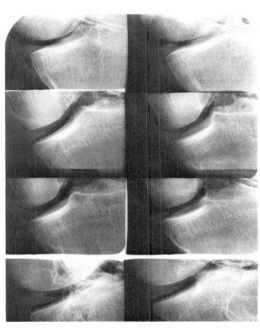

Pneumoarthrogram.

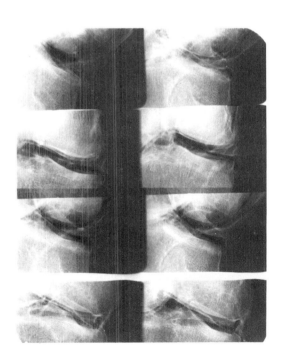

Double-contrast arthrogram.

Contrast arthrograms of knee courtesy Dr. Karl Witt.

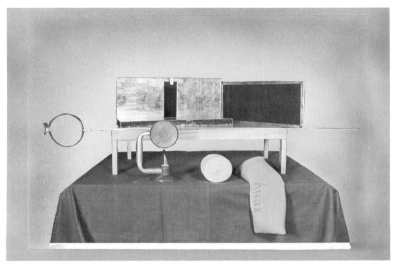

Equipment used for performing horizontal-ray, double-contrast arthrography of knee. Metal film holder allows six exposures on one 7" x 17" film. Low wooden table supports leg during examination of lateral meniscus. Long aluminum pointer is attached to x-ray tube to aid in accurate direction of central beam.

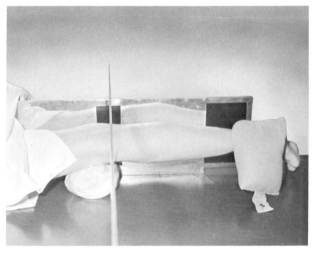

Position for initial exposure of medial meniscus.

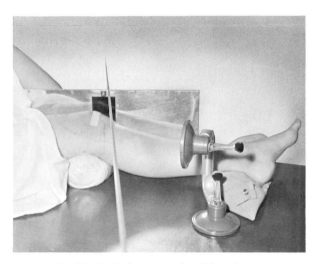

Position for final exposure of medial meniscus.

Above illustrations courtesy Dr. Robert H. Freiberger.

DOUBLE-CONTRAST ARTHROGRAPHY OF KNEE

Horizontal ray method

The horizontal ray method of performing double-contrast arthrography of the knee was first described by Andrén and Wehlin,[1] and more recently by Freiberger and associates.[2] It was found that by using horizontal ray projection and a comparatively small amount of each of the two contrast agents, improved double-contrast delineation of the knee joint structures could be obtained. This is because excess of the heavy iodinated solution drains into the dependent part of the joint, leaving only the desired thin opaque coating on the gas-enveloped uppermost part, the part then under investigation.

The radiologist, with the use of a metal ruler under radioscopic observation, draws a line on each side of the laterally placed and maximally extended knee. The lines are drawn so that they superimpose the articular margin of the respective tibial plateau, the slope of which coincides with the plane of that side of the joint space. This is done for the purpose of demonstrating an unobstructed view of each side of the joint space by directing the central ray parallel with its plane.

Freiberger[2] recommends that six views be taken of each meniscus, these being consecutively exposed on one 7" × 17" film. The accessory equipment used for this procedure is shown in the upper left photograph. The cotton pillow, cut from a roll of cotton, is 5 inches in diameter and about 6 inches in length.

Medial meniscus

1. The patient is adjusted in the semiprone position (central photograph) that places the posterior aspect of the medial meniscus uppermost.

2. To widen the joint space, the cylindrical cotton pillow is placed under the lower end of the femur and a sandbag is placed across the ankle.

3. The central ray is directed along the line that is drawn on the medial side of the knee and centered to the meniscus.

4. The vertical film holder is placed between the patient's legs and adjusted to center the exposure window to the central ray.

With rotation toward the supine position, the leg is turned 30 degrees for each of the succeeding five exposures. The central ray is directed along the localization line. For the last three exposures, the pillow is adjusted under the knee to center the meniscus to the film. In order to prevent undue flexion of the knee, the sandbag is placed under the ankle, as shown in the lower photograph.

[1]Andrén, L., and Wehlin, L.: Double-contrast arthrography of knee with horizontal roentgen ray beam, Acta Orthop. Scand. **29:**307-314, 1960.
[2]Freiberger, Robert H., Killoran, P.J., and Cardona, G.: Arthrography of the knee by double contrast method, Amer. J. Roentgen. **97:**736-747, 1966.

DOUBLE-CONTRAST ARTHROGRAPHY OF KNEE

Horizontal ray method—cont'd

Lateral meniscus

1. The patient is adjusted in the semiprone position that places the posterior aspect of the lateral meniscus uppermost. The wooden table is then placed under the affected extremity and astride the unaffected one, as shown in the opposite photograph.

2. To widen the joint space, the cotton pillow is placed under the lower end of the femur and a sandbag is placed across the ankle.

3. The x-ray tube is adjusted so as to direct the central ray along the line drawn on the lateral side of the knee.

4. The vertical film holder is now placed on the wooden table and adjusted to center the exposure aperture to the central ray.

As for the medial meniscus, six studies are made on one 7" × 17" film. With movement toward the supine position, the leg is rotated 30 degrees for each of the consecutive exposures, from the initial prone oblique position to the supine oblique position shown in the lower photograph. The central ray angulation is adjusted as required to direct it along the localization line. For the last three exposures, the cotton pillow is placed under the knee, and the sandbag is placed under the ankle.

A soft tissue technique and a focal-film distance of at least 40 inches (preferably 48 inches) are used for these studies.

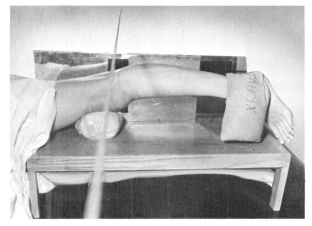

Position for initial exposure of lateral meniscus.

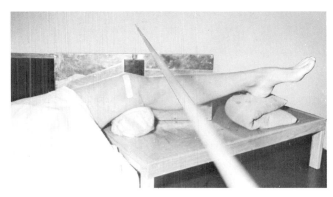

Position for final exposure of lateral meniscus.

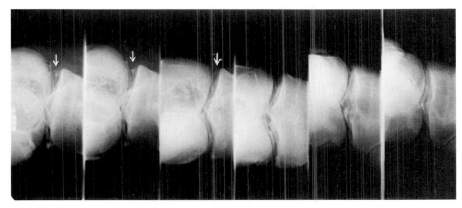

Medial meniscus. Tear in posterior half. Note irregular streaks of positive-contrast material within meniscal wedge (arrows).

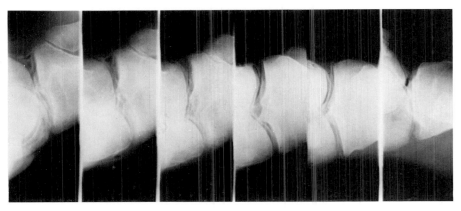

Normal lateral meniscus on above patient.

All illustrations and diagnostic information courtesy Dr. Robert H. Freiberger.

Anatomy and positioning
of the
shoulder girdle

The shoulder girdle

The shoulder girdle is formed by the clavicles and scapulae, and serves to connect the upper extremities to the trunk. While the alignment of these four bones is considered a girdle, it is incomplete both in front and behind. The girdle is completed in front by the sternum, which articulates with the medial ends of the clavicles, but the scapulae are widely separated in the back. Because the upper extremity of the humerus is included in the shoulder joint, it seems logical to consider its anatomy with that of the shoulder.

CLAVICLE

The clavicle is classified as a long bone, has a body, or shaft, and two articular extremities. It lies in an obliquely transverse plane just above the first rib, forming the anterior part of the shoulder girdle. Its lateral extremity articulates with the acromion process of the scapula, and its medial extremity with the upper segment of the sternum. The clavicle serves as a fulcrum for the movements of the arm and is doubly curved for strength. The curvature is more acute in the male than in the female.

The acromioclavicular articulation is a diarthrodial joint, permitting both gliding and rotary movements. The sternoclavicular articulation, which is the only bony union between the upper extremity and the trunk, is a diarthrodial joint adapted to circumduction, elevation, depression, and forward and backward movements of the clavicle. The clavicle carries the scapula with it through any movement.

SCAPULA

The scapula is classified as a flat bone. It forms the posterior part of the shoulder girdle. It is triangular in shape and has two surfaces, three borders, and three angles. It lies on the upper posterior thorax between the second and seventh ribs, with its vertebral border parallel with the vertebral column. The body of the bone is arched from above downward for greater strength, and its surfaces serve for the attachment of numerous muscles.

The anterior, or costal, surface of the scapula is slightly concave and almost entirely filled by the subscapularis muscle, which arises from it. The serratus anterior muscle attaches to the vertebral border of the costal surface from the medial to the inferior angles.

The posterior, or dorsal, surface is divided into two portions by a prominent spinous process. The spine arises at the upper third of the vertebral border from a smooth,

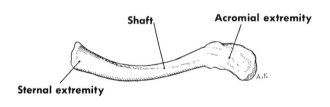

ANTERIOR ASPECT OF CLAVICLE

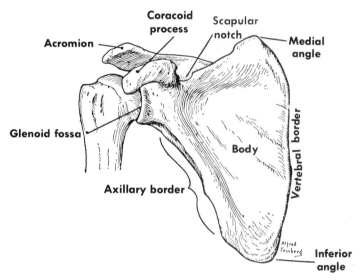

ANTERIOR ASPECT OF SCAPULA

triangular area and runs obliquely upward to end in a flattened triangular projection called the acromion. The area above the spine is called the supraspinatus fossa, and gives origin to the supraspinatus muscle. The infraspinatus muscle arises from the portion below the spine, which is called the infraspinatus fossa. The teres minor muscle arises from the upper two-thirds of the axillary border of the dorsal surface, and the teres major from the lower third and from the inferior angle. The dorsal surface of the vertebral border affords attachment for the levator scapulae, the rhomboideus major, and the rhomboideus minor muscles.

The superior border extends from the medial angle to the coracoid process and presents a deep depression, the scapular notch, at its lateral end. The vertebral border extends from the medial to the inferior angles. The axillary border extends from the glenoid fossa to the inferior angle.

The medial angle is formed by the junction of the superior and vertebral borders. The inferior angle is formed by the junction of the vertebral and axillary borders. The lateral angle, the thickest part of the scapula, ends in a shallow, oval depression called the glenoid fossa. The glenoid fossa articulates with the head of the humerus. The constricted region around the glenoid fossa is called the neck of the scapula. The coracoid process arises from a thick base that extends from the scapular notch to the upper part of the neck of the scapula. It projects first forward and medialward and then curves on itself to project lateralward. The coracoid process can be palpated just below, and slightly medial to, the acromioclavicular articulation.

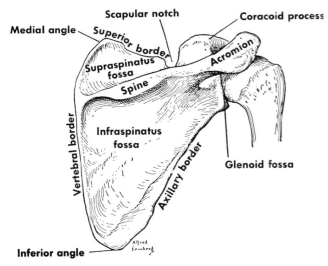

POSTERIOR ASPECT OF SCAPULA

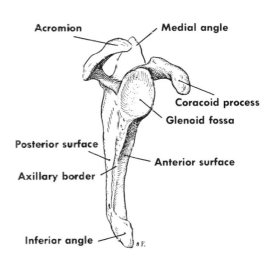

LATERAL ASPECT OF SCAPULA

HUMERUS

The upper end of the humerus consists of a head, an anatomic neck, two prominent processes termed the greater and lesser tuberosities, or tubercles, and a surgical neck. The head is large, smooth, and rounded, and lies in an oblique plane on the upper medial side of the humerus. It articulates with the glenoid fossa of the scapula. Just below the head, lying in the same oblique plane, is the narrow constricted area called the anatomic neck. The constriction of the shaft just below the tuberosities is called the surgical neck.

The lesser tuberosity is situated on the anterior surface of the bone immediately below the anatomic neck. The tendon of the subscapularis is inserted at the lesser tuberosity. The greater tuberosity is located on the lateral surface of the bone just below the anatomic neck and is separated from the lesser tuberosity by a deep depression called the bicipital, or intertubercular, groove. The upper surface of the greater tuberosity slopes backward at an angle of approximately 25 degrees and presents three flattened impressions for muscle insertions. The anterior impression is the highest of the three and affords attachment to the tendon of the supraspinatus. The middle impression is the point of insertion of the infraspinatus muscle. The tendon of the upper fibers of the teres minor is inserted at the posterior impression; its lower fibers are inserted into the shaft of the bone immediately below this point.

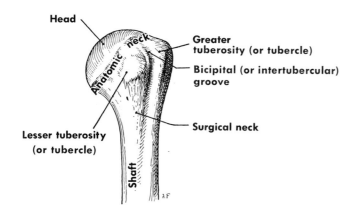

ANTERIOR ASPECT OF UPPER END OF HUMERUS

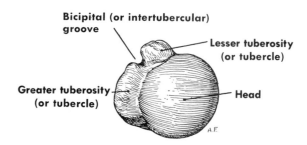

SUPERIOR ASPECT OF HUMERUS

SHOULDER JOINT

The articulation between the glenoid fossa and the head of the humerus forms a diarthrodial joint of the ball-and-socket type, which allows movement in all directions. While many muscles connect with, support, and enter into the function of the shoulder joint, technologists are chiefly concerned with the insertion points of the short rotators. The insertion points of these muscles—the subscapularis, the supraspinatus, the infraspinatus, and the teres minor—have already been stated.

An articular capsule completely encloses the shoulder joint. The tendon of the long head of the biceps muscle, which arises from the upper margin of the glenoid fossa, passes through the capsule of the shoulder joint, arches over the head of the humerus, and descends through the bicipital groove. The short head of the biceps arises from the coracoid process and, with the long head of the muscle, is inserted at the radial tuberosity. Because it is connected with both the shoulder and the elbow joints, the biceps synchronizes their action.

Important bursae are located under the deltoid (between it and the capsule), under the tendon of the subscapularis, and in the bicipital groove under the tendon of the long head of the biceps.

The interaction of movement between the wrist joint and the elbow and shoulder joints makes the position of the hand important in the radiography of these parts. Any rotation of the hand also rotates these joints. The best approach to the study of the mechanics of joint and muscle action is to perform all the movements ascribed to each joint and carefully note the reaction in remote parts.

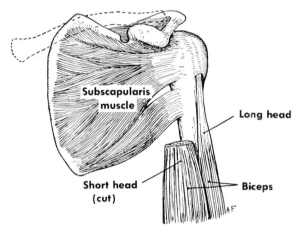

MUSCLES ON ANTERIOR SURFACE OF SCAPULA AND UPPER HUMERUS

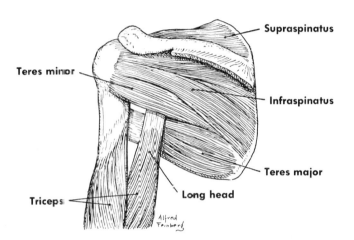

MUSCLES ON POSTERIOR SURFACE OF SCAPULA AND UPPER HUMERUS

123

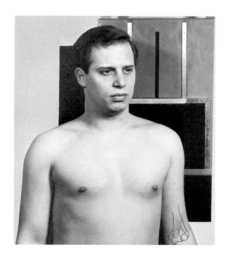

External rotation.

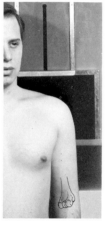

Neutral rotation.

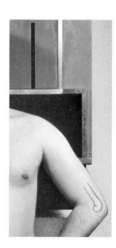

Internal rotation.

SHOULDER
Anteroposterior projections
Posteroanterior views

Film: $8'' \times 10''$ or $10'' \times 12''$ crosswise or lengthwise, according to the area to be included.

Position of patient

The patient may be examined in either the erect or the supine position. It must be kept in mind, however, that shoulder and arm lesions, whether traumatic or pathologic in origin, are extremely sensitive to movement and to pressure. For this reason, the erect position should be used whenever possible so that the patient's body position can be adjusted so as to require little or no manipulation of the arm.

Position of part

Adjust the position of the cassette and of the patient's body so as to center the film to the coracoid process. In order to overcome the curve of the back and the resultant obliquity of the shoulder structures, rotate the patient enough to place the blade of the scapula parallel with the plane of the film; when the patient is in the supine position support the elevated shoulder and hip on sandbags. When the patient is in this basic body position, locate the epicondyles and, while holding them between the thumb and index fingers of one hand, adjust the arm as follows:

1. Ask the patient to turn the palm of his hand forward. Abduct the arm slightly and adjust it so as to place the coronal plane of the epicondyles parallel with the plane of the film; when the patient is erect, the arm may be immobilized by having him rest the hand against a standard or the back of a chair. This adjustment of the arm, referred to as the *external rotation position*, places it in the true anteroposterior, or anatomic, position. The external rotation position is used to demonstrate the bony and soft structures of the shoulder and upper humerus in their anatomic position. It shows the glenohumeral joint relationship and the region of the subacromial bursa, and gives a profile view of the greater tuberosity of the humerus, the site of the insertion of the supraspinatus tendon.

2. Ask the patient to rest the palm of his hand against his thigh. This position of the arm rolls the head of the humerus into a *neutral position*, placing the epicondyles at an angle of about 45 degrees to the plane of the film. The resultant projection shows the posterior part of the supraspinatus insertion site, sometimes profiling small calcific deposits not otherwise visualized.

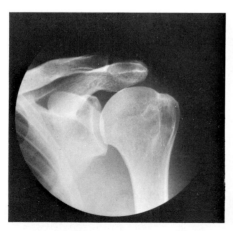

External rotation.

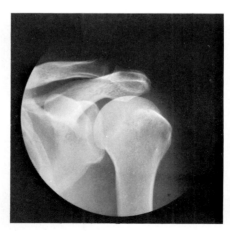

Neutral rotation.

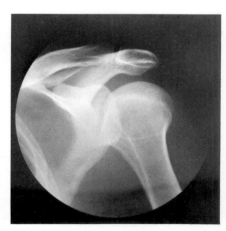

Internal rotation.

SHOULDER
Anteroposterior projections
Posteroanterior views

Position of part—cont'd

3. Ask the patient to flex his elbow somewhat, rotate the arm internally, and rest the back of the hand on his hip. Adjust the arm so as to place the coronal plane of the epicondyles perpendicular to the plane of the film. (When the shoulder is too painful for adequate internal rotation of the arm, the patient may turn somewhat away from the film, but if the part-film distance becomes too great, he should be turned for adjustment from the posteroanterior position.) This adjustment of the arm, referred to as the *internal rotation position*, rolls the humerus into the true lateral position. The internal rotation position demonstrates the region of the subdeltoid bursa and, when the arm can be abducted enough to clear the lesser tuberosity of the head of the scapula, a profile view of the site of the insertion of the subscapularis tendon.

Central ray

The central ray is directed perpendicularly to the coracoid process.

Infraspinatus insertion. With the patient's arm in the anteroposterior position (external rotation), direct the central ray to the coracoid process at an angle of 25 degrees toward the feet. The resultant projection profiles the second impression on the greater tuberosity, the site of insertion of the infraspinatus tendon, and also opens up the subacromial space.

Subacromial space. Berens and Lockie[1] recommend an anteroposterior projection, with the central ray directed to the coracoid process at an angle of 15 degrees toward the feet, to open up the subacromial space and thus to demonstrate ossification of the coracoacromial ligament or other lesions of the subacromial space. They state that ossification of the coracoacromial ligament shows as a tongue of bone projecting from the anteroinferior aspect of the acromion process.

[1]Berens, D. L., and Lockie, L. M.: Ossification of the coracoacromial ligament Radiology **74:**802-805, 1960.

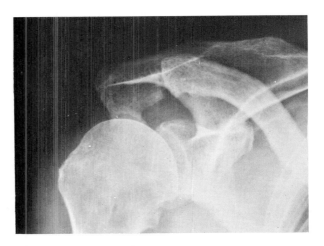

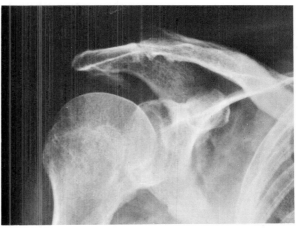

Two cases showing ossification of coracoacromial ligament.
Radiographs and diagnostic information courtesy Dr. David L. Berens.

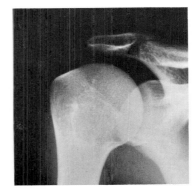

Central ray 25 degrees toward the feet.

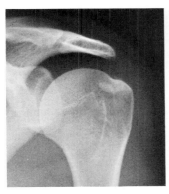

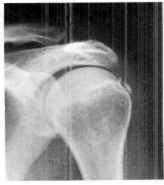

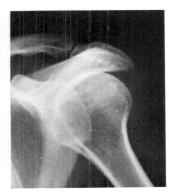

External rotation.   Neutral rotation.   Internal rotation.

Calcareous peritendinitis.
Above radiographs and diagnostic information courtesy Dr. Hudson J. Wilson, Jr.

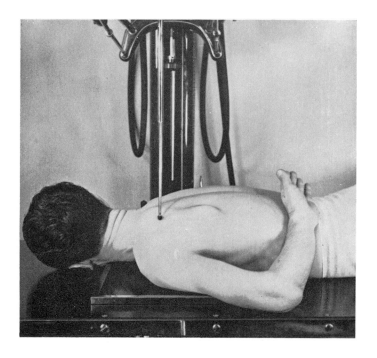

SHOULDER
Teres minor insertion
Blackett-Healy position
Film: $8'' \times 10''$ crosswise.

Position of patient

Adjust the patient in the prone position, his arms along the sides of the body and his head resting on the cheek of the affected side. Place a long sandbag under the ankles for the patient's comfort.

Position of part

Place the cassette under the shoulder and center it to a point about 1 inch distal to the coracoid process. Turn the arm to a position of extreme internal rotation and, if possible, flex the elbow and place the hand on the patient's back.

Respiration is suspended at the end of exhalation for a more uniform density.

Central ray

Direct the central ray vertically to the head of the humerus.

Structures shown

This position rotates the head of the humerus so that the third impression of the greater tuberosity is brought forward, giving a tangential view of the insertion of the teres minor at the outer edge of the bone just below the articular surface of the head.

NOTE: Blackett[1] states that this view of the teres minor insertion can be obtained with the patient in the anteroposterior position by turning the arm to a position of extreme internal rotation.

[1]Blackett, Charles W.: Personal communication.

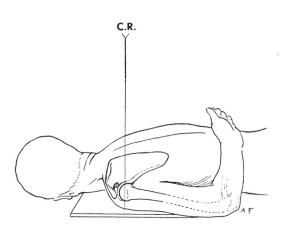

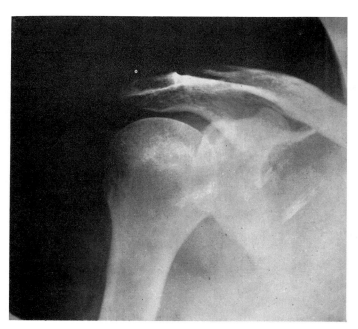

Courtesy Dr. Charles W. Blackett.

SHOULDER
Subscapularis insertion
Blackett-Healy position

Film: $8'' \times 10''$ or $10'' \times 12''$ crosswise.

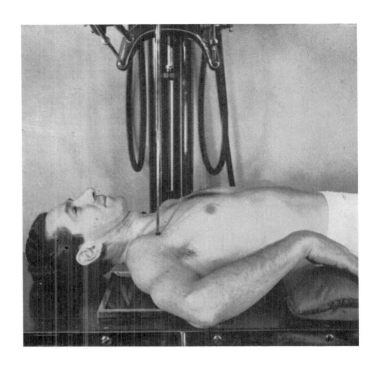

Position of patient

Place the patient in the supine position, his arms along the sides of the body and his head resting on the table.

Position of part

When using Potter-Bucky technique, align the body so that the affected shoulder joint is centered to the midline of the table. For non-Bucky technique, place the cassette under the shoulder and center to the joint.

Elevate the opposite shoulder approximately 15 degrees and support it with a sandbag. Abduct the affected arm to a right angle to the long axis of the body, flex the elbow, and rotate the arm internally by pronating the hand.

Place one sandbag under the hand and another on top of it. Respiration is suspended at the end of exhalation for a more uniform density.

Central ray

Direct the central ray vertically to the shoulder joint.

Structures shown

A tangential view of the insertion of the subscapularis at the lesser tuberosity, which forms the inferior edge of the bone in this projection, and the axillary area over which the subscapularis tendon passes.

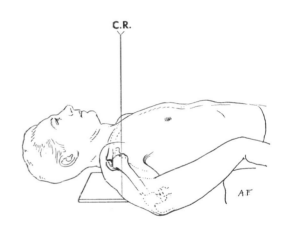

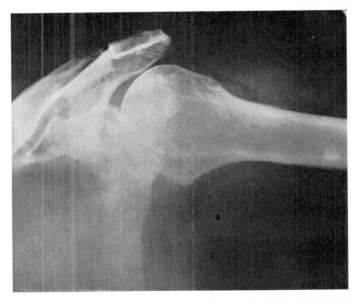

Courtesy Dr. Charles W. Blackett.

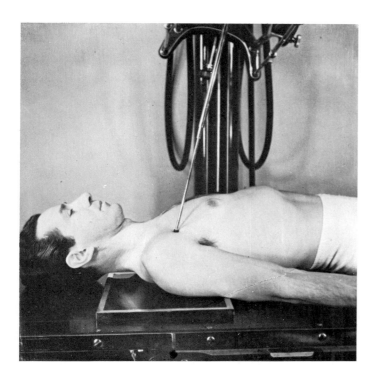

SHOULDER
Coracoid process
Inferosuperior projection
Film: $8'' \times 10''$ or $10'' \times 12''$ crosswise.

Position of patient

Place the patient in the supine position, his arms along the sides of the body and his head resting on the table.

Position of part

When using Potter-Bucky technique, adjust the position of the body so as to center the affected coracoid process to the midline of the table. For non-Bucky technique, place the cassette under the shoulder and center it to a point 1 to 2 inches proximal to the coracoid process, according to the central ray angulation to be used.

Adjust the shoulders to lie in the same transverse plane. Abduct the arm of the affected side slightly, and supinate the hand and immobilize it with a sandbag across the palm. Respiration is suspended at the end of exhalation for a more uniform density.

When using Potter-Bucky technique, adjust the cassette so that the midpoint of the film will coincide with the central ray.

Central ray

Direct the central ray to the coracoid process at an angle of from 15 to 30 degrees toward the head. The degree of angulation depends upon the shape of the patient's back; round-shouldered patients will require a greater angulation than those who have a straight back.

Structures shown

A slightly inferosuperior view of the coracoid process projected free of self-superimposition. Because the coracoid is curved on itself, it casts a small, oval shadow in the direct anteroposterior projection of the shoulder. The scapular notch is also clearly demonstrated in this projection.

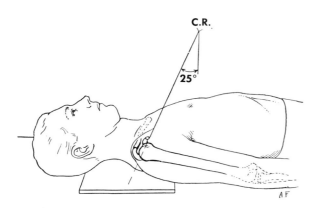

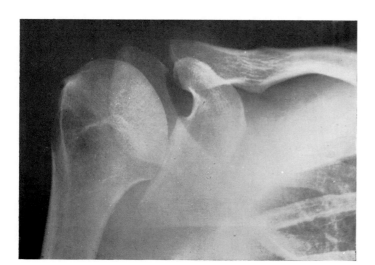

SHOULDER
Glenoid fossa
Grashey position
Film: $8'' \times 10''$ or $10'' \times 12''$ crosswise.

Position of patient

While this projection can be made with the patient in either the supine or the erect position, the latter is more comfortable for the patient and facilitates accurate adjustment of the part.

Position of part

Center the film to the shoulder joint. Rotate the body approximately 45 degrees toward the affected side. If the patient is in the supine position, support the elevated shoulder and hip on sandbags.

Adjust the degree of rotation to place the scapula parallel with the plane of the film and the head of the humerus in contact with it. Abduct the arm slightly in internal rotation and place the hand against the side of the body.

Respiration is suspended at the end of exhalation for a more uniform density.

Central ray

Direct the central ray perpendicularly to a point 2 inches medial and 2 inches distal to the upper outer border of the shoulder.

Structures shown

The joint space between the humeral head and the glenoid fossa. This projection shows the glenoid fossa in profile.

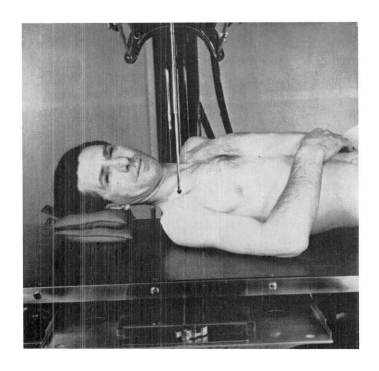

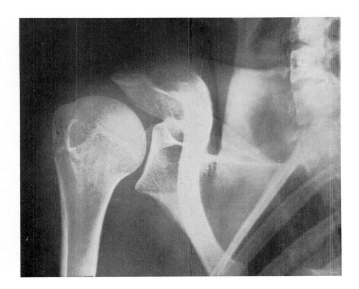

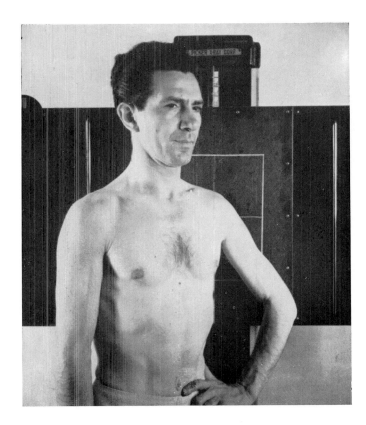

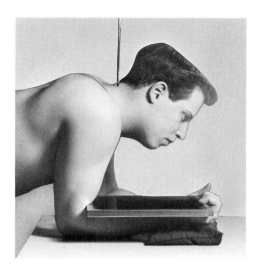

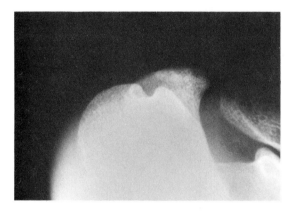

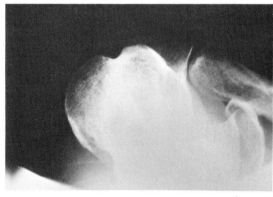

Superoinferior projections.

BICIPITAL GROOVE
Superoinferior projection
Fisk position[1]
Film: 8″ × 10″.

Position of patient

The patient is asked to stand facing the end of the table. When necessary, this position can be easily adapted to the seated position; when this is done, a local gonadal shield should be applied.

Position of part

Ask the patient to flex his elbow, lean forward, and rest his forearm on the table with the hand supinated.

Place the cassette on the forearm, with its longitudinal midline parallel with the long axis of the forearm, and ask the patient to close his fingers over the end of it. Adjust a sandbag under the hand and wrist so as to place the cassette in the horizontal position. When the opposite bicipital groove is to be examined for comparison, mask the outer half of the film.

Have the patient lean forward or backward as required to place the humerus at an angle of 10 to 15 degrees, open backward, to the vertical. Palpate and mark the location of the bicipital groove; it is the easily palpable depression between the greater and lesser tuberosities.

Central ray

Direct the central ray vertically through the previously marked bicipital groove.

Structures shown

This projection shows an axial view of the acromioclavicular joint as well as of the bicipital groove. The bicipital groove is often superimposed but not obscured by the acromion process.

NOTE: With the use of a shock-proof tube head that can be lowered enough for an *inferosuperior projection*, the patient may be examined in the erect position. The arm may be retracted, or the patient may be asked to lean forward 10 to 15 degrees to place the bicipital groove in a tangential position. The palm of the hand is rested against the thigh. After localizing and marking the bicipital groove, place a 5″ × 7″ cassette on the shoulder and ask the patient to hold it in position with his opposite hand. The central ray is directed vertically through the bicipital groove.

[1]Fisk, Charles: Adaptation of the technique for radiography of the bicipital groove, Radiol. Techn. **37**:47-50, 1965.

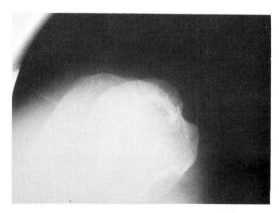

Inferosuperior projection.

SHOULDER
Rolled-film axial projection
Cleaves position

Cleaves[1] devised this method of obtaining an axial view of the shoulder joint for use with patients who cannot or should not abduct the arm enough for one of the routine axial projections.

Film

This projection requires that a 5″ × 7″ film be enclosed in a light-proof envelope and then curved around a small tube so that it can be placed as high in the axilla as possible. This requirement can be met by obtaining a mailing tube measuring 2 inches in diameter and 7½ inches in length, and dismantling a 5″ × 7″ cardboard film holder for the lead foil backing and the envelope. The lead foil is glued around the mailing tube for backing; because it does not go all the way around the tube, the center point must be prominently marked, as shown in the adjacent photograph. The envelope is used to enclose the film and, because of the thickness of the shoulder, a pair of flexible fluorescent screens. The loaded envelope is centered to the lead foil backing, curved around the tube and then secured at each end with an elastic band. Since the screens are loose in the envelope, special care must be used to avoid damaging them when loading and unloading.

Position of patient

The patient is seated sideways at the end of the table. When necessary, this projection can be adapted to the supine position.

Position of part

Ask the patient to supinate his hand and rest it on his lap. Place the film roll as high in the axilla as possible, adjust it so that it is horizontal, and have the patient brace his arm against the table to hold the roll in position.

Central ray

Direct the central ray vertically to the acromioclavicular joint.

Variations. Direct the central ray to the acromioclavicular articulation (1) at a 5-degree medial angulation to bring out the lesser tuberosity and the bicipital groove, and (2) at a 5-degree lateral angulation to bring out the coracoid process.

Structures shown

An axial view of the glenohumeral joint, the greater and lesser tuberosities, the bicipital groove, and the coracoid process.

[1]Cleaves, Edwin N.: A new film holder for roentgen examination of the shoulder, Amer. J. Roentgen. 45:288-290, 1941.

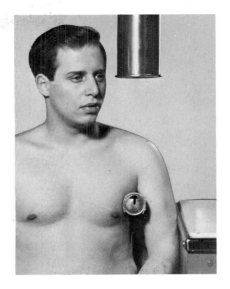

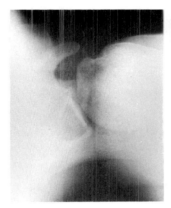
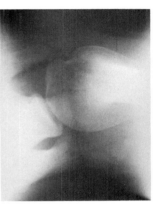

Central ray vertical.   Central ray 5 degrees medialward.

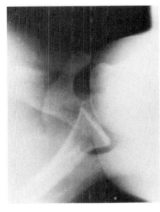

Central ray 5 degrees lateralward.

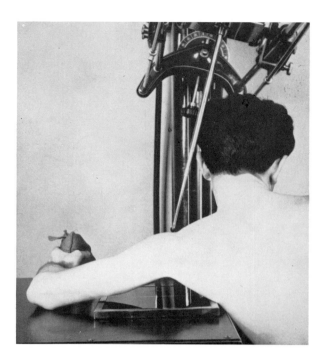

SHOULDER JOINT
Superoinferior axial projection

The patient's ability to abduct his arm to a near right angle to the long axis of his body, and the advisability of his doing so, should be verified before this position is undertaken.

Film

An 8″ × 10″ film placed lengthwise or crosswise as required for accurate centering to the shoulder joint. A curved cassette or, if the shoulder is small, a flexible film holder may be used for this position.

Position of patient

Seat the patient sideways at the end of the table, the shoulder at the midline of the table, on a stool or chair high enough to enable him to extend the affected shoulder well over the cassette.

Position of part

Place the cassette near the end of the table and parallel with its long axis.

Ask the patient to hold the hand of the affected side and raise the arm to a position as near as possible at right angles to the long axis of his body. Have him then lean lateralward over the cassette until the shoulder joint is over the midpoint of the film and bring the elbow to rest on the table. Have the patient's elbow flexed 90 degrees, and place the thumb side of his hand up. Immobilize the extremity with a sandbag across the forearm. In order to obtain a direct lateral view of the head of the humerus, adjust any forward or backward leaning of the body so as to place the humeral epicondyles in the vertical position.

When abduction is limited, seat the patient higher, and use a 5″ × 7″ cassette elevated on sandbags to place it as far as possible up in the axilla.

Respiration is suspended for the exposure.

Central ray

Have the patient lean his head toward the unaffected shoulder. Direct the central ray to the shoulder joint at an angle of 5 to 15 degrees toward the elbow.

Structures shown

A superoinferior projection showing the joint relationship of the upper end of the humerus and the glenoid fossa. The acromioclavicular articulation, the outer portion of the coracoid process, and the points of insertion of the subscapularis and the teres minor are well demonstrated. Depending upon the flexibility of the patient, a greater or lesser portion of the medial structures is shown.

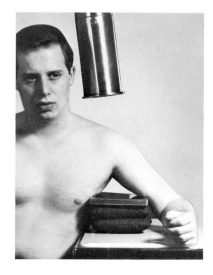

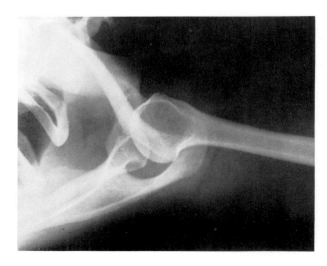

SHOULDER JOINT
Inferosuperior axial projection
Lawrence position

When abduction is limited, inferosuperior projections of the shoulder are better and more easily done with a mobile unit and, when possible, with the patient in the seated position.

Film: 8″ × 10″ placed in the vertical position above the shoulder.

Position of patient

With the patient in the supine position, elevate the head and shoulders about 3 or 4 inches with folded sheets or small, firm pillows.

Position of part

As nearly as possible, abduct the arm of the affected side at right angles to the long axis of the body. Flex the elbow and adjust a support under the arm. Keeping the arm in external rotation, adjust the forearm and hand in a comfortable position, either grasping a vertical support or extended on sandbags or a firm pillow.

Have the patient turn his head away from the side being examined. Place the cassette on edge above the shoulder and as close as possible to the neck. Support the cassette in position with sandbags.

Respiration is suspended for the exposure.

Central ray

Direct the central ray horizontally through the axilla to the region of the acromioclavicular articulation. The degree of medial angulation of the central ray depends upon the degree of abduction of the arm.

Structures shown

An inferosuperior projection showing the glenohumeral joint, the lateral portion of the coracoid process, and the acromioclavicular articulation. The insertion site of the subscapularis tendon on the anterior border of the head of the humerus, and the point of insertion of the teres minor tendon on the posterior border of the humeral head are also shown.

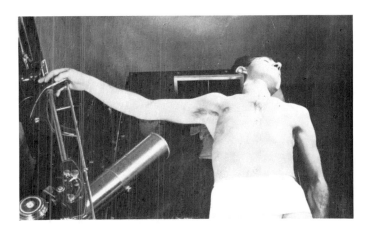

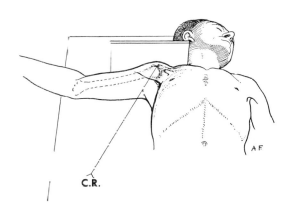

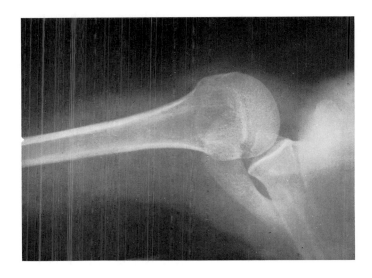

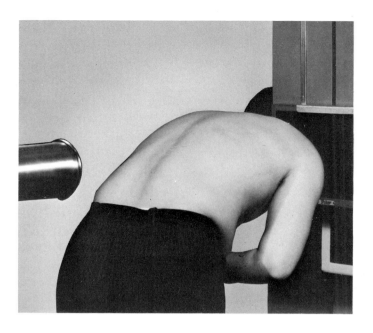

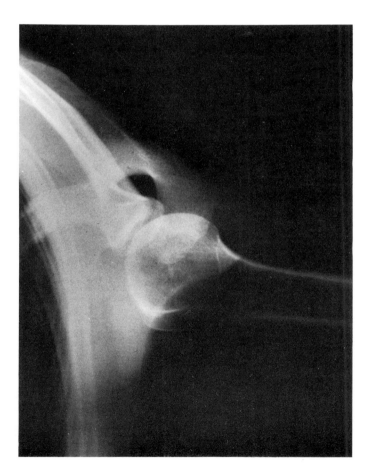

SHOULDER JOINT
Horizontal transaxilla projection

This projection and the one on the facing page are particularly useful in examining the patient with a recent injury whose arm cannot be moved, and the patient whose arm is held to the side by a dressing.

Film

An 8″ × 10″ film placed crosswise on the side of a vertical cassette holder that will accommodate the patient's head and neck beside the stand. This projection requires the use of a grid-front cassette or a wafer grid.

Position of patient

The patient is placed in the erect position, either standing or seated, with the affected shoulder centered to the vertically placed cassette.

Position of part

Ask the patient to lean directly forward and rest the upper border of the shoulder against the cassette.

Central ray

Direct the central ray horizontally through the region of the axilla.

Structures shown

An axial projection taken especially to show the relationship of the head of the humerus to the glenoid fossa, usually in cases of posterior dislocation.

GLENOHUMERAL JOINT

Semiaxial anteroposterior projection

This position is used to demonstrate the relationship of the head of the humerus to the glenoid fossa when the arm cannot be abducted, usually in cases of posterior dislocation. This condition is demonstrated when the shadow of the head of the humerus is cast distal to the shadow of the glenoid fossa.

This position is also used to obtain a semiaxial view of the clavicle and of the scapular spine. For this purpose, and in order to obtain less distortion, the cassette is adjusted at an angle of 45 degrees (as indicated by the broken lines in the upper photograph), so as to place the film at right angles to the central ray.

Film

Select an 8″ × 10″ film and place it lengthwise behind the shoulder. A grid-front cassette or a stationary grid should be used for this projection and, if possible, a 72-inch focal-film distance.

Position of patient

The patient is seated with his back toward, and resting against, the end of the table.

Position of part

Ask the patient to sit erect. Since most of the patients for whom this position is used have a dislocation, provide whatever support needed for the forearm, but make no attempt to change the position of the arm.

Place the cassette on the table and center it in line with the glenohumeral joint. When necessary, support the cassette on sandbags to elevate it to the middorsal area.

Central ray

Direct the central ray to the region of the coracoid process at a caudal angle of 40 to 45 degrees.

Structures shown

The relationship of the head of the humerus to the glenoid fossa and, depending upon the size of the exposure field, a semiaxial view of the clavicle and the spine of the scapula.

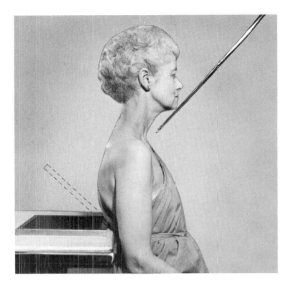

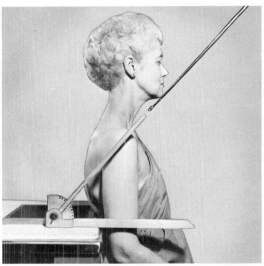

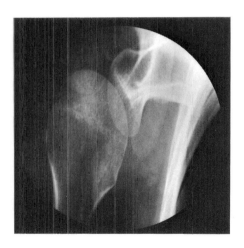

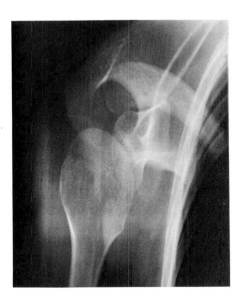

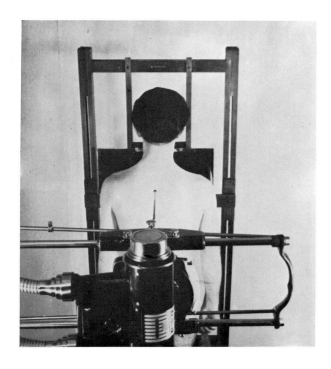

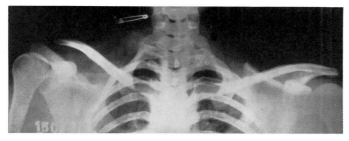

Courtesy Dr. William H. Shehadi.

SHOULDER
Acromioclavicular articulations
Bilateral frontal projection
Pearson position

Film

Select a 7″ × 17″ film and place it crosswise, or, for broad-shouldered subjects, select two 8″ × 10″ films and place them crosswise for simultaneous exposure. In the latter case, each film must carry an identification marker.

Position of patient

Because a dislocation, partial or complete, of the acromioclavicular joint tends to reduce itself in the recumbent position, the demonstration of this condition depends upon the erect position. This projection must, therefore, be made with the patient in the erect position, either seated or standing.

Position of part

Place the patient in either the anteroposterior or the posteroanterior position before a vertical cassette stand and adjust the height of the cassette so that the midpoint of the film will lie at the level of the acromioclavicular joints. Center the median sagittal plane of the body to the midline of the cassette. The weight of the body must be equally distributed on the feet to avoid rotation.

Rest the chest against the cassette for support, and with the arms hanging by the sides, adjust the shoulders to lie in the same transverse plane. It is important that the arms hang unsupported and, if possible, that the patient hold in each hand one of a pair of sandbags of equal weight.

Central ray

Direct the central ray perpendicularly to the midline of the body at the level of the acromioclavicular joints.

Structures shown

A bilateral frontal projection of the acromioclavicular joints. This position is used to demonstrate dislocation, separation, and function of the joints.

SHOULDER
Acromioclavicular articulation
Anteroposterior and lateral projections
Alexander positions

Alexander[1] suggested that these positions be used in cases of suspected acromioclavicular subluxation or dislocation.

Film: 8″ × 10″ lengthwise.

Position of patient

The patient is placed in the erect position, either standing or seated.

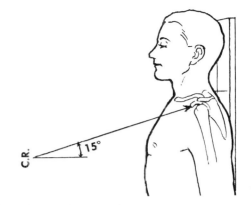

Anteroposterior projection
Position of part

Have the patient turn his back toward the cassette holder, and ask him to sit or stand erect. Center the affected shoulder to the cassette holder. Adjust the height of the cassette so that the midpoint of the film is at the level of the acromioclavicular joint. Adjust the patient's position or that of the cassette so that the center of the film will coincide with the region of the coracoid process.

Central ray

Direct the central ray to the coracoid process at an angle of 15 degrees toward the head. This angulation projects the shadow of the acromioclavicular joint above that of the acromion.

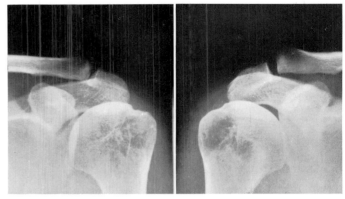

Normal and abnormal acromioclavicular joints on same patient.

Radiographs courtesy Dr. Ramsay Spillman.

Lateral projection
Position of part

Turn the patient to the posteroanterior position, and ask him to place the hand of the affected side well up under the opposite axilla. Rotate the unaffected side 30 to 35 degrees away from the film, and adjust the patient's position so as to center the acromioclavicular joint (the region of the medial border of the head of the humerus) to the midline of the film.

Just before making the exposure, have the patient grasp the side of the cassette stand and pull the affected shoulder firmly against it. Placing the arm across the chest draws the scapula lateralward and forward. The slight obliquity of the chest and the pressure against the glenohumeral joint further rotate the scapula outward and forward. The scapula and the acromioclavicular joint are thus placed in the lateral position, that is, at right angles to the plane of the film.

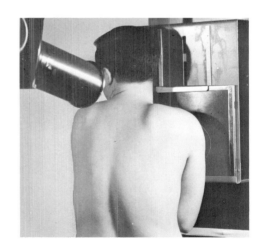

Central ray

Direct the central ray through the coracoid process at an angle of 15 degrees toward the feet.

Structures shown

Frontal and lateral views of the acromioclavicular joint and of the relationship of the bones entering into its formation.

[1]Alexander, O. M.: Radiography of the acromioclavicular articulation, Med. Radiogr. Photogr. **30**:34-39, 1954.

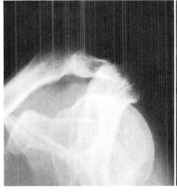
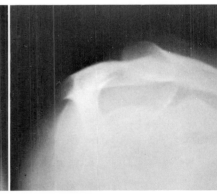
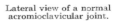

Lateral view of a normal acromioclavicular joint.

Lateral view of abnormal acromioclavicular joint on above patient.

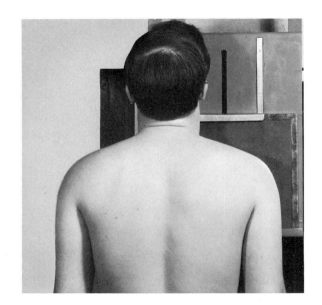

CLAVICLE
Posteroanterior projection
Anteroposterior view

Film: $10'' \times 12''$ crosswise.

Position of patient

The patient may be placed in either the prone or the erect position. However, if the clavicle is being examined for either a fracture or a destructive disease, and if the patient cannot be placed in the erect position, the anteroposterior position is used in order to obviate the possibility of fragment displacement or injury.

Position of part

Adjust the body so as to center the clavicle to the midline of the table or cassette stand. Place the arms along the sides of the body and adjust the shoulders to lie in the same transverse plane. Center the film to a point midway between the median sagittal plane of the body and the outer border of the shoulder at the level of the coracoid process.

Respiration is suspended at the end of exhalation for a more uniform density.

Central ray

Direct the central ray perpendicularly to the midpoint of the film.

Structures shown

A frontal projection of the clavicle, showing better detail when made in the posteroanterior direction.

NOTE: For a semiaxial projection of the clavicle, direct the central ray to the supraclavicular fossa at an angle of 25 to 30 degrees toward the feet; the angulation of the central ray is reversed when the patient is in the supine position.

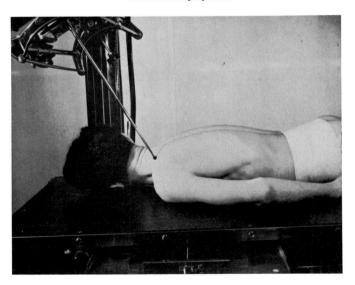

Posteroanterior projection.

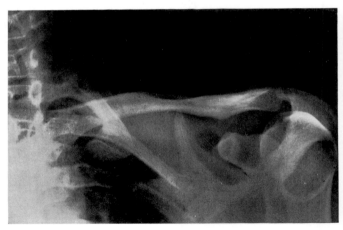

Semiaxial projection.

CLAVICLE
Axial projection
Supine position

Film: $8'' \times 10''$ placed in vertical position at the top of shoulder.

Position of patient

With the patient in the supine position, elevate the head and shoulders 2 or 3 inches on folded sheets or on small, firm pillows. Place the arms along the sides of the body.

Position of part

Depress the shoulder, if possible, to place the clavicle, as nearly as possible, in a transverse plane. Have the patient turn his head away from the side being examined. Place the cassette on edge at the top of the shoulder, close to the neck, and support it in position with sandbags. Respiration is suspended for the exposure.

Central ray

Tilt the tube so that the central ray will pass between the clavicle and the chest wall as nearly as possible at right angles to the plane of the film.

If the medial third of the clavicle is in question, it is also necessary to angle the central ray outward; from 15 to 25 degrees usually proves sufficient.

Structures shown

An inferosuperior view of the clavicle projected clear of superimposed shadows.

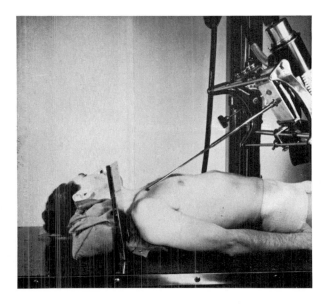

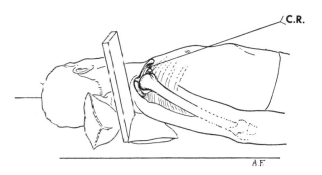

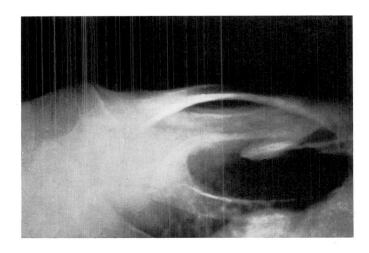

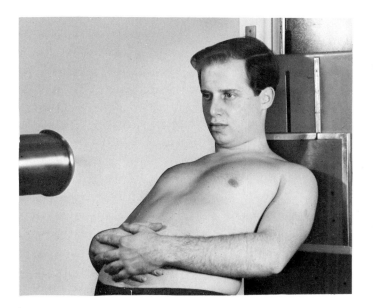

CLAVICLE
Axial projection
Anterior lordotic position

An axial projection of the clavicle can be obtained with far less discomfort to the patient when he can be adjusted from the erect position. This is particularly true of small children, who assume the lordotic position with ease.

Film: $10'' \times 12''$ for adults.

Position of patient

Place the patient in the anteroposterior position, either standing or seated, before, and depending upon his height, approximately 1 foot away from, the cassette stand.

Position of part

Adjust the patient's position so as to center the affected shoulder to the film. Assist the patient in assuming the lordotic position, center the film to the clavicle, estimate any required angulation of the central ray, and then have the patient reassume the erect position while the tube is being adjusted for any necessary angulation.

Before the patient assumes the lordotic position, ask him to place his arms in a comfortable position (which, for most patients, is achieved by clasping the hands over the abdomen). Place one hand against the lumbar region to give the patient support, and then have him lean backward in a position of extreme lordosis and rest his neck and shoulder against the cassette; the neck will be in extreme flexion.

Adjust the degree of leaning so as to place the coronal plane of the clavicle as nearly as possible at right angles to the plane of the film.

Respiration is suspended at the end of full inhalation in order to further elevate and angle the clavicle.

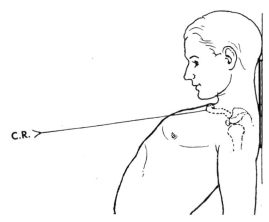

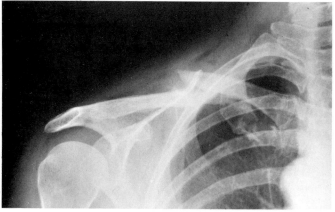

Posteroanterior projection.

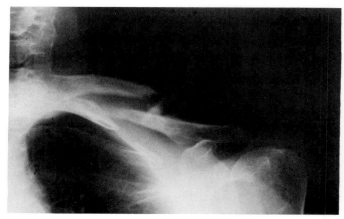

Lordotic projection on opposite patient.

Radiographs courtesy Dr. Hudson J. Wilson, Jr.

CLAVICLE
Axial projection
Anterior lordotic position—cont'd

Central ray

Direct the central ray to the inferior border of the clavicle at right angles to its coronal plane.

Structures shown

An exact axial view of the clavicle is obtained when the anterior and posterior ends of the first rib are seen to be exactly superimposed.

NOTE: When a patient cannot assume the lordotic position, the transthoracic axial projection may be used. Have him turn and lean forward, as shown in the adjacent photograph. Adjust the degree of leaning so as to place the coronal plane of the clavicle at right angles to the plane of the film. Direct the central ray horizontally, and make the exposure on full inhalation for better delineation of the clavicle. The transthoracic axial projection requires exposure factors comparable to those used for a lateral projection of the chest.

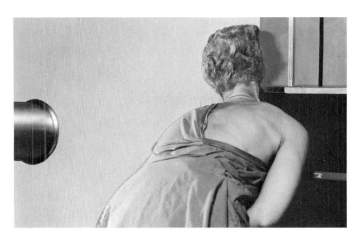

Position for transthoracic axial projection of clavicle (see note).

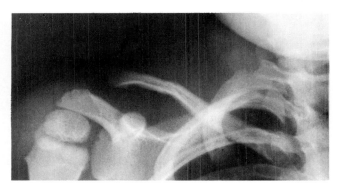

Posteroanterior projection.

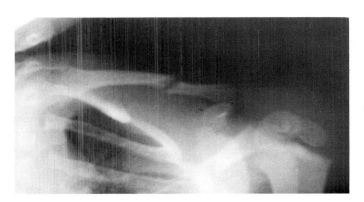

Lordotic view on opposite patient, 3 years of age.

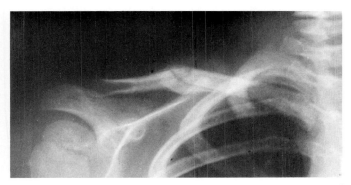

Posteroanterior projection.

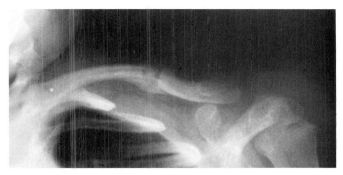

Lordotic view of opposite patient, 3½ years of age.

Radiographs courtesy Dr. Edward M. Winant.

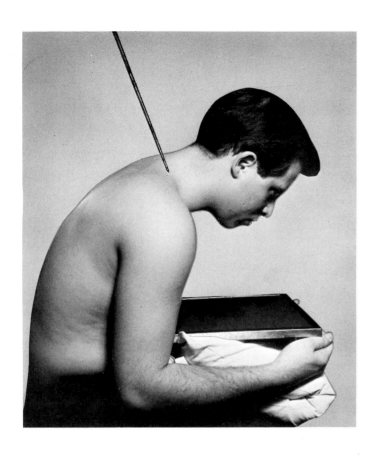

CLAVICLE
Axial projection
Tarrant position

The Tarrant position[1] is particularly useful with aged patients and with patients who have multiple injuries or who, for some other reason, cannot assume the lordotic position.

Film: $10'' \times 12''$ crosswise.

Position of patient

The patient is examined in the sitting position.

Position of part

Adjust a sheet of leaded rubber over the gonadal area, and then place a folded pillow or blankets on the patient's lap to support the horizontally placed cassette at about the level of the diaphragm. Center the cassette to the affected shoulder and, if possible, have the patient hold it in position.

Ask the patient to lean slightly forward. Tarrant[1] suggested that sandbags be placed on the end of the table to support the patient's head when he is seated so that this aid is possible.

Central ray

Direct the central ray anteriorly at right angles to the coronal plane of the clavicle.

Because of the considerable part-film distance, a long focal-film distance should be used to reduce magnified distortion.

Structures shown

An axial or a near axial view of the clavicle projected above the thoracic cage.

[1]Tarrant, R. M.: The axial view of the clavicle, Xray Techn. **21**:358-359, 1950.

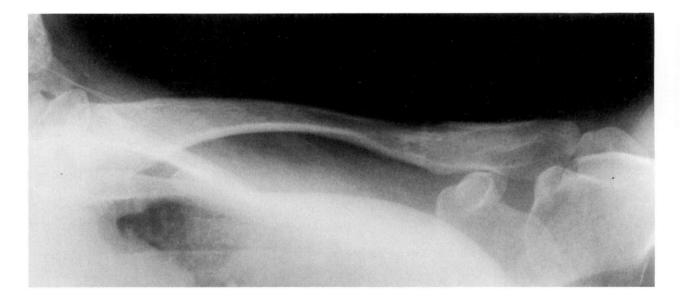

CLAVICLE
Right-angle projections
Quesada method

Film: $10'' \times 12''$ crosswise for each exposure.

Position of patient

Place the patient in the prone position and adjust the body so as to center the clavicle to the midline of the table or to the midpoint of the cassette-changing tunnel.

Position of part

With the patient's clavicle centered to the midline of the table or to the midpoint of the cassette-changing tunnel, place the arms along the sides of the body and adjust the shoulders to lie in the same transverse plane. Rest the head on the cheek of the affected side.

When using Potter-Bucky technique, adjust the cassette so that the center point of the film will coincide with the central ray.

In order to obtain better delineation of the clavicle, instruct the patient to hold his breath at the end of inhalation for the transthoracic exposure.

Central ray

As the centering must be accurate, it is advisable to make a mark on the table or cassette tunnel for use as a guide in directing the central ray; the mark is made beside the shoulder at a point in line with the midpoint of the clavicle.

1. Direct the central ray to the midpoint of the clavicle at an angle of 45 degrees toward the feet.

2. Change the cassette; direct the central ray 45 degrees toward the head and center to the midpoint of the clavicle.

Structures shown

Quesada[1] recommends that this method of obtaining exact right-angle views of the clavicle be used as a preoperative procedure for patients with a comminuted fracture.

[1]Quesada, Fortunato: Technique for the roentgen diagnosis of fractures of the clavicle, Surg. Gynec. Obstet. **42:**424-428, 1926.

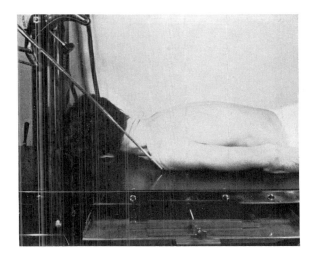

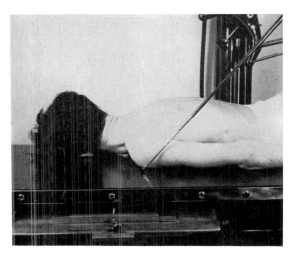

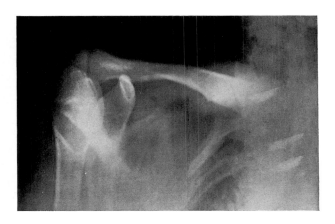

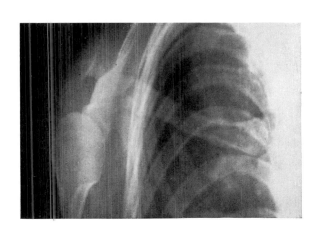

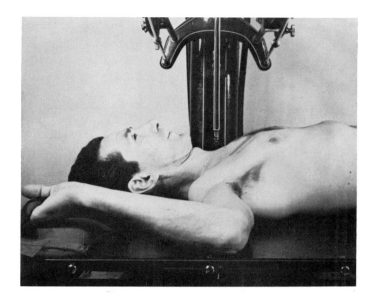

SCAPULA
Anteroposterior projection
Posteroanterior view
Film: $10'' \times 12''$ lengthwise.

Position of patient

The patient may be placed in either the erect or the supine position, the erect position being preferable if the shoulder is tender.

Position of part

Adjust the body so as to center the affected scapula to the midline of the Potter-Bucky diaphragm. Abduct the arm to a right angle to the body so as to draw the scapula outward, and then flex the elbow and support the hand in a comfortable position. Do not rotate the body toward the affected side for this projection because the resultant obliquity would offset the effect of drawing the scapula outward.

This view of the scapula should be made during quiet breathing in order to obliterate lung detail.

Central ray

Direct the central ray perpendicularly to the mid-scapular area.

Structures shown

An anteroposterior projection of the scapula, with the outer portion of its body free of superimposition.

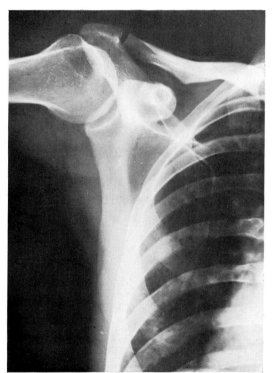

SCAPULA

Lateral projections

Film: $10'' \times 12''$ lengthwise.

Position of patient

The patient is placed in the erect position, either standing or seated, facing a vertical Potter-Bucky stand.

When a patient cannot be placed in the erect position, a lateral projection of the scapula can be easily obtained by adjusting the degree of body rotation and the placement of the arm from either the prone or the supine position.

Position of part

Adjust the patient in an oblique position, with the affected scapula approximately centered to the film. The arm is placed according to the area of the scapula to be demonstrated.

1. For the delineation of the wing of the scapula, the elbow is flexed and the hand rested on the side of the body at a level that will prevent the shadow of the humerus from overlapping that of the scapula.

As suggested by Mazujian,[1] the arm may be adjusted across the upper chest. For this placement, the patient is instructed to grasp the opposite shoulder to hold the arm in position.

2. For the demonstration of the acromion and coracoid processes, ask the patient to extend the arm upward and rest the forearm on his head.

3. For the demonstration of the glenohumeral joint, to prove or disprove posterior dislocation, McLaughlin[2] recommends that the arm hang beside the body and be adjusted so as to have it superimposed by the wing of the scapula.

After the placement of the arm for any one of the above projections, grasp the axillary and vertebral borders of the scapula between the thumb and index fingers of one hand and adjust the body rotation so as to place the wing of the scapula perpendicular to the plane of the film.

Central ray

Direct the central ray horizontally to the medial border of the protruding scapula.

[1]Mazujian, Mary: Lateral profile view of the scapula, Xray Techn. **25**:24-25, 1953.
[2]McLaughlin, H. L.: Posterior dislocation of the shoulder, J. Bone Joint Surg. **34-A**:584-590, 1952.

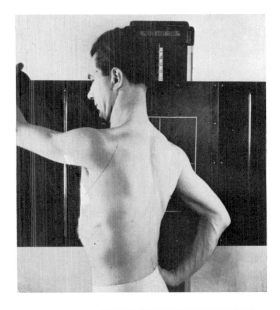

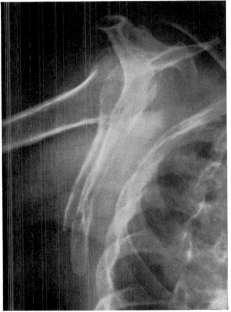

Courtesy Dr William H. Shehadi.

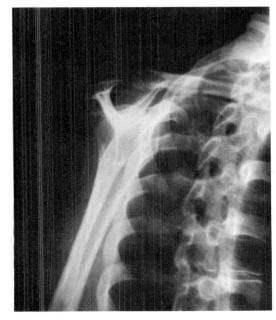

Scapula and arm superimposed.

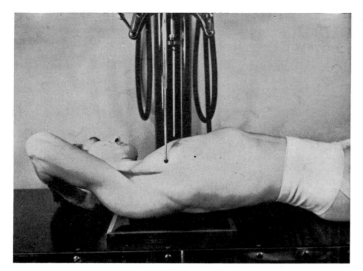

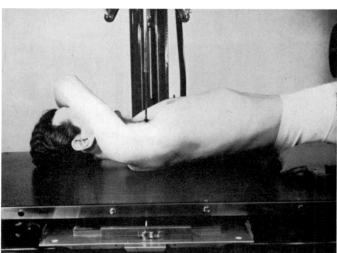

SCAPULA
Anterior oblique projections

Film: $10'' \times 12''$ lengthwise.

Position of patient

The patient may be examined in either the supine or the erect position, although the latter should be used when the shoulder is painful.

Position of part

Have the patient in the anteroposterior position, either supine or erect. Align the body so as to center the affected scapula to the midline of the Potter-Bucky diaphragm.

1. For an oblique anteroposterior projection, ask the patient to extend his arm upward, flex the elbow, and place the supinated hand under his head. Have him turn away from the affected side enough to oblique the shoulder slightly.

2. For an oblique lateral projection, ask the patient to extend his arm and rest the flexed elbow on his forehead. Rotate the body away from the affected side. Grasp the axillary and vertebral borders of the scapula between the thumb and index fingers of one hand and adjust the rotation of the body so as to project the scapula free of the rib cage.

3. For a direct lateral projection, draw the arm across the chest and adjust the body rotation so as to place the scapula perpendicular to the plane of the film.

Central ray

Direct the central ray perpendicularly to the lateral border of the rib cage at the mid-scapular area.

Structures shown

An oblique (or a lateral) view of the scapula projected free or nearly free of rib superimposition. Compare the delineation of the different parts of the bone in the two oblique studies shown.

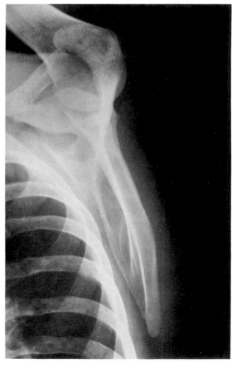

Oblique anteroposterior projection.

Oblique lateral projection.

SCAPULA
Posterior oblique projections
Lorenz and Lilienfeld positions
Film: $10'' \times 12''$ lengthwise.

Position of patient

The patient may be placed in either the erect or the lateral recumbent position. When the shoulder is painful, the erect position should be used if possible.

Position of part

With the patient in the lateral position, either erect or recumbent, align the body so as to center the scapula to the midline of the Potter-Bucky diaphragm. Adjust the arm according to the view desired.

1. For the Lorenz position, adjust the arm at a right angle to the long axis of the body, flex the elbow, and rest the hand against the patient's head. Rotate the body slightly forward and have the patient grasp the side of the table or the stand for support.

2. For the Lilienfeld position, extend the arm of the affected side obliquely upward and have the patient rest the hand on his head. Rotate the body slightly forward and have the patient grasp the side of the table or the stand for support.

For either position, grasp the axillary and vertebral borders of the scapula between the thumb and index fingers of one hand and adjust the rotation of the body so that the scapula will be projected free of the rib cage.

Central ray

With the central ray perpendicular to the plane of the film, direct it between the chest wall and the mid-area of the protruding scapula.

Structures shown

An oblique view of the scapula, the degree of obliquity depending upon the position of the arm. Compare the delineation of the different parts of the bone in the two oblique studies shown.

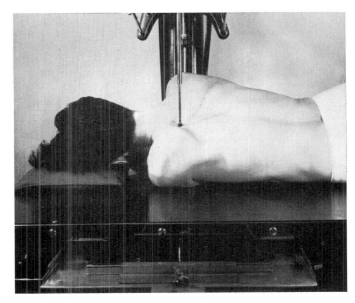

Lorenz position.

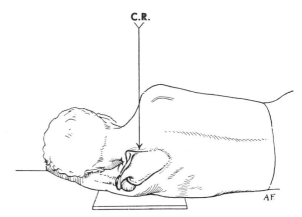

Lilienfeld position.

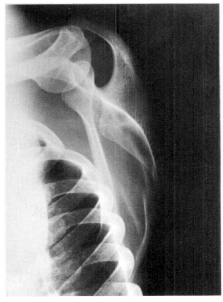

Lorenz position.

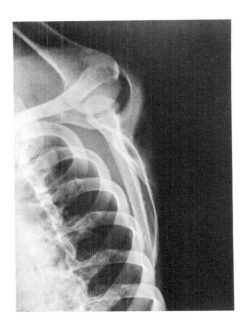

Lilienfeld position.

147

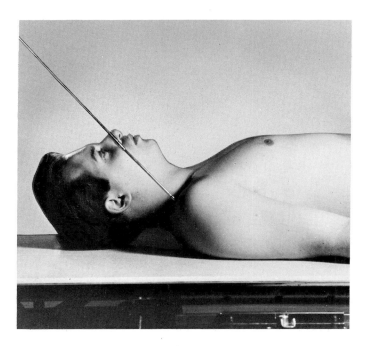

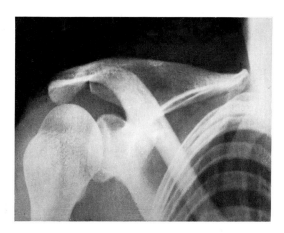

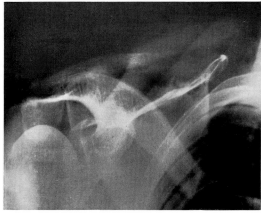

Courtesy Dr. Hudson J. Wilson, Jr.

SCAPULAR SPINE
Tangential projection
Laquerriere-Pierquin position
Film: $8'' \times 10''$ crosswise.

Position of patient

As described by the originators,[1] the patient is placed in the supine position.

Position of part

Center the shoulder to the midline of the table. Adjust the patient's rotation so as to place the wing of the scapula in a horizontal position. When this requires that the opposite shoulder be elevated, support it on sandbags. Turn the head away from the affected shoulder enough to prevent superimposition.

Funke[2] found that in the examination of flat-chested patients, clavicular superimposition can be prevented by inserting a 15-degree radioparent wedge under the shoulder to angle it caudally.

Central ray

The central ray is directed through the posterosuperior region of the shoulder at an angle of 45 degrees toward the feet; a 35-degree angulation suffices for obese and round-shouldered subjects.

After the adjustment of the x-ray tube, position the grid tray so as to center the film to the central ray.

Structures shown

The spine of the scapula is projected in profile and free of bony superimposition except for the outer end of the clavicle. Laquerrière and Pierquin[1] suggested that this superimposition be overcome by shifting the central ray several inches off center, medially or laterally, as required, for the demonstration of a laterally located lesion.

NOTE: When the shoulder is too painful to tolerate the pressure of the supine position, the tangential view of the spine of the scapula can be equally well obtained with the patient in either the prone position[3] or the erect position. These are described on the facing page.

[1]Laquerrière and Pierquin: De la nécessité d'employer une technique radiographique spéciale pour obtenir certains détails squelettiques, J. Radiol. Electr. **3:**145-148, 1918.

[2]Funke, Thomas: Tangential view of the scapular spine, Med. Radiogr. Photogr. **34:**41-43, 1958.

[3]Voorhis, Mary W.: The spine of the scapula, Du Pont X-ray News, no. 42.

SCAPULAR SPINE
Tangential projection
Prone and erect positions

Film: 8″ × 10″ crosswise.

PRONE POSITION

Position of part

Place the patient in the prone position and center his shoulder to the midline of the table. Place the arms along the sides of his body and adjust the shoulders to lie in the same transverse plane. In order to prevent undue lateral rotation of the scapula, have the patient rest his head on the chin and supinate the hand of the affected side. A radioparent wedge may be adjusted under the side of the shoulder and upper arm to place the scapula in the horizontal position.

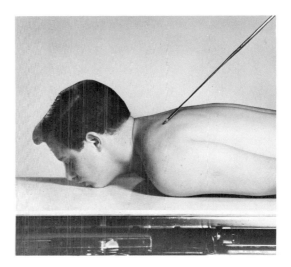

Central ray

The central ray is directed through the scapular spine at an angle of 45 degrees toward the head; it exits at the anterosuperior aspect of the shoulder.

ERECT POSITION (STANDING)

A grid-front cassette or a stationary grid is recommended. Place the cassette in a vertical holder that will accommodate the patient's head at the side of the stand.

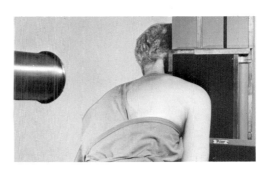

Position of part

Adjust the patient's position so as to center the shoulder to the film and have him stand at a distance that will enable him to lean forward at an angle of 45 degrees and rest his shoulder against the cassette.

Central ray

Direct the central ray horizontally through the scapular spine.

ERECT POSITION (SEATED)

A grid-front cassette or a stationary grid is recommended. A long focal-film distance, preferably 72 inches, should be used because of the increased part-film distance.

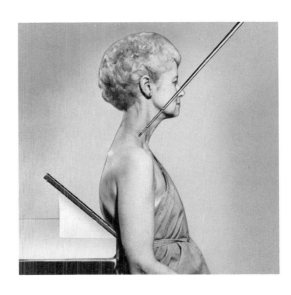

Position of part

Seat the patient with his back toward, and resting against, the end of the table. Place the cassette on the table, center it in line with the shoulder, and adjust it on sandbag supports so as to place it at an angle of 45 degrees.

Central ray

Direct the central ray through the anterosuperior aspect of the shoulder at a posteroinferior angle of 45 degrees; it will be at right angles to the plane of the film.

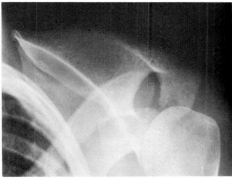

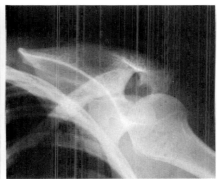

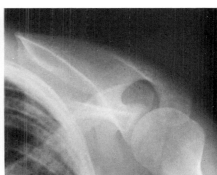

Prone position.   Leaning position.   Seated position.

Anatomy and positioning of the bony thorax

Sternum and ribs

The bony thorax

The bony thorax is formed by the sternum, the twelve pairs of ribs, and the twelve thoracic vertebrae. It is more or less conical in shape, being narrower above than below, its width is greater than its depth, and it is longer in back than in front.

THE STERNUM

The sternum, or breastbone, is directed forward and downward in the median sagittal plane of the anterior thorax. It is a narrow, flat bone about 6 inches long, and consists of three parts—the manubrium, the gladiolus, or body, and the xiphoid, or ensiform, cartilage. The sternum supports the clavicles at the upper manubrial angles and affords attachment to the costal cartilages of the first seven pairs of ribs at its lateral borders.

The manubrium, which is the upper part of the sternum, is quadrilateral in shape and is the broadest part of the sternum. It has a depression on its upper border termed the jugular, or manubrial, notch. On each side of the manubrial notch the bone slants lateralward and backward and bears an articular surface for the reception of the sternal end of the clavicle. On its lateral borders, immediately below the articular notches for the clavicles, are shallow depressions for the attachment of the cartilages of the first pair of ribs. The manubrial notch is easily palpable, and in the thorax of average form, it lies anterior to the interspace between the second and third thoracic vertebrae when the body is erect.

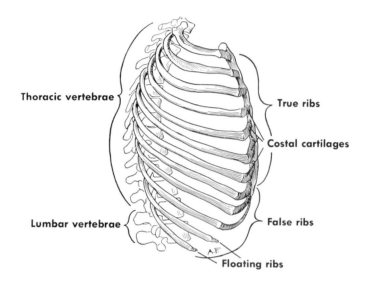

ANTERIOR ASPECT OF BONY THORAX

LATERAL ASPECT OF BONY THORAX

152

The gladiolus, or body, which is the longest part of the sternum, is joined to the manubrium at an obtuse angle, called the sternal angle, at the level of the junction of the second costal cartilage. Both the manubrium and the gladiolus contribute to the attachment of the second costal cartilage. The succeeding five pairs of costal cartilages are attached to the lateral borders of the gladiolus. The sternal angle is palpable and, in the normally formed thorax, lies anterior to the interspace between the fourth and fifth thoracic vertebrae when the body is erect.

The xiphoid process, which forms the distal part of the sternum, is variable in shape. It is a cartilaginous structure in early life but ossifies, at least in part, in later life.

The xiphoid often deviates from the median sagittal plane of the body.

THE STERNOCLAVICULAR JOINTS

The sternoclavicular joints, which are the only points of articulation between the upper extremities and the trunk, are diarthroses that permit limited movement in almost all directions. These joints are formed by the articulation between the sternal ends of the clavicles and the clavicular notches of the manubrium. A circular disk of fibrocartilage is interposed in each joint between the articular ends of the bones, and the joints are enclosed in articular capsules.

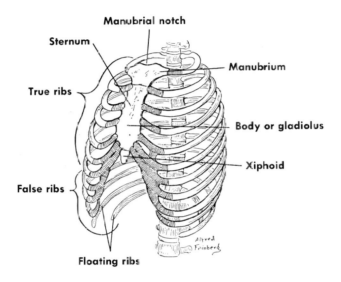

ANTEROLATERAL ASPECT OF BONY THORAX

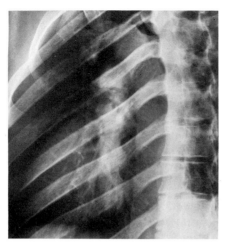

40-inch focal-film distance.

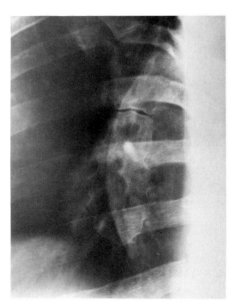

Contact focal-film distance.

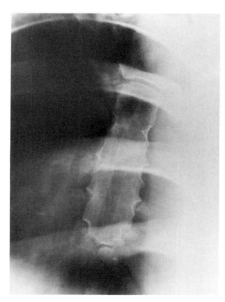

Contact focal-film distance plus breathing motion.

The sternum

The position of the sternum with respect to the denser thoracic structures, both bony and soft, makes it one of the more difficult organs to radiograph satisfactorily. Few problems are involved in obtaining a lateral view, but the sternum's anteroposterior relationship to the thoracic vertebrae makes it impossible to make a direct frontal view of the sternum without the aid of tomography. In order to separate the shadows cast by the vertebrae and the sternum, it is necessary either to rotate the body from the posteroanterior position or to angle the central ray medially. The exact degree of angulation required depends upon the depth of the chest, deep chests requiring less angulation than shallow chests.

While angulation of the body or of the central ray clears the sternum of the vertebral shadow, it superimposes the shadows of the posterior ribs and the lung markings; if the sternum is placed to the left of the thoracic vertebrae, it is also overshadowed by the heart and other mediastinal structures. The superimposition of the homogeneous density of the heart shadow can be used to advantage, as will be seen by comparing the radiographs on the opposite page.

The rib shadows can be blurred by using the shortest possible focal-film distance.[1] If a *shock-proof* tube is used, the tube carriage can be placed in contact with the patient's back. The resulting short focal-spot-rib distance with the comparatively long rib-film distance will greatly diffuse the rib shadows and thereby afford excellent delineation of the sternum. Care must be exercised to obviate the need for repeat exposures at contact distance, however, because the radiation exposure to the patient is considerable.

The pulmonary markings, particularly of elderly persons and of heavy smokers, cast confusing shadows on that of the sternum unless the motion of shallow breathing is utilized to eliminate them. The exposure time, preferably five to ten seconds, should be long enough to cover several phases of respiration. The milliamperage must be relatively low in order to maintain the desired milliampere-second factor.

If the female patient has large, pendulous breasts, they should be drawn to the sides and held in position with a wide bandage to prevent their shadows from overlapping that of the sternum and to obtain closer proximity of the sternum to the film. This is particularly important in the lateral view, where the breast shadows often obscure the lower portion of the sternum.

[1]Zimmer, E. A.: Das Brustbein und seine Gelenke, Fortschr. Roentgenstr., supp. vol. 58, Leipzig, 1939, Georg Thieme.

STERNUM
Right posterior oblique projection
Right anterior oblique view
Film: $10'' \times 12''$ lengthwise.

Position of patient

With the patient in the prone position, adjust his body in the right posterior oblique position in order to utilize the heart shadow. Have the patient support himself on the forearm and the flexed knee.

Position of part

Align the patient's body so that the long axis of the sternum is centered to the midline of the table. Adjust the elevation of the shoulder and hip so that the thorax is rotated just enough to prevent superimposition of the vertebral and sternal shadows. The required degree of rotation can be estimated with sufficient accuracy by placing one hand on the patient's sternum and the other hand directly above it on his thoracic vertebrae to act as guides while adjusting the position.

Place the film in the Potter-Bucky tray and center it to the midsternal area.

When breathing motion is to be utilized, apply a compression band across the thorax and tighten it just enough to restrict rib movement. Instruct the patient to breathe softly during the exposure.

When a short exposure time is to be used, instruct the patient to hold his breath at the end of exhalation in order to obtain a more uniform density.

Central ray

Direct the central ray perpendicularly to the midpoint of the film.

Structures shown

A slightly oblique posteroanterior projection of the sternum. The detail demonstrated depends largely upon the technical procedure employed. When breathing motion is utilized, the pulmonary markings will be obliterated. A short focal-film distance will further aid in the demonstration of the sternum by minimizing the detail of the rib shadows.

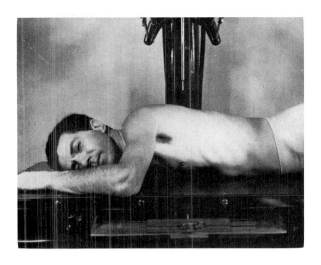

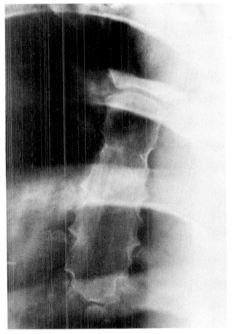

Right posterior oblique projection.

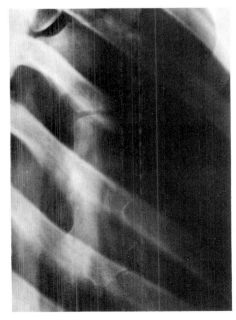

Left posterior oblique projection.

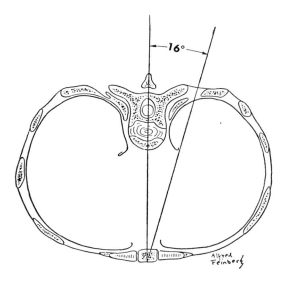

SCHEMATIC DRAWING OF 26cm. CHEST

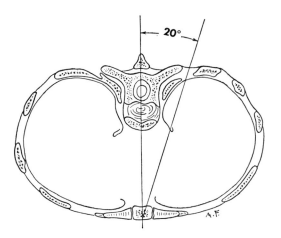

SCHEMATIC DRAWING OF 18cm. CHEST

Thickness-tilt guide for posteroanterior sternum

Depth of thorax (centimeters)	Degree of tube angulation
15.0	22
16.5	21
18.0	20
19.5	19
21.0	18
22.5	17
24.0	16
25.5	15
27.0	14
28.5	13
30.0	12

STERNUM

Lateromedial projection

The tube-tilt method of radiographing the sternum produces a more accurate projection than that produced by the body-rotation method, there being considerably less magnification and distortion of the projected image since the sternum is in closer contact with, and parallel to, the film. The patient is placed in a true posteroanterior position, and the sternal and vertebral shadows are separated by medial angulation of the central ray. The degree of angulation necessary to separate the two shadows depends upon the depth of the chest and therefore varies from patient to patient. For this reason, a specific angulation is not in keeping with the aim to obtain, as nearly as possible, a true frontal view of the sternum on each subject. The angulation required for each patient is estimated by measuring the depth of the thorax in the median plane at the level of the sternal angle. If immobilization is to be used, the measurement should be made after the compression band is applied. The degree of central ray angulation needed to project the sternum free of the vertebral shadow at "contact distance" for the different chest thicknesses is given in the accompanying Thickness-Tilt Guide.

It is customary to use non-Bucky technique in this method of examining the sternum because of the transverse angulation of the central ray. If Potter-Bucky technique is preferred, either a portable Potter-Bucky, a stationary grid, or a grid-front cassette can be used. However, care must be exercised in placing the grid so that the lead strips will be parallel with the angulation of the central ray. When using a portable Potter-Bucky, place the tray side to the head end of the patient in order to have access to the tray in changing cassettes.

Holly[1] described a practical, platformlike device for use with a portable Potter-Bucky. The device serves as a headrest and at the same time leaves the tray side of the Potter-Bucky unobstructed so that cassettes can be changed without disturbing the position of the patient. The platform is 4 inches wide, and is the same length and height as the tray side of the grid.

Runge[2] recommended a nonscreen, non-Bucky technique. He has devised a wooden box 5 inches high with slightly projecting upper edges to immobilize the film holder. The box is placed transversely on the table, and the patient leans on it so that his sternum is in close proximity to the film holder. If the sternum is tender, the patient can partially support his weight on his forearms.

[1]Holly, E. W.: Some radiographic techniques in which movement is utilized. Radiogr. Clin. Photogr. **18**:78-83, 1942.
[2]Runge, R. K.: A technique for roentgenography of the sternum, Xray Techn. **13**:153-154, 1942.

STERNUM
Lateromedial projection—cont'd

Film: 10″ × 12″ lengthwise.

Position of patient

Place the patient in the prone position and center the median sagittal plane of his body to the mid-line of the cassette or *portable* Potter-Bucky diaphragm.

Position of part

Adjust the placement of the cassette or Potter-Bucky diaphragm so that the manubrial notch will lie about 2 inches below the upper border of the film. With the long axis of the sternum centered to the midline of the film, adjust the body in a true posteroanterior position.

Rest the patient's head on his cheek and have him face the tube so that the slight rotation of the vertebral column caused by turning the head will coincide with the direction of the central ray.

Measure the depth of the chest after compression has been applied (the spinous process of the fifth or sixth thoracic vertebra will lie at the level of the sternal angle) and refer to the Thickness-Tilt Chart for the degree of central ray angulation required to project the sternum free of the vertebral shadow.

Breathing instruction depends upon the technical method being employed—cessation of breathing for a short exposure time or continued quiet breathing for a long exposure time.

Central ray

The central ray is directed to the midpoint of the film, preferably from the left side of the body in order to project the heart shadow on that of the sternum.

Structures shown

A slightly oblique posteroanterior projection of the sternum, the detail demonstrated in the bone depending largely upon the technical procedure employed.

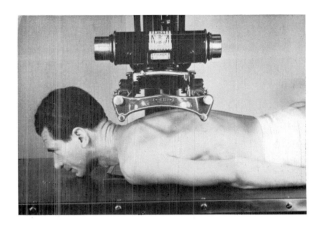

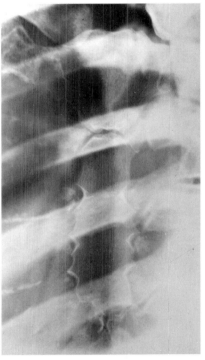

Central ray projected from left side.

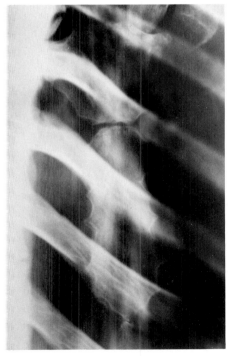

Central ray projected from right side.

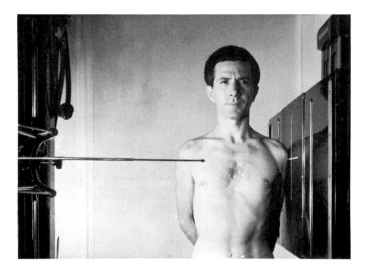

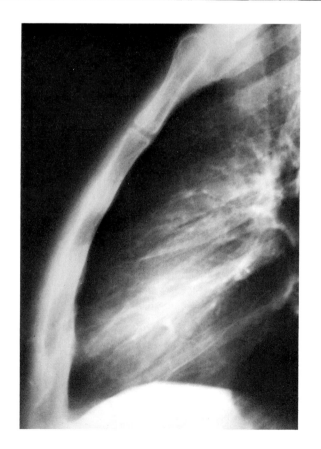

STERNUM
Lateral projection
Erect position

Film: $10'' \times 12''$ lengthwise.

Position of patient

Place the patient in a lateral position, either seated or standing, before a vertical Potter-Bucky stand.

Position of part

Have the patient sit or stand straight and then adjust the height of the film so that its upper border will be about $1\frac{1}{2}$ inches above the manubrial notch.

Rotate the shoulders backward, have the patient lock his hands behind his back, and center the sternum to the midline of the grid. Being careful to keep the median sagittal plane of the body vertical, place the patient close enough to the stand so that he can rest his shoulder firmly against it. Adjust the patient so that the broad surface of the sternum is at right angles to the plane of the film.

The breasts of the female patients should be drawn to the sides and held in position with a wide bandage so that their shadows will not obscure the lower portion of the sternum.

Respiration is suspended at the end of deep inhalation in order to obtain sharper contrast between the posterior surface of the sternum and the adjacent structures.

For a direct lateral view of the sternoclavicular region only, center a vertically placed $8'' \times 10''$ cassette at the level of the manubrial notch.

Central ray

Direct the central ray horizontally to the midpoint of the film.

Structures shown

A lateral view of the entire length of the sternum and/or of the superimposed sternoclavicular joints and medial ends of the clavicles.

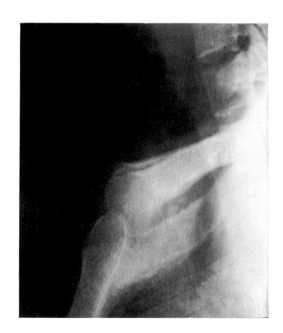

STERNUM
Lateral projection
Recumbent position

Film: $10'' \times 12''$ lengthwise.

Position of patient

Place the patient in the lateral recumbent position and center the long axis of the sternum to the midline of the table.

Position of part

Flex the patient's hips and knees to a comfortable position and support the lower knee and ankle on sandbags. Extend the arms upward enough to prevent their shadows from overlapping that of the sternum. Rest the patient's head on the dependent arm, and have him grasp the end of the table with the hand of the upper side to aid in stabilizing the position.

Place a folded sheet or a loofah sponge under the lower thoracic region and adjust the support to place the long axis of the sternum horizontal. Adjust the rotation of the body so that the broad surface of the sternum is at right angles to the plane of the film.

A compression band may be applied across the hips. Respiration is suspended at the end of deep inhalation in order to obtain sharper contrast between the posterior surface of the sternum and the adjacent structures.

With the cassette in the Potter-Bucky tray, center to the midsternal area.

Central ray

Direct the central ray vertically to the midpoint of the film. The focal-film distance should be at least 36 inches because of the great part-film distance.

Structures shown

A lateral view of the entire length of the sternum.

NOTE: In cases of severe injury, the patient can be examined in the supine position by cross table or horizontal ray projection. In this case, a grid-front cassette or a stationary grid should be used.

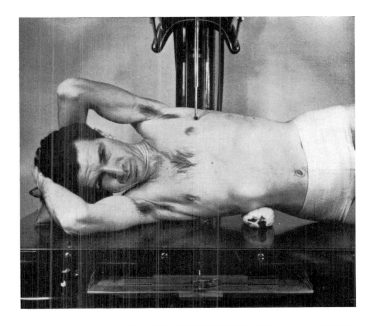

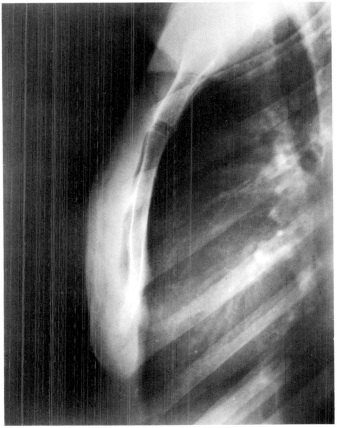

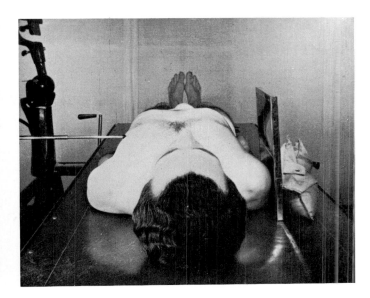

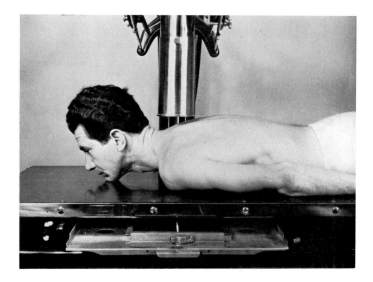

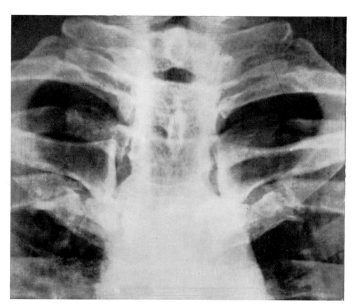

Long focal-film distance.

Short focal-film distance.
Bilateral projections.

STERNOCLAVICULAR ARTICULATIONS
Posteroanterior projection
Anteroposterior view
Film: $8'' \times 10''$ crosswise.

Position of patient

Place the patient in the prone position and center the median sagittal plane of the body to the midline of the table. The following procedure can be adapted for use with the patient who is standing or seated erect. Casualty patients who cannot be turned from the supine position can be equally well examined with the under-table tube and a grid-front cassette.

Position of part

For non-Bucky technique, center the film to the manubrial notch.

Place the arms along the sides of the body with the palms facing upward, and adjust the shoulders to lie in the same transverse plane.

1. For a bilateral examination, rest the patient's head on the chin and adjust it so that the median sagittal plane is vertical.

2. For a unilateral examination, ask the patient to turn his head to face the affected side and then to rest his head on his cheek. The rotation of the head rotates the spine slightly away from the side being examined and thus gives a better view of the lateral portion of the manubrium.

For Potter-Bucky technique, center the film at the level of the spinous process of the third thoracic vertebra, which lies posterior to the manubrial notch.

Respiration is suspended at the end of exhalation in order to obtain a more uniform density.

Central ray

Direct the central ray perpendicularly to the midpoint of the film.

Structures shown

A posteroanterior projection of the sternoclavicular joints, and of the medial portions of the clavicles.

NOTE: If *shock-proof* equipment is available, better detail of the sternoclavicular joints can be obtained by diffusing of the vertebral shadow with a short focal-film distance. "Contact distance," which will almost completely obliterate the vertebral shadow, can be used by removing the cone from the head of a *shock-proof* dental or mobile unit. Because of the extremely short focal-film distance over a thin part, the small radiation aperture of the x-ray tube sharply delimits the exposure field. Precision centering is required in order to prevent repeated exposure to the patient.

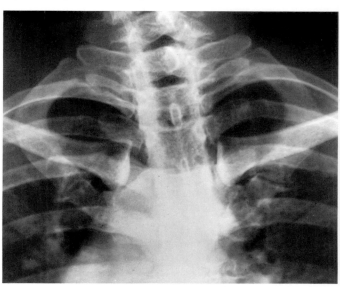

Unilateral projection.

STERNOCLAVICULAR ARTICULATIONS
Unilateral projections
Film: $8'' \times 10''$ crosswise.

Body rotation method
Position of patient

The patient may be placed in either a prone position or in a seated erect position.

Position of part

Keeping the affected side adjacent to the film, oblique the patient enough to project the vertebral shadow well behind that of the sternoclavicular joint, and then adjust his position so as to center the joint to the cassette or to the midline of the Potter-Bucky diaphragm. Adjust the shoulders to lie in the same transverse plane. Center the film at the level of the sternoclavicular joint.

Central ray

Direct the central ray perpendicularly to the midpoint of the film.

Central ray angulation method
Position of patient

The patient is placed in the prone position. Adjust the cassette under his upper chest so as to center the film to the affected sternoclavicular joint.

Position of part

Extend the arms along the sides of the body with the palms of the hands facing upward, and adjust the shoulders to lie in the same transverse plane. Ask the patient to rest his head on his chin, and then adjust the head so that its median sagittal plane is vertical.

Central ray

From the side being examined, the central ray is directed to the midpoint of the film at an angle of 15 degrees toward the median sagittal plane of the body.

A specific angle is satisfactory in examinations of the sternoclavicular articulations because there is only a slight anteroposterior overlapping of the vertebrae and these joints.

Structures shown

A slightly oblique view of the sternoclavicular joint by either method. Due to the fact that the joint is closer to, and parallel with, the plane of the film, less distortion is obtained with the central ray angulation method than with the body rotation method.

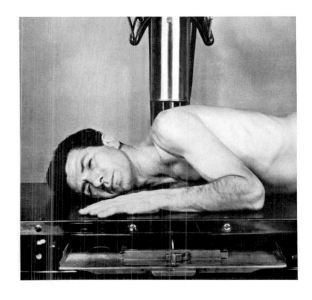

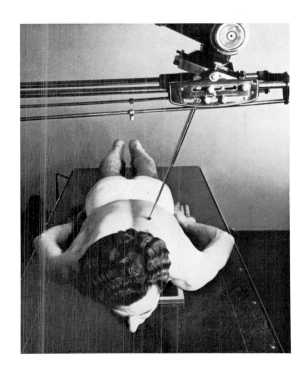

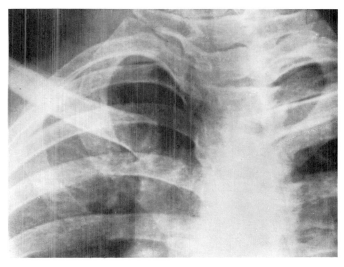

Central ray angulation method.

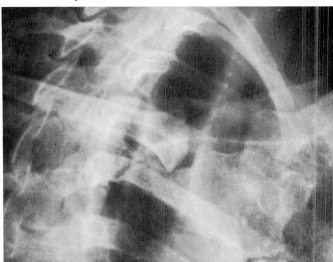

Body rotation method.

161

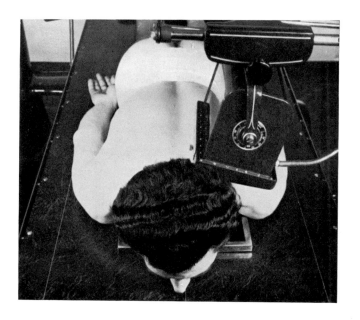

STERNOCLAVICULAR ARTICULATIONS
Lateromedial projection
Zimmer method

Film: $8'' \times 10''$ crosswise.

Position of patient

Adjust the patient in the prone position, with the median sagittal plane of the body centered to the midline of the table.

Position of part

Place a cassette or a cassette-changing tunnel under the chest and center it to the manubrial notch.

Extend the arms along the sides of the body with the hands facing upward. Adjust the shoulders to lie in the same transverse plane. Rest the head on the tip of the chin, with the median sagittal plane vertical.

Locate the spinous process of the third thoracic vertebrae and make a wax-pencil mark 6 cm. to each side of it to indicate the centering points.

When using the 15-degree angulation of the central ray recommended by Zimmer,[1] place the cassette in the tunnel and shift it 1½ inches toward the contralateral side. Alternately mask one-half of the film with a piece of sheet lead. It is not necessary to shift the film when using a 5-degree angulation of the central ray.

Respiration is suspended for the exposures.

Central ray

Direct the central ray either 5 or 15 degrees toward the median sagittal plane, first from one side and then from the opposite side. The central ray is directed to the previously marked localization points.

If *shock-proof* equipment is available, contact distance should be used; if not, use the smallest possible cone and as short a focal-film distance as is safe.

Structures shown

A slightly oblique view of both sternoclavicular joints on one film. The vertebral shadow is absent.

[1]Zimmer, E. A.: Das Brustbein und seine Gelenke, Fortschr. Roentgenstr., supp. vol. 58, Leipzig, 1939, Georg Thieme.

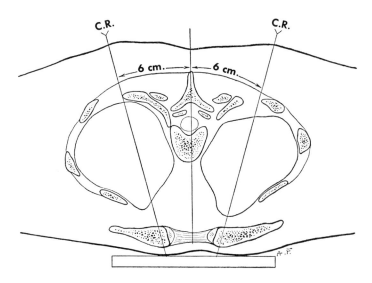

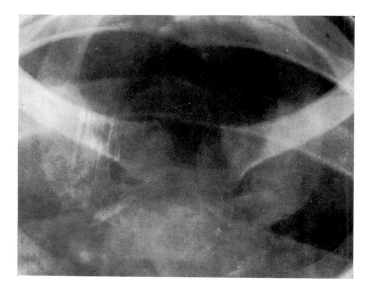

STERNOCLAVICULAR ARTICULATION
Lateral projection
Kurzbauer position[1]
Film: 8″ × 10″ lengthwise.

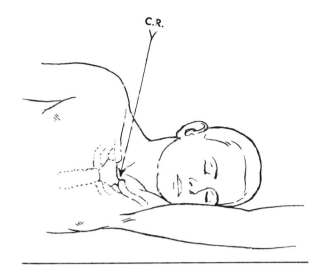

Position of patient

The patient lies in the lateral recumbent position on the side being examined, with the sternoclavicular region approximately centered to the midline of the table. Flex the patient's hips and knees to a comfortable position.

Position of part

Have the patient fully extend the dependent arm and grasp the end of the table for support. Make any necessary adjustment to center the sternoclavicular articulation to the midline of the table. Place the uppermost arm along the side of the body and have the patient grasp the dorsal surface of his hip to hold the shoulder in a depressed position. The extension of the dependent shoulder, coupled with the depression of the uppermost shoulder, prevents the superimposition of the shadows of the articulations.

Adjust the thorax so as to place the anterior surface of the manubrium at right angles to the plane of the film.

Adjust the position of the film so that its midpoint will coincide with the central ray.

Respiration is suspended at the end of full inhalation.

Central ray

Direct the central ray through the lowermost sternoclavicular articulation at an angle of 15 degrees toward the feet.

Structures shown

An unobstructed lateral view of the sternoclavicular articulation adjacent to the film.

While the best result is obtained with the patient in the recumbent position, a comparable view can be obtained with the erect position when the shoulder is too tender for pressure.

[1]Kurzbauer, Robert: The lateral projection in the roentgenography of the sternoclavicular articulation, Amer. J. Roentgen. 56:104-105, 1946.

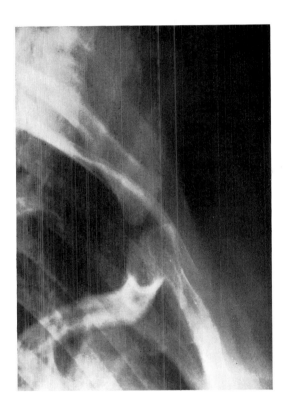

The ribs

The twelve pairs of ribs are simply numbered from above downward. With the exception of the last two pairs, in which the cartilage is absent, each rib consists of a long, slender, arched bone and a costal cartilage. The ribs are attached posteriorly to the bodies of the thoracic vertebrae. The first, tenth, eleventh, and twelfth ribs each articulates with one vertebral body, and the others articulate with two bodies. Anteriorly, the cartilages of the first seven pairs of ribs are attached directly to the sternum and are called true ribs, or vertebrosternal ribs. The succeeding three pairs of ribs are attached cartilage to superjacent cartilage and are called false, or vertebrochondral, ribs. The last two pairs have no anterior attachment and are called floating, or vertebral, ribs. The term false rib is applied to both the vertebrochondral and the floating ribs.

The ribs are situated in an oblique plane slanting forward and downward so that their anterior ends lie from 3 to 5 inches below the level of their vertebral ends. The degree of obliquity gradually increases from the first to the ninth rib, and then decreases to the twelfth rib. The spaces between the ribs are referred to as the intercostal spaces. The ribs vary in breadth and length. From the first rib, which is the shortest and broadest, the breadth gradually decreases to the twelfth rib, which is the narrowest rib. The length increases from the first to the seventh, then gradually decreases to the twelfth rib.

A typical rib consists of (1) a head that articulates with the vertebral bodies, (2) a flattened neck, (3) a tubercle that articulates with the transverse process of a thoracic vertebra, except in the eleventh and twelfth ribs, and (4) a shaft. From the point of articulation with the vertebral body, the rib projects obliquely backward to the point of articulation with the transverse process, and then it turns lateralward to the angle of the shaft, where the bone arches forward and medialward in an oblique plane from above downward.

The heads of the ribs are closely bound to the vertebral bodies and are permitted only slight gliding movements, these articulations being called costovertebral joints. The articulations between the necks and tubercles of the ribs and the transverse processes of the vertebrae, the costotransverse joints, permit only slight upward and downward movements of the first six pairs, but greater freedom of movement is permitted in the succeeding four pairs. With the exception of the first pair, which are rigidly attached to the sternum, the sternocostal articulations permit gliding movements.

RESPIRATORY EXCURSION

The normal oblique position of the ribs is changed very little during quiet respiratory movements; however, the degree of obliquity is decreased with deep inhalation and is increased with deep exhalation. The first pair of ribs, which are rigidly attached to the manubrium, rotate at their vertebral ends and move with the sternum as one structure during respiratory movements.

On deep inhalation the anterior ends of the ribs are carried forward, upward, and outward, while their necks are rotated downward. On deep exhalation the anterior ends are carried downward, backward, and inward, while the necks are rotated upward. The last two pairs of ribs are depressed and held in position by the action of the diaphragm when the anterior ends of the upper ribs are elevated during respiration.

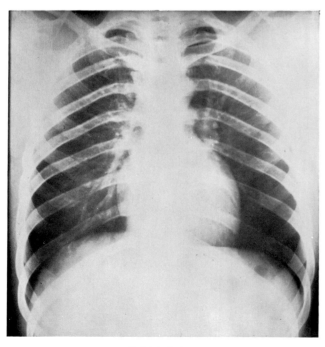

Full inhalation.

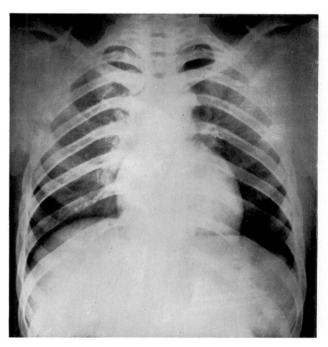

Full exhalation.

THE DIAPHRAGM

The ribs situated above the diaphragm are examined through the air-filled lungs, while those situated below the diaphragm must be examined through the upper abdomen. Because of the difference in penetration required for the two regions, the position and respiratory excursion of the diaphragm play a large part in radiography of the ribs.

The position of the diaphragm varies with bodily habitus, being at a higher level in short, broad subjects and at a lower level in tall, thin subjects. In the subject of average size and shape, the right side of the diaphragm arches backward from the level of about the sixth or seventh costal cartilage to the level of the ninth or tenth thoracic vertebra when the body is in the erect position. The left side of the diaphragm will lie at a slightly lower level. Because of the oblique position of both the ribs and the diaphragm, several pairs of ribs lie partially above and partially below the diaphragm.

The position of the diaphragm changes considerably with the position of the body, being at its lowest level when the body is erect and at its highest level when the body is supine. For this reason, it is desirable to place the patient in the erect position when examining the ribs above the diaphragm, and in a recumbent position when examining the ribs below the diaphragm. When the body is in a lateral recumbent position, the diaphragm lies in an oblique plane, the lower half being higher in position than the upper half. This point must be remembered and utilized when radiographing the axillary portion of the ribs; a prone oblique position is used for a transthoracic projection, and a supine oblique position is used for a transabdominal projection.

The respiratory excursion of the diaphragm averages about 1½ inches between deep inhalation and deep exhalation. The excursion will be less in obese subjects and more in thin subjects. Deeper inhalation or exhalation, and therefore greater depression or elevation of the diaphragm, is achieved on the second respiratory movement than is achieved on the first. This point should be utilized when examining the ribs that lie at the diaphragmatic level.

When the body is placed in the supine position, the anterior ends of the ribs are displaced upward, outward, and backward. For this reason, the anterior ends of the ribs are poorly visualized when the patient is radiographed in the supine position.

BODY POSITION

While it is desirable in rib examinations to take advantage of the effect that body position has on the position of the diaphragm, the effect is not of sufficient importance to justify subjecting a patient to a painful change in position from the erect to the recumbent or vice versa. Rib injuries, minor as well as extensive, are painful, and even slight movement frequently causes the patient considerable distress. Therefore, unless the change can be effected with a tilt-table, patients with recent injury should be examined in the position in which they arrive in the department. The ambulatory patient can be positioned for recumbent projections with a minimum of discomfort by bringing the tilt-table to the vertical position for each position change. With the patient standing on the footboard, he can be comfortably adjusted and then lowered to the horizontal position.

CASUALTY PATIENTS

The first, and usually the only, requirement in the initial radiographic examination of the casualty patient who has sustained severe trauma to the rib cage is to take frontal (posteroanterior or anteroposterior) and lateral projections of the chest. These projections are made not only to demonstrate the site and extent of rib injury but to investigate the possibility of injury to the underlying structures by depressed rib fractures. The patient is examined in the position in which he arrives, usually recumbent on a stretcher. This body position necessitates a horizontal ray projection for the detection of fluid and/or air levels.

Less seriously injured patients sometimes arrive after adhesive strapping has been applied around the lower thorax to restrict rib movement and thus to make breathing less painful. Fractures having appreciable fragment separation or displacement are readily detected through smooth, recently applied strapping. Undisplaced transverse fractures frequently are not discernible before the appearance of callus formation, even without strapping. Failure to demonstrate fissure fractures of this type is not of great importance since surgical intervention is not required.

It is desirable to radiograph ribs before the application of adhesive strapping, but no patient need be subjected to the discomfort of having freshly applied strapping removed since no fracture of clinical significance will be missed as a result of its presence. It is, however, necessary to remove old, wrinkled strapping for progress examinations. Fortunately, the patient will have recovered enough in the two- or three-week interval to tolerate the removal without too much discomfort. Unless the technologist is fully qualified to do so, dressings should be removed by a physician or a nurse.

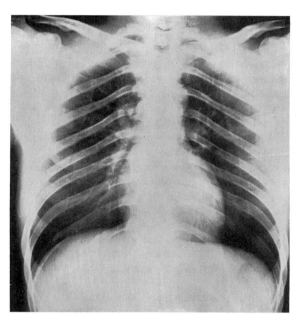

Posteroanterior projection.

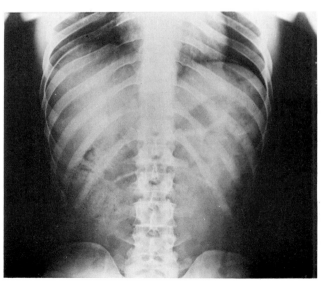

Anteroposterior projection.

RADIOGRAPHY OF THE RIBS

In radiography of the ribs, unless the affected area is definitely localized near one end of the thorax, where either the first or the last rib will be included on a smaller film, a 14″ × 17″ scout film should be made first to identify the rib or ribs involved and to establish the extent of the suspected trauma or pathology.

After localizing the lesion, determine (1) the position required to place the affected rib region parallel with the plane of the film, and (2) whether the projection should be made from above or below the diaphragm.

The anterior portions of the ribs, usually referred to simply as the anterior ribs, are examined in the posteroanterior position. The posterior portions of the ribs or more simply the posterior ribs, are examined in the anteroposterior position if the focal-film distance is less than 36 inches, but they are well shown in the posteroanterior position if the distance is 36 inches or more. The axillary portions of the ribs are best shown in an oblique position. Because the lateral position results in superimposition of the two sides, it is usually used only in the investigation of fluid and/or air levels.

When the ribs that are overshadowed by the heart are involved, the body must be rotated so as to project the ribs free of the heart shadow, or the exposure must be

Anteroposterior projection.

increased to compensate for the density of the heart. While their anterior and posterior ends are superimposed, the left ribs are cleared of the heart shadow in either the left posterior oblique projection (left anterior oblique view) or the right anterior oblique projection (right posterior oblique view). These two positions place the right-sided ribs parallel with the plane of the film and are reversed to obtain comparable views of the left-sided ribs.

When ribs above the diaphragm are examined, particularly on elderly patients and heavy smokers, better detail can be obtained by utilizing shallow breathing movement to diffuse the lung markings.[1] In order to restrict rib movement, an immobilization band should be applied across the thorax with moderate pressure. It is advisable for the patient to practice shallow breathing before the exposure is made. For this procedure, the milliampere-second factor must be converted to a low current–long exposure time combination; the time should be long enough to cover two or three phases of respiration.

When a patient is unable to breathe smoothly and evenly for the time required for the exposure, vibratory movement from the pulsating heart during suspended respiration for an exposure of five to seven seconds will greatly diffuse if not obliterate pulmonary markings.

[1]Bloom, Arthur R.: A new technique of taking roentgenographs of the upper ribs, Radiology 33:648-649, 1939.

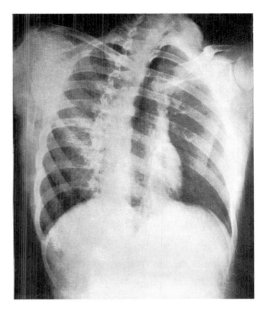

Left anterior oblique view.

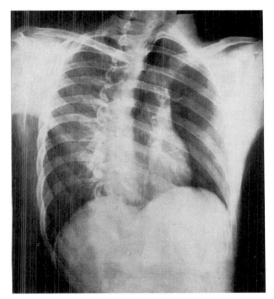

Right posterior oblique view.

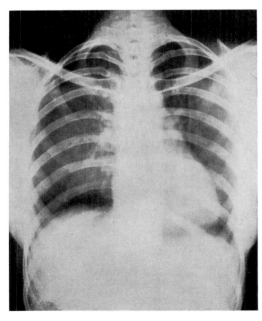

Quiet breathing.

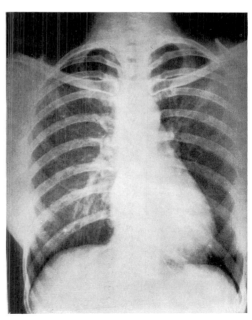

Suspended respiration.

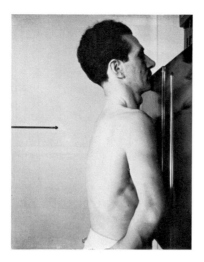

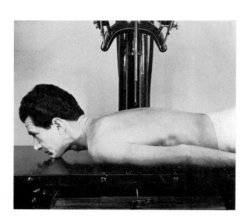

UPPER ANTERIOR RIBS
Posteroanterior projection
Anteroposterior view

Film: $14'' \times 17''$ lengthwise.

Position of patient

The patient is placed in the posteroanterior position, either erect or recumbent. Because the diaphragm descends to its lowest level in the erect position, the standing or the seated-erect position should be used for projections of the upper ribs when the patient's condition permits.

Position of part

Center the median sagittal plane of the body to the midline of the Potter-Bucky grid. Adjust the position of the film so that it projects approximately $1\frac{1}{2}$ inches above the upper border of the shoulders.

Rest the patient's hands against his hips with the palms turned outward in order to rotate the scapulae away from the rib cage. Adjust the shoulders to lie in the same transverse plane, and if the patient is erect, instruct him to keep them in contact with the stand. Rest the head on the chin and adjust it so that its median sagittal plane is vertical.

Unless breathing movement is to be utilized, respiration is suspended at the end of full inhalation to depress the diaphragm as much as possible.

Central ray

With the central ray perpendicular to the plane of the film, center (1) to the midpoint of the film for the upper ribs, or (2) approximately 5 inches proximal to the midpoint of the film for the seventh, eighth, and ninth ribs. In the latter case, high centering aids in projecting the shadow of the diaphragm below that of the affected rib.

Structures shown

A posteroanterior projection of the ribs above the diaphragm.

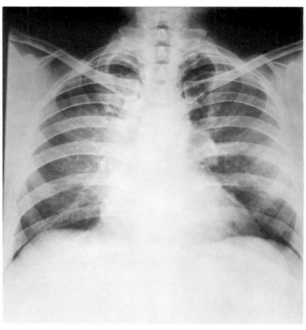

High centering.   Normal centering.

POSTERIOR RIBS
Anteroposterior projection
Posteroanterior view

Film: $14'' \times 17''$ lengthwise for ribs above the diaphragm, and crosswise for those below the diaphragm.

Position of patient

The patient is placed in the anteroposterior position, either erect or recumbent. When the patient's condition permits, the erect position should be used for ribs above the diaphragm, and the supine position for ribs below the diaphragm.

Position of part

Center the median sagittal plane of the body to the midline of the Potter-Bucky grid.

Ribs above diaphragm. Place the film lengthwise and center at the level of the sixth thoracic vertebra; the film will project about $1\frac{1}{2}$ inches above the upper border of the shoulders.

Rest the patient's hands, palms outward, against the hips. Adjust the shoulders to lie in the same transverse plane and rotate them forward to draw the scapulae away from the rib cage. The angle of the ribs can be decreased somewhat by having the patient extend his arms to the vertical position, the hands being supported on or under the head.

Unless respiratory movement is to be utilized, have the patient suspend respiration at the end of full inhalation in order to depress the diaphragm.

Ribs below diaphragm. Place the film crosswise and center it at the level of the twelfth thoracic vertebra; the film will project approximately $1\frac{1}{2}$ inches below the crests of the ilia.

Adjust the shoulders to lie in the same transverse plane and place the arms in a comfortable position.

Respiration is suspended at the end of full exhalation for the purpose of elevating the diaphragm.

Central ray

With the central ray perpendicular to the plane of the film, center (1) 4 or 5 inches above the midpoint of the film for ribs above the diaphragm, or (2) 4 or 5 inches below the midpoint of the film for ribs below the diaphragm.

This centering projects the shadow of the diaphragm either below or above ribs that it would otherwise partially overlap.

Structures shown

An anteroposterior projection of the posterior ribs above or below the diaphragm, according to the region examined.

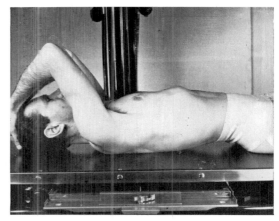

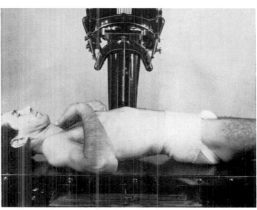

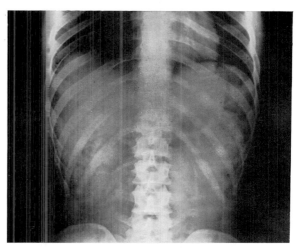

Full inhalation.

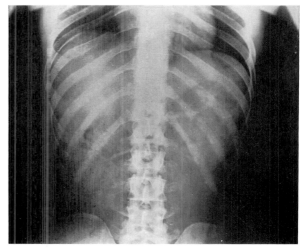

Full exhalation.

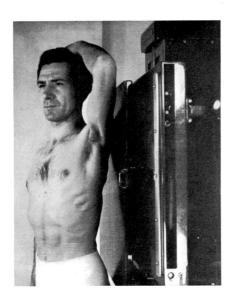

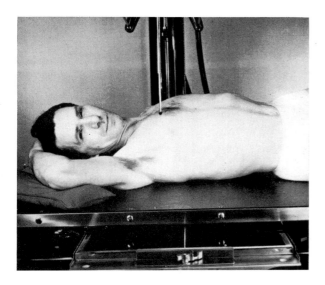

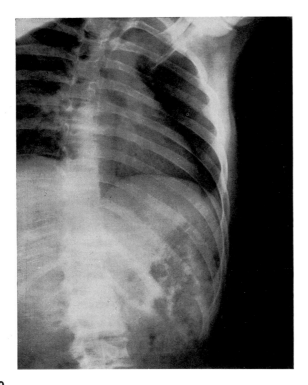

AXILLARY PORTION OF THE RIBS
Anterior oblique projection
Posterior oblique view

Film: 14″ × 17″ lengthwise for ribs above the diaphragm, crosswise for ribs below the diaphragm.

Position of patient

The patient may be examined in either the erect or the recumbent position. Unless contraindicated by the patient's condition, the erect position is preferable for ribs above the diaphragm, and the recumbent position for ribs below the diaphragm.

Position of part

From the anteroposterior position, rotate the body to an angle of approximately 45 degrees, the affected side toward the film. Center a plane midway between the median sagittal plane and the lateral surface of the body to the midline of the Potter-Bucky grid. If the patient is in the recumbent position, support the elevated hip on sandbags.

Abduct the arm of the affected side and elevate it to carry the scapula away from the rib cage. Rest the hand on the patient's head if he is in the erect position, or place it under or above the head if he is in the recumbent position. The opposite extremity may be placed along the side of the body.

Center the film at the level of the sixth thoracic vertebra for ribs above the diaphragm, and at the level of the twelfth thoracic vertebra for ribs below the diaphragm. The film, placed lengthwise, may be centered midway between these points for a scout projection.

Breathing instructions

Respiration is suspended at the end of deep exhalation for ribs below the diaphragm and, unless breathing movement is to be utilized, at the end of full inhalation for ribs above the diaphragm.

Central ray

With the central ray directed perpendicularly to the plane of the film, center 4 or 5 inches above the midpoint of the film for the upper ribs, and 4 or 5 inches below the midpoint for ribs below the diaphragm.

Structures shown

The axillary portion of the ribs projected free of self-superimposition.

AXILLARY PORTION OF THE RIBS
Posterior oblique projection
Anterior oblique view

Film: 14″ × 17″ lengthwise for scout examination and ribs above the diaphragm, and crosswise for ribs below the diaphragm.

Position of patient

The patient may be examined in either the erect or the recumbent position. Unless contraindicated by the patient's condition, the erect position should be used for ribs above the diaphragm, and the recumbent position for ribs below the diaphragm.

Position of part

From the posteroanterior position, rotate the body to an angle of approximately 45 degrees, with the affected side away from the film. If the patient is in the recumbent position, have him rest on the forearm and the flexed knee of the elevated side. Align the body so that a longitudinal plane midway between the median sagittal plane and the lateral surface of the body is centered to the midline of the Potter-Bucky grid.

Center the film at the level of the sixth thoracic vertebra for ribs above the diaphragm, at the level of the twelfth thoracic vertebra for ribs below the diaphragm, or, placed lengthwise, midway between these points for a scout projection.

Breathing instructions

Respiration is suspended at the end of full exhalation for ribs below the diaphragm and, unless breathing movement is to be utilized, at the end of full inhalation for ribs above the diaphragm.

Central ray

With the central ray perpendicular to the plane of the film, center 4 or 5 inches above the midpoint of the film for the upper ribs, and 4 or 5 inches below the midpoint of the film for the lower ribs.

Structures shown

The axillary portion of the ribs free of bony superimposition. When this position is used, the target-film distance should be at least 36 inches because of the great part-film distance.

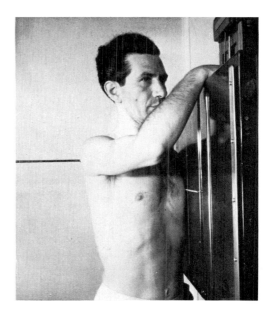

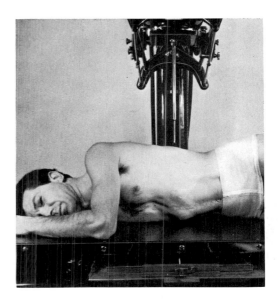

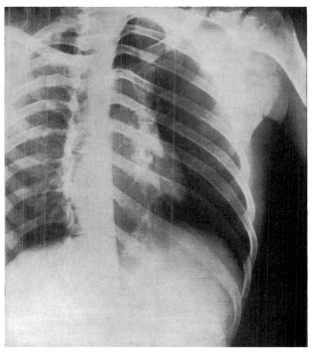

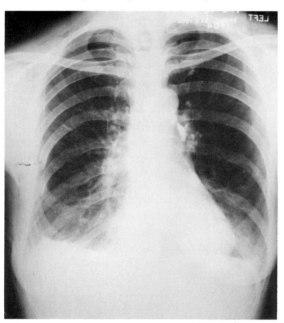

Axial view of patient in position before angled cassettes.

RIBS
Wide-angle frontal projection
Corbin technique

Wide-angle roentgenography was devised by Corbin[1] for the purpose of obtaining frontal plane separation (1) of anatomic structures and lesions that are poorly shown due to foreshortening, and (2) of those that are usually obscured by superimposition in conventional frontal projections.

Two cassettes are placed in a frame so constructed that the films form an angle of 90 degrees to each other, and that each film forms an angle of 45 degrees to the central ray. The patient is positioned before the imaginary base of the triangle so formed. Due to the progressive increase in the part-film and focal-film distances, the resultant simultaneous bilateral projections give a panoramic view showing separation and magnification of the shadows of the structures composing the part.

The pair of cassettes can be held in position with a commercially available wide-angle cassette holder that can be hooked onto any conventional cassette stand or with a similar homemade device. In the absence of grid-front cassettes, the homemade frame should be so constructed as to accommodate stationary grids, as does the commercial frame.

Wide-angle projections require an exposure increase equivalent to 6 to 10 kilovolts.

[1]Berlin, H. S., Unger, S. M., Corbin, L. J., Jacobson, H. G., and Poppel, M. H.: Wide-angle roentgenography, Amer. J. Roentgen. **90**:189-197, 1963.

Conventional projection.

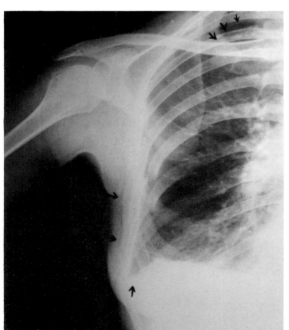

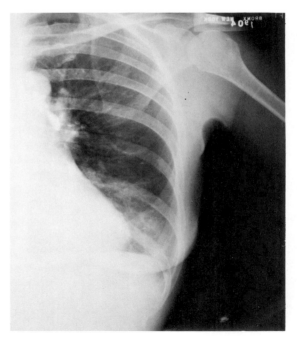

Wide-angle projections on the above patient.

Radiographs courtesy Dr. Leon J. Corbin.

COSTAL JOINTS
Semiaxial anteroposterior projection
Williams position

Williams[1] recommends this position for the demonstration of the costal joints in cases of rheumatoid (Marie-Strümpell) spondylitis.

Film: 11″ × 14″ lengthwise.

Position of patient

Place the patient in the supine position. Let the head rest directly on the table in order to avoid accentuating the dorsal kyphosis.

Position of part

Adjust the body in a true anteroposterior position, with its median sagittal plane centered to the midline of the table. If the patient has an accentuated dorsal kyphosis, extend the arms over the head; otherwise, the arms may be placed along the sides of the body. Adjust the shoulders to lie in the same transverse plane.

With the cassette in the Potter-Bucky tray, adjust its position so that the midpoint of the film will coincide with the central ray; the film will project approximately 4 inches beyond the upper border of the shoulders.

Compression may be applied across the thorax. Respiration is suspended at the end of full inhalation because the lung markings are less prominent at this phase of breathing.

Central ray

Direct the central ray through the sixth thoracic vertebra at an average angle of 20 degrees toward the head. Increase the central ray angulation slightly (5 to 10 degrees) when examining patients who have an accentuated dorsal kyphosis.

Structures shown

The costovertebral and costotransverse joints.

NOTE: Williams[1] states that in large-boned subjects it may be necessary to examine the two sides separately in order to demonstrate the costovertebral joints. This is done by alternately rotating the body approximately 10 degrees medially.

Williams, A. Justin: Personal communication.

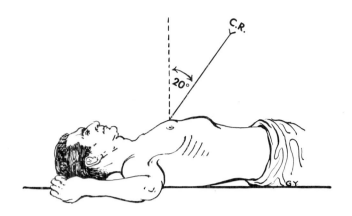

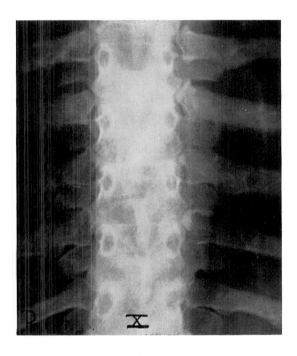

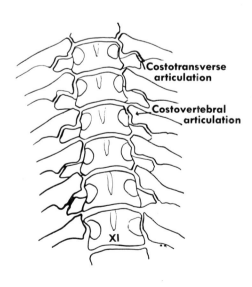

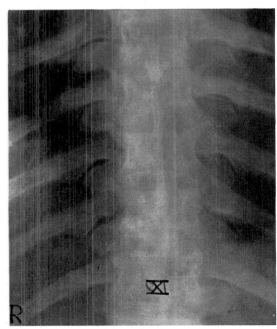

Radiographs and drawing courtesy Dr. A. Justin Williams.

Anatomy and positioning of the pelvic girdle and the upper femora

The pelvis

The pelvis serves as a base for the trunk and as a girdle for the attachment of the lower extremities. The pelvic girdle is formed by the two hipbones in front and at the sides, and by the sacrum and coccyx behind. The pubes of the hipbones articulate with each other anteriorly at the midline of the body, forming a joint called the symphysis pubis. The ilia articulate with the sacrum posteriorly, and these joints are called the sacroiliac joints. The pubic symphysis, and the sacroiliac joints are amphiarthroses, which allow only a little movement.

THE HIP

The hipbone, also called the os coxae and os innominatum, consists of three parts—the ilium, the pubis, and the ischium. All three bones enter into the formation of the acetabulum, the cup-shaped socket that receives the head of the femur, where they are separated by cartilage in youth but become fused into one bone in adulthood.

The ilium. The ilium consists of a body and a broad, curved, winglike portion called the ala. The body of the ilium forms the upper portion of the acetabulum. The ala projects upward from the body to form the prominence of the hip. The ala has three margins, or borders—anterior, posterior, and superior. The anterior and posterior borders each present two prominent projections, which are separated from each other by a notch. These projections are termed the superior and inferior spines, respectively. The superior margin extends from the anterior to the posterior superior iliac spines and is termed the crest of the ilium. The medial surface of the ala is divided into anterior and posterior portions. The anterior portion is called the iliac fossa, and is separated from the body of the bone by a smooth, arc-shaped ridge, the arcuate line, which forms a part of the circumference of the pelvic brim. The arcuate line passes obliquely downward and medialward to its junction with the pubis, where there is a slight, rounded elevation called the iliopectineal eminence. The lower part of the posterior portion of the ala presents a large facet, the auricular surface, for articulation with the sacrum.

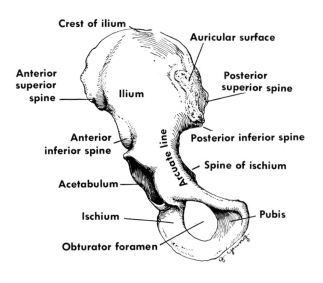

ANTERIOR ASPECT OF RIGHT HIP BONE

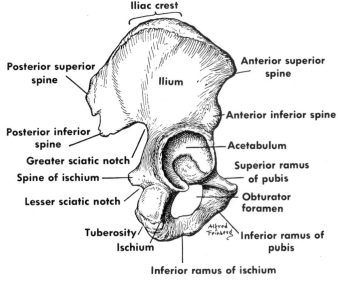

LATERAL ASPECT OF RIGHT HIP BONE

The pubis. The pubic bone consists of a body and two rami—the superior, or ascending, ramus, and the inferior, or descending, ramus. The body of the pubis forms the lower anterior portion of the acetabulum. (The flattened portion of the pubis at the midline was formerly called the body of the bone.) The superior ramus projects downward and medialward from the acetabulum to the midline of the body. Here the bone curves downward and then backward and lateralward to join the ischium. The lower prong is termed the inferior ramus. The upper surface of the superior ramus presents a ridge, the pectin, or pectineal line, which is continuous with the arcuate line of the ilium.

The ischium. The ischium, like the pubis, consists of a body and two rami. The body of the ischium forms the lower posterior portion of the acetabulum. Its superior ramus projects backward and downward from the acetabulum to an expanded portion called the ischial tuberosity. The inferior ramus projects forward and medialward from the tuberosity to its junction with the inferior ramus of the pubis. By this posterior union, the rami of the pubis and the ischium enclose the obturator foramen. At the upper posterior border of the superior ramus, there is a prominent projection called the ischial spine.

The greater sciatic notch begins just below the posterior inferior iliac spine and extends to the ischial spine. The lesser sciatic notch lies between the ischial spine and the ischial tuberosity.

THE FEMUR

The proximal end of the femur consists of a head, a neck, and two large processes termed the greater and lesser trochanters. The head is smooth and rounded, and is received into the acetabular cavity of the hip. It is connected to the shaft by a pyramid-shaped neck. The neck is constricted near the head but expands to a broad base at the shaft of the bone. The neck projects medialward, upward, and forward from the shaft. The trochanters are situated at the junction of the shaft and the base of the neck, the greater trochanter at the upper lateral part of the shaft, and the lesser trochanter at the posterior medial part. The prominent ridge extending between the trochanters at the base of the neck on the posterior surface of the shaft is called the intertrochanteric crest. The less prominent ridge connecting the trochanters anteriorly is called the intertrochanteric line.

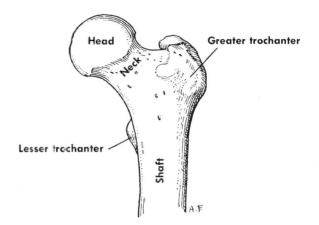

ANTERIOR ASPECT OF UPPER END OF FEMUR

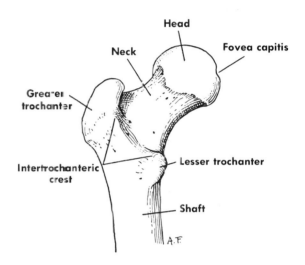

POSTERIOR ASPECT OF UPPER END OF FEMUR

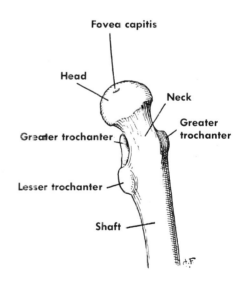

MEDIAL ASPECT OF UPPER END OF FEMUR

THE FEMUR—cont'd

The upper portion of the greater trochanter projects above the neck and curves slightly backward and medialward. The most prominent point of the lateral surface of the greater trochanter is always in direct line with the upper border of the neck of the femur. The angulation of the neck of the femur varies considerably with age, sex, and stature. In the adult of average form, the neck projects forward from the shaft at an angle of approximately 15 to 20 degrees, and upward at an angle of approximately 120 to 130 degrees to the long axis of the shaft. In youth the latter angle is wider, that is, the neck is more vertical in position. The angle is narrower—the neck is more horizontal in position—in wide pelves.

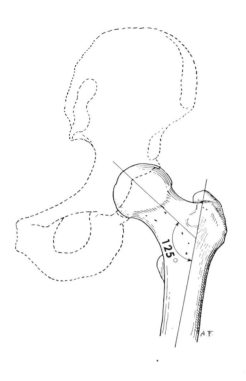

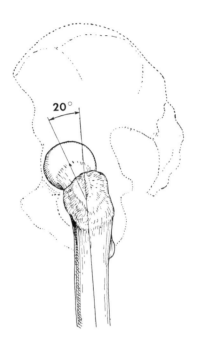

THE HIP JOINT

The articulation between the acetabulum and the head of the femur is a diarthrosis of the ball-and-socket type, which permits free movement in all directions. The knee and ankle joints are hinge joints, so that the wide range of movements of the lower extremity depend upon the ball-and-socket joint of the hip. Because the knee and ankle joints are hinge joints, inversion and eversion of the foot causes rotation of the entire extremity and, if carried far enough, of the pelvis. This makes the position of the feet important in radiography of the hip and pelvis; they must be immobilized in the correct position in order to avoid rotation resulting in distortion of the upper end of the femur.

The two palpable bony points of localization for the hip joint are the anterior superior iliac spine and the upper margin of the pubic symphysis. The midpoint of a line drawn between these two points will lie directly above the center of the dome of the acetabular cavity. A line drawn at right angles to the midpoint of the first line will lie parallel with the long axis of the neck of the femur in the adult of average form when the extremity is extended in the anatomic position. For accurate localization of the femoral neck in atypical subjects, or when the extremity is not in the anatomic position, (1) draw a line between the anterior superior iliac spine and the upper margin of the pubic symphysis, and (2) palpate the greater trochanter of the femur and draw a line from a point 1 inch below its most prominent part to the midpoint of the first line.

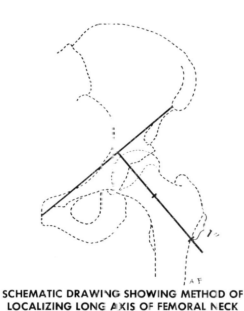

SCHEMATIC DRAWING SHOWING METHOD OF
LOCALIZING LONG AXIS OF FEMORAL NECK

The pelvic girdle

The female pelvis is lighter in structure than the male pelvis. It is broader and shallower, and the inlet is larger and more rounded. The sacrum is wider, it curves more sharply backward, and the sacral promontory is flatter. The width and depth of the pelvis vary with stature as well as with sex.

The pelvis is divided into two portions by an oblique plane that extends from the upper anterior margin of the sacrum to the upper margin of the symphysis pubis. The boundary line of this plane is called the brim of the pelvis. The region above the brim is called the greater or false pelvis, and the region below the brim is called the lesser or true pelvis.

The brim forms the superior strait, or inlet, of the true pelvis, and is measured in three directions in pelvimetry. Its anteroposterior, or conjugate, diameter is measured from the upper anterior margin of the sacrum to the upper margin of the symphysis pubis; its transverse diameter, across the widest region; and its oblique diameter, from the iliopectineal eminence of one side to the sacroiliac joint of the opposite side. The inferior strait, or outlet, of the true pelvis is measured from the tip of the coccyx to the lower margin of the pubic symphysis in the anteroposterior direction, and between the ischial tuberosities in the transverse direction. The region between the inlet and the outlet is called the pelvic cavity.

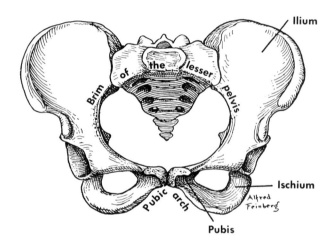

FEMALE PELVIS

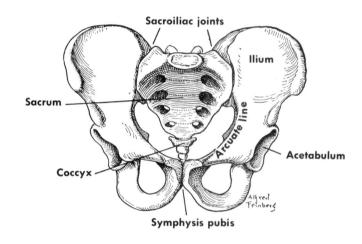

MALE PELVIS

When the body is in the erect or seated position, the pelvic brim forms an angle of approximately 60 degrees to the transverse plane. This angle varies with other body positions, the degree and direction of the variation depending upon the lumbar and sacral curves.

The bony landmarks used in radiography of the pelvis and hips are the iliac crests, the anterior superior iliac spines, the symphysis pubis, the greater trochanters of the femora, the ischial tuberosities, and the tip of the coccyx. Most of these points are easily palpable even in obese subjects. However, because of the heavy muscles immediately above the iliac crest, care must be exercised in locating this structure in order to avoid centering too

high. It is advisable to have the patient inhale deeply, and while the muscles are relaxed during exhalation, palpate for the highest point of the iliac crest.

The highest point of the greater trochanter, which can be palpated immediately below the depression in the soft tissues of the lateral surface of the hip, is in the same transverse plane as the midpoint of the hip joint and the coccyx. The most prominent point of the greater trochanter is in the same transverse plane as the symphysis pubis. To avoid embarrassment to the patient by palpation of the symphysis pubis, it is advisable to use the greater trochanter instead of the symphysis when localizing structures in this plane.

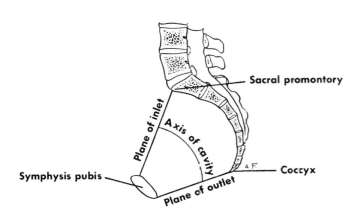

MIDSAGITTAL SECTION SHOWING INLET AND OUTLET OF TRUE PELVIS

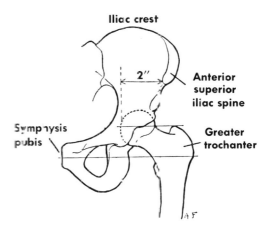

BONY LANDMARKS AND LOCALIZATION PLANES OF PELVIS

PELVIC GIRDLE AND UPPER FEMORA
Anteroposterior projection
Posteroanterior view

For all examinations of the pelvis and the upper femora, local gonadal shielding should be applied when it will not overlap the area under investigation.

Film: 14″ × 17″ crosswise.

Position of patient

Place the patient on the table in the supine position.

Position of part

Center the median sagittal plane of the body to the midline of the table and adjust it in a true anteroposterior position. Adjust the shoulders to lie in the same transverse plane, flex the elbows, and rest the hands on the upper chest. In order to relieve strain, support the knees on small sandbags.

Place a long sandbag under the ankles and adjust them so that the ankle joints are in the same transverse plane. If the extremities are of unequal length, make the adjustment at the joints above the abnormality. That is, if one leg is shorter than the other, adjust the knee joints in the same transverse plane; if the femora are of unequal length, make the adjustment at the pelvis so as to place the greater trochanters in the same transverse plane.

Place a small sandbag between the ankles, and unless otherwise requested, invert the feet about 15 degrees to overcome the anteversion of the femoral necks and thus place their long axis parallel with the plane of the film. (Because the ankle and knee joints are hinge joints, inversion of the foot rotates the entire extremity medially. Inversion of the foot is performed by grasping the heel and turning the foot medially until the position of the longitudinal axis of the heel indicates that the desired degree of extremity-rotation has been obtained.) Immobilize with a sandbag across the ankles.

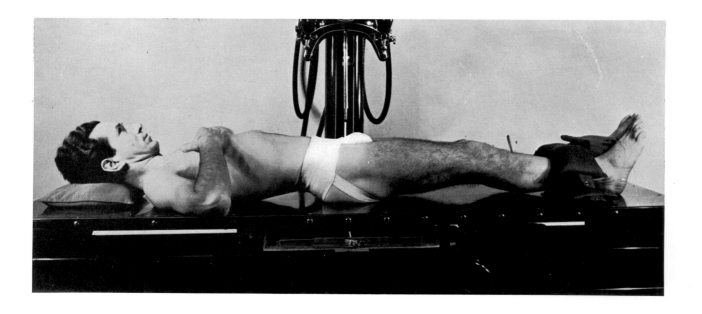

PELVIC GIRDLE AND UPPER FEMORA
Anteroposterior projection
Posteroanterior view

Position of part—cont'd

Measure the distance from the anterior superior iliac spine to the tabletop on each side to be sure there is no rotation of the pelvis. If a soft tissue abnormality (swelling or atrophy) is causing rotation of the pelvis, elevate one side on a radioparent pad to overcome the rotation.

With the cassette in the Potter-Bucky tray, center at the level of the soft tissue depression just above the greater trochanter. This centering will include the entire pelvic girdle and the upper fourth of the femora on pelves of average size and shape.

If the pelvis is deep, palpate for the crest of the ilium and, depending upon the focal-film distance, adjust the position of the film so that its upper border will project 1 to 1½ inches above the crest of the ilium.

Unless breathing is labored, respiration need not be suspended for the exposure.

Central ray

Direct the central ray perpendicularly to the midpoint of the film.

Structures shown

A posteroanterior view (anteroposterior projection) of the pelvic girdle, and of the head, neck, trochanters, and upper third or fourth of the shaft of the femora.

Congenital dislocation of the hip

Martz and Taylor[1] recommend two anteroposterior projections of the pelvis for the demonstration of the relationship of the femoral head to the acetabulum in patients with congenital dislocation of the hip. The first projection is made with the central ray directed vertically to the symphysis pubis to detect any lateral or superior displacement of the femoral head. The second projection is made with the central ray directed to the symphysis pubis at a cranial angulation of 45 degrees. This angulation will cast the shadow of an anteriorly displaced femoral head above that of the acetabulum, and the shadow of a posteriorly displaced head below that of the acetabulum.

[1]Martz, Carl D., and Taylor, Clifford C.: The 45-degree angle roentgenographic study of the pelvis in congenital dislocation of the hip, J. Bone Joint Surg. **36-A**:528-532, 1954.

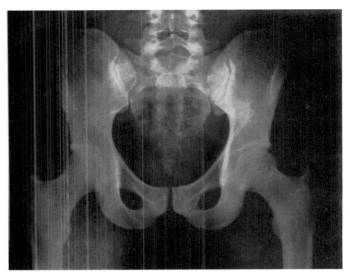

Male pelvis.

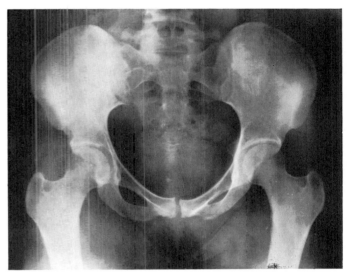

Female pelvis.

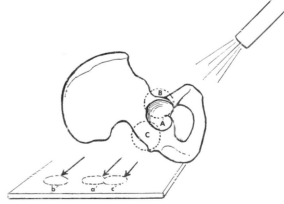

Drawing adapted from Dr. Carl D. Martz and Dr. Clifford C. Taylor.

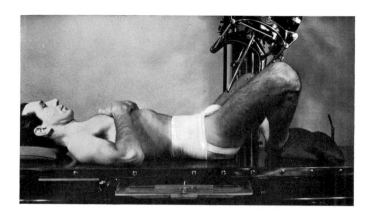

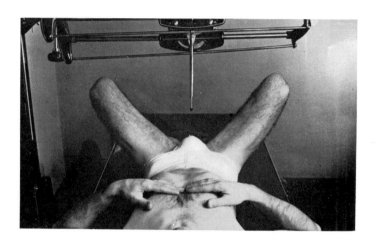

FEMORAL NECKS
Bilateral inferosuperior projection
Cleaves position
Film: $14'' \times 17''$ crosswise.

Position of patient

Place the patient in the supine position. Center the median sagittal plane of the body to the midline of the table. Adjust the shoulders to lie in the same transverse plane, flex the elbows, and rest the hands on the upper chest.

Position of part

Adjust the pelvis in a true anteroposterior position. A compression band may be placed well above the hip joints so that it will not interfere with their flexion.

1. Have the patient flex his hips and knees and draw his feet up as much as possible, that is, enough to place the femora in a near vertical position if the affected side will permit. Instruct the patient to hold this position, which is relatively comfortable, while you adjust the tube and film.

2. Angle the tube so as to direct the central ray parallel with the long axes of the femoral shafts and center to the symphysis pubis.

3. With the cassette in the Potter-Bucky tray, adjust its position so that the midpoint of the film will coincide with the central ray.

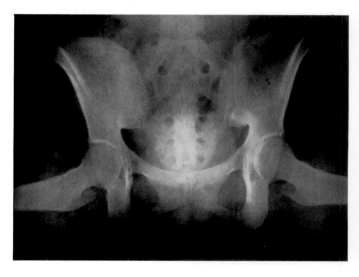

FEMORAL NECKS
Bilateral inferosuperior projection
Cleaves position

Position of part—cont'd

4. Abduct the thighs and have the patient turn his feet inward so as to brace the soles against each other for support. Center the feet to the midline of the table and immobilize them with sandbags. Recheck the position of the thighs, being careful to abduct them to the same degree. If possible, abduct the thighs approximately 40 degrees from the vertical to place the long axis of the femoral necks parallel with the plane of the film.

This position is adapted for a unilateral examination by adjusting the body position so as to center the anterior superior iliac spine of the affected side to the midline of the table. Fully extend the unaffected extremity and support it on sandbags placed under the knee and ankle. Have the patient flex the hip and knee of the affected side and draw the foot up to the opposite knee. After adjusting the central ray angulation and the position of the cassette tray, have the patient brace the sole of the foot against the opposite knee and lean the thigh lateralward approximately 40 degrees.

Structures shown

An axiolateral view of the femoral heads, necks, and trochanteric areas projected onto one film for comparison.

This projection is popularly known as the "frog" position.

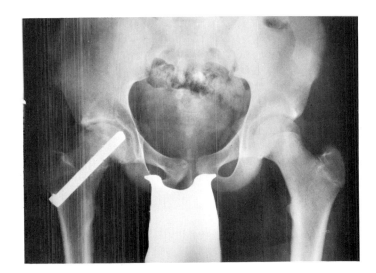

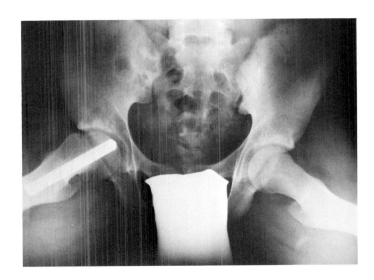

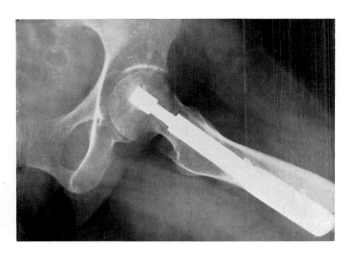

Radiographs courtesy Dr. Hudson J. Wilson, Jr.

PELVIS AND UPPER FEMORA
Lateral projection

Film: 14″ × 17″ lengthwise.

Position of patient

The patient may be examined in either the recumbent or the erect position. If the recumbent position is used, the thighs should be fully extended so that the femora will not obscure the shadow of the pubic arch.

Position of part

Recumbent position. When the patient can be placed in the lateral position, center the midaxillary plane of the body to the midline of the table. Have the patient grasp the side of the table to aid in stabilizing the position. Place a folded sheet or loofah sponges under the lower thorax and adjust the support so as to place the vertebral column parallel with the tabletop. If the vertebral column is allowed to sag, it will rotate the pelvis in the longitudinal plane.

Support the fully extended extremities at hip level on sandbags; place sandbags under the knee and ankle of the dependent leg and adjust them so that the long axis of the extremity is parallel with the table, and then support the upper leg at hip level by placing sandbags between the knees and ankles.

Adjust the pelvis in a true lateral position, with the anterior superior iliac spines lying in the same vertical plane.

Immobilize with a compression band applied across the trochanteric region of the pelvis or by placing sandbags against the anterior and posterior aspects of the lower thighs and across the ankles.

Berkebile and associates[1] recommend a cross-table lateral projection of the pelvis for the demonstration of the gull-wing sign in cases of fracture dislocation of the acetabular rim and posterior dislocation of the femoral head. This study requires the use of a grid-front cassette or a stationary grid.

Erect position. Place the patient in the lateral position before a vertical Potter-Bucky diaphragm and center the midaxillary plane of the body to the midline of the diaphragm. Have the patient stand straight, with the weight of the body equally distributed on the feet. Adjust the position of the body so that its median sagittal plane is parallel with the plane of the film.

If the extremities are of unequal length, place a support of suitable height under the foot of the short side. Have the patient grasp the side of the stand for support.

[1]Berkebile, R. D., Fischer, D. L., and Albrecht, L. F.: The gull-wing sign; value of the lateral view of the pelvis in fracture dislocation of the acetabular rim and posterior dislocation of the femoral head, Radiology 84:937-939, 1965.

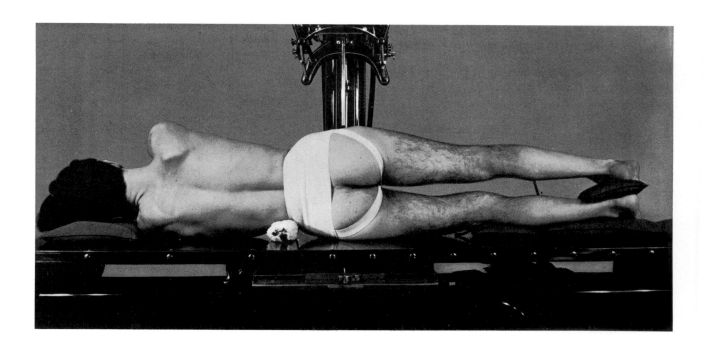

PELVIS AND UPPER FEMORA

Lateral projection—cont'd

Centering point

With the film in the Potter-Bucky tray, center at the level of the soft tissue depression just above the greater trochanter.

Central ray

Direct the central ray perpendicularly to the midpoint of the film.

Structures shown

A lateral view of the lumbosacral junction, the sacrum and coccyx, and the superimposed hipbones and upper femora.

If the position is exact, the acetabular shadows will be perfectly superimposed. The larger circle of the fossa farther from the film will be equidistant from the smaller circle of the fossa nearer the film throughout their circumference.

NOTE: Donaldson, Badgley, and Hunsberger[1] recommend the erect lateral view of the pelvis for the demonstration of femoral head-to-acetabulum relationship in cases of hip dislocation. They state that if the patient must be examined in the recumbent position, he is often more comfortable on the injured side, but that an adequate view can be obtained if he lies on the uninjured side.

[1]Donaldson, S. W., Badgley, C. E., and Hunsberger, W. G.: Lateral view of the pelvis in examination for hip dislocation, J. Bone Joint Surg. **30-A**:512-514, 1948.

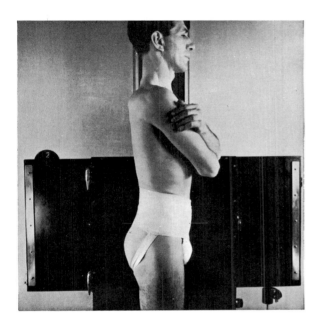

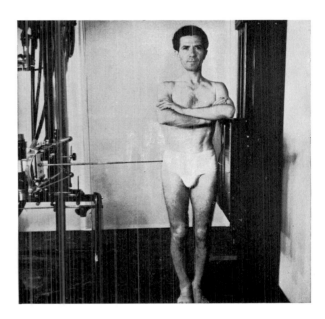

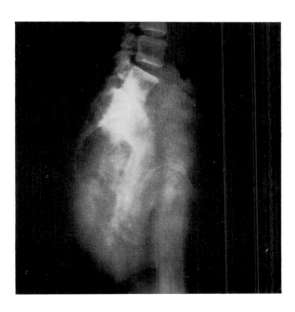

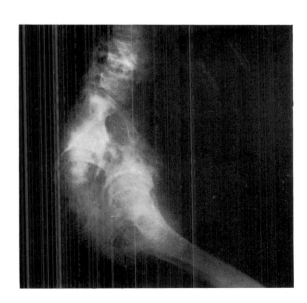

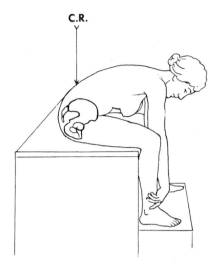

C.R.

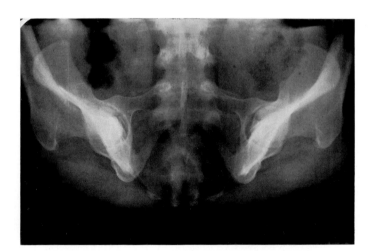

PELVIS AND HIP JOINTS
Semiaxial projection
Chassard-Lapiné position

Chassard and Lapiné[1] devised this position for the purpose of measuring the transverse, or biischial, diameter in pelvimetry. It is now being utilized by Broderick[2] for determining the relationship of the femoral head to the acetabulum, and by Rapp[3] and many others for the demonstration of the opacified rectosigmoid. Rapp suggested that it be used in cystography to show the anterior and posterior surfaces of the opacified bladder, and in uterosalpingography to gain added information about the uterine cavity.

Film: 14″ × 17″ crosswise for adult pelvis and upper femora; to size for children or for a smaller area.

Position of patient

Seat the patient well back on the side or end of the table so that the posterior surface of the knees is in contact with the edge of the table.

Position of part

When the subject is too short for this position to center the midaxillary plane of the body to the midline of the Potter-Bucky grid, shift the cassette forward in the tray. Center the longitudinal axis of the film to the median sagittal plane of the body, or if the patient is seated on the end of the table, center the median sagittal plane of the body to the midline of the table. Place a bench or other suitable support under the feet.

In order to prevent the thighs from limiting flexion of the body too greatly, have the patient abduct them as far as the edge of the table permits. The patient is then instructed to lean directly forward until the symphysis pubis is in close contact with the table; the vertical axis of the pelvis will be tilted forward approximately 45 degrees. Unless he is obese, the average patient can achieve this degree of flexion without strain.

Have the patient grasp his ankles to aid in maintaining the position. Respiration is suspended for the exposure.

The exposure factors required for this projection are approximately the same as those required for a lateral view of the pelvis.

Central ray

Direct the central ray vertically through the lumbosacral region at the level of the greater trochanters.

When flexion of the body is restricted, direct the central ray anteriorly at right angles to the coronal plane of the symphysis pubis.

Structures shown

A semiaxial projection of the pelvis, demonstrating the relationship between the femoral heads and the acetabula, the pelvic bones, and any opacified structure within the pelvis.

[1]Chassard and Lapiné: Étude radiographique de l'arcade pubienne chez la femme enceinte; une nuovelle méthode d'appréciation du diamètre bi-ischiatique, J. Radiol. Electr. 7:113-124, 1923.
[2]Broderick, T. F.: Complementary roentgenographic view of the hip, J. Bone Joint Surg. 37-A:295-298, 1955.
[3]Raap, Gerard: A position of value in studying the pelvis and its contents, Southern Med. J. 44:95-98, 1951.

HIP
Anteroposterior projection
Posteroanterior view

Film: $10'' \times 12''$ lengthwise.

Position of patient

Place the patient in the supine position and support the knees and ankles on long sandbags.

Position of part

Center the sagittal plane passing 2 inches medial to the anterior superior iliac spine to the midline of the table, and then adjust the body in a true anteroposterior position. Flex the elbows and place the arms in a comfortable position. Adjust the shoulders to lie in the same transverse plane.

Unless otherwise instructed by the radiologist or the attending doctor, grasp the heels and invert the feet approximately 15 degrees to overcome the anteversion of the femoral neck and thereby place its long axis parallel with the plane of the film. Place a small sandbag between the feet and immobilize with a long sandbag across the ankles.

With the cassette in the Potter-Bucky tray, center at the level of the highest point of the greater trochanter.

Central ray

Direct the central ray vertically to the midpoint of the film.

Structures shown

An anteroposterior projection of the hipbone, and of the head, neck, trochanters, and upper third of the shaft of the femur.

In the initial examination of a hip lesion, whether traumatic or pathologic in origin, the frontal projection is usually made on a film large enough to include the entire pelvic girdle and upper femora. Progress studies may be restricted to the affected side.

NOTE: Accident patients who have sustained severe injury are not usually transferred to the radiographic table but are radiographed on the stretcher or bed. After the localization point has been established and marked, one assistant should be stationed on each side of the stretcher to grasp the sheet and lift the pelvis just enough for the placement of the cassette, while a third person supports the injured extremity. Any necessary manipulation of the extremity must be made by the attending surgeon or by the radiologist, never by the technologist.

If a wafer grid or a grid-front cassette is not available, use the smallest possible cone in order to minimize secondary radiation.

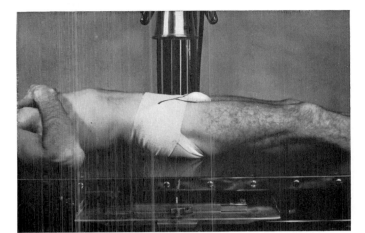

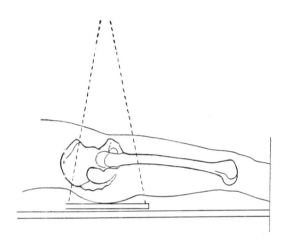

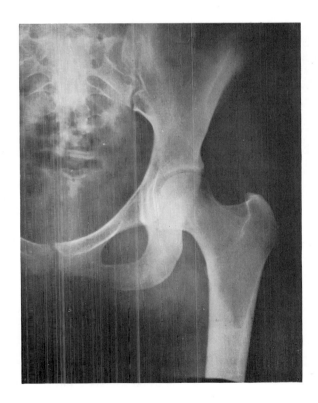

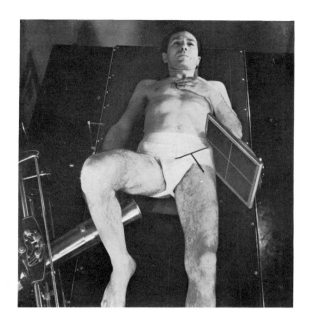

FEMORAL NECK
Inferosuperior projection
Danelius-Miller modification of Lorenz[1] position
Film: $8'' \times 10''$ lengthwise.

Position of patient

Adjust the patient in the supine position. When examining a subject who is thin or is lying on a bed that sags, elevate the pelvis on a firm pillow or folded sheets enough to center the most prominent point of the greater trochanter to the film. The support must not extend beyond the lateral surface of the body or it will interfere with the placement of the cassette. Support the affected extremity at hip level on sandbags or firm pillows.

Localization point

In order to localize the long axis of the femoral neck, first draw a line between the anterior superior iliac spine and the upper border of the symphysis pubis and mark its center point; second, palpate for the most prominent lateral projection of the greater trochanter and mark a point 1 inch distal to it. A line drawn between these two points will parallel the long axis of the femoral neck regardless of the position of the extremity.

Position of part

Flex the knee and hip of the unaffected side and adjust the extremity in a position that will not interfere with the projection of the central ray. If possible, rest the leg on a suitable support, with the thigh in a vertical position. Adjust the pelvis in a true anteroposterior position.

Grasp the heel and invert the foot of the affected side about 15 or 20 degrees and immobilize it with sandbags. The manipulation of patients with unhealed fractures should be done by either the attending surgeon or the radiologist, never by the technologist.

[1]Lorenz: Die röntgenographische Darstellung des subskapularen Raumes und des Schenkelhalses im Querschnitt, Fortschr. Roentgenstr. **25:**342-343, 1917-1918.

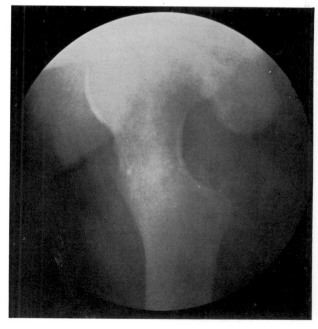

Nongrid film.

FEMORAL NECK
Inferosuperior projection
Danelius-Miller modification of
Lorenz position—cont'd

Position of film

Place the cassette in the vertical position and with its upper border in contact with the lateral surface of the body at, or just above, the level of the crest of the ilium. Angle the lower border away from the body until the cassette is exactly parallel with the long axis of the femoral neck. The cassette is supported in position with sandbags.

When using a wafer grid, be careful to place it so that the lead strips will be in the horizontal position.

Central ray

Direct the central ray at right angles to the long axis of the femoral neck, and center it about 2½ inches below the point of intersection of the localization lines.

Structures shown

An axiolateral view of the head, neck, and trochanters of the femur.

NOTE: The thickness of the part traversed by the central ray is almost comparable to that of the lateral lumbar spine. It is essential, therefore, to use as small a cone as possible, in order to minimize secondary radiation, particularly if a wafer grid or a grid-front cassette is not used. However, when the projection is being used as a guide in fracture reduction in the operating room, it is advisable to hold the exposure time to a minimum by eliminating the grid.

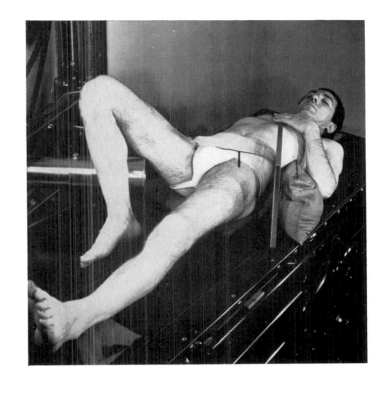

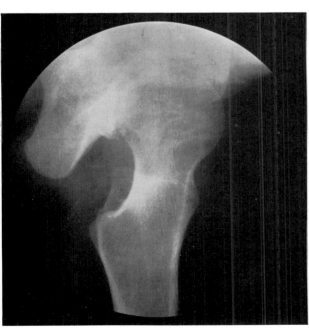

Stationary grid film.

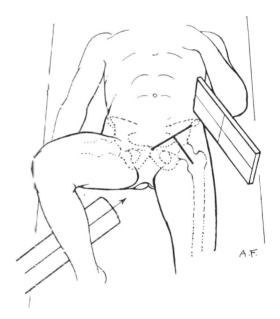

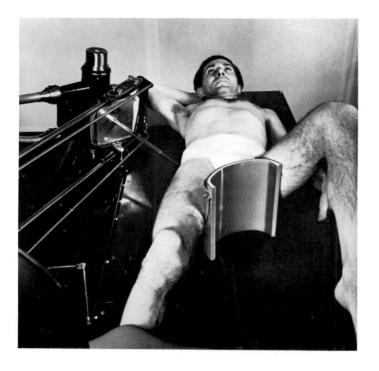

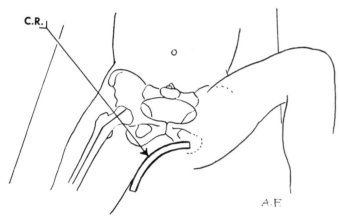

C.R.

A.F.

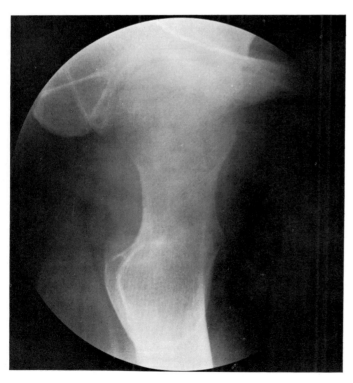

FEMORAL NECK
Superoinferior projection
Leonard-George position
Film: $8'' \times 10''$ with a curved cassette.

Position of patient

With the patient in the supine position, elevate the pelvis on a small, firm pillow or folded sheets enough to place the greater trochanters 4 inches above the tabletop in order to center the hip to the vertically placed cassette. Support the affected extremity at hip level on pillows or sandbags.

Position of part

Flex the hip and knee of the unaffected side, if they are not immobilized, and abduct the thigh enough to accommodate the position of the curved cassette.

The affected extremity is usually in abduction in either a cast or a splint; if not, and it is possible, abduct it enough for accurate placement of the curved cassette in the groin.

Place the cassette in the vertical position well up between the thighs and center it to the crease of the groin of the affected side. With the leg in abduction, this center point will be at right angles to the femoral neck.

If the extremity is not immobilized, grasp the heel and invert the foot about 15 or 20 degrees to overcome the anteversion of the femoral neck and thus place its long axis parallel with the horizontal and its lateral aspect at right angles to the plane of the film. Immobilize with a sandbag placed across the ankle.

Central ray

Direct the central ray from above downward and medialward at right angles to the long axis of the femoral neck; it enters the lateral surface of the hip just above the soft tissue depression.

Structures shown

An axiolateral view of the head, neck, and trochanteric area of the femur. Due to the convexity of the cassette, the femoral head and the trochanteric areas are somewhat distorted.

FEMORAL NECK

Mediolateral projection

Johnson position[1]

This method of obtaining an axiolateral view of the femoral neck is employed when the opposite femur cannot be adjusted for one of the two preceding positions.

Film: 8″ × 10″ placed lengthwise in a vertical position.

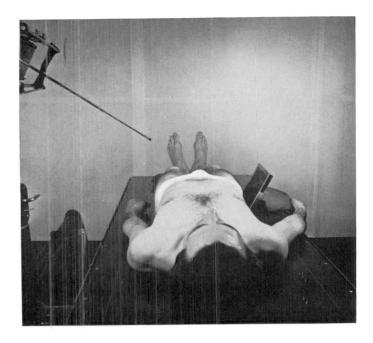

Position of part

When necessary, elevate the pelvis on folded sheets or a firm pillow so as to place the greater trochanters about 6 inches above the tabletop (2 inches above the center line of the film). This is to allow for the laterodorsal angle of the central ray. Support the extremities at hip level on pillows or sandbags. Adjust the body in a true anteroposterior position.

Place the cassette in the vertical position along the lateral surface of the hip and center the transverse line of the cassette to the greater trochanter, which should be approximately 2 inches above the longitudinal line. Tilt the cassette backward 25 degrees from the vertical and support it in position with sandbags or other suitable support.

Central ray

The central ray is directed to the greater trochanter at a double angle—25 degrees toward the head plus 25 degrees posteriorly. It enters at about the midsagittal plane of the thigh.

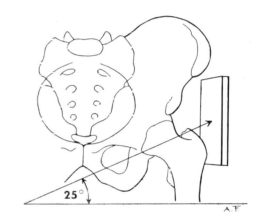

Structures shown

An axiolateral view of the head, neck, and trochanteric region of the femur.

[1]Johnson, C. R.: A new method for roentgenographic examination of the upper end of the femur, J. Bone Joint Surg. **30**:859-866, 1932.

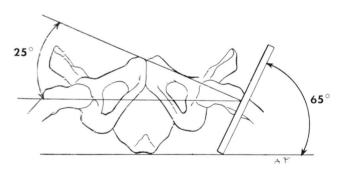

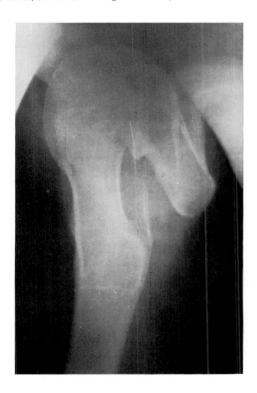

Drawings adapted from Dr. C. R. Johnson.

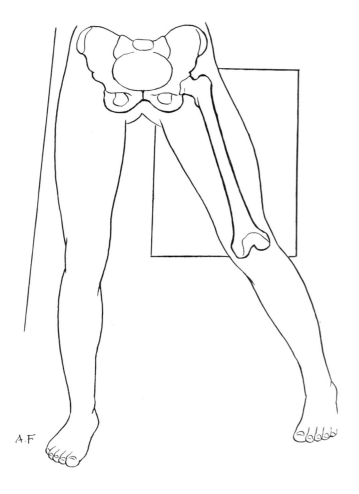

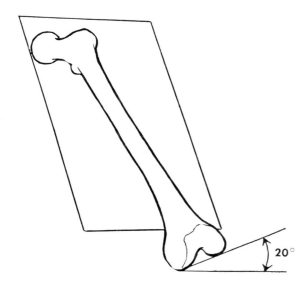

Drawings adapted from Dr. E. A. Dooley, Dr. C. W. Caldwell, and Dr. G. A. Glass.

A.F

20°

FEMORAL NECK
Anteroposterior projection
Dooley, Caldwell, and Glass method[1]
Film

Select a film large enough to include at least 6 inches of the femoral shaft for calculation of the shaft-neck angle, usually an 11″ × 14″.

Position of patient

The patient is adjusted in the supine position. Center the sagittal plane that lies 1 inch medial to the anterior superior iliac spine to the midline of the table. Adjust the body in a true anteroposterior position.

Position of part

Moderately abduct the leg, rotate the thigh internally about 20 degrees, and immobilize it with sandbags.

Localize the femoral neck and mark its midpoint (a point on the bisecting line about 2 inches below the intersection of the two localization lines).

With the cassette in the Potter-Bucky tray, adjust its position to include at least 6 inches of the shaft of the femur.

Central ray

Direct the central ray vertically and center to the femoral neck, irrespective of the position of the film.

Structures shown

An anteroposterior projection of the hip bone, and of the femoral head, neck, trochanters, and upper shaft.

The shaft-neck angle is calculated from a tracing of the anteroposterior projection.

[1]Dooley, E. A., Caldwell, C. W., Jr., and Glass, G. A.: Roentgenography of the femoral neck, Amer. J. Roentgen. **39**:834-837, 1938.

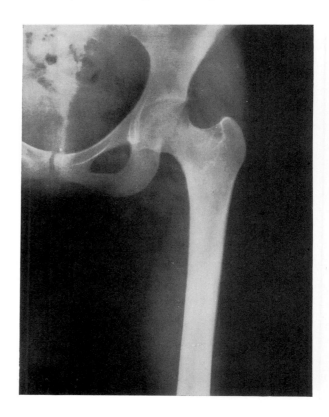

FEMORAL NECK
Inferosuperior projection
Dooley, Caldwell, and Glass method
Shaft-neck angle

1. Draw a line P from a point 1 inch below the most prominent lateral projection of the greater trochanter through the long axis of the femoral neck.

2. Draw a line C through the mid-neck at right angles to the line P.

3. Draw a line F through the long axis of the shaft of the femur.

The line C bisects the femoral neck, and the line PC forms the axis of the femoral neck, which, in conjunction with the femoral axis F, forms the shaft-neck angle.

Film: 8″ × 10″ or 10″ × 12″ crosswise.

Position of part

With the patient in the supine position, flex the hip and knee and adjust the thigh at right angles to the horizontal. Abduct the thigh the difference in degrees between the shaft-neck angle and 90 degrees to place the femoral neck parallel to the horizontal. Support the leg in the horizontal position.

With the cassette in the Potter-Bucky tray, center to the femoral neck.

Central ray

Direct the central ray perpendicularly to the midpoint of the film.

Structures shown

An axiolateral view of the head, neck, and trochanteric area of the femur.

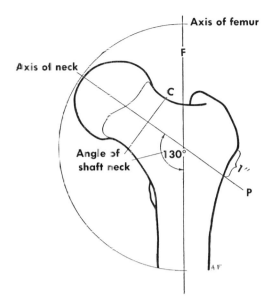

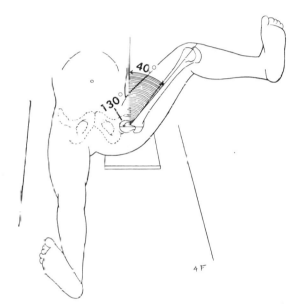

Drawings adapted from Dr. E. A. Dooley, Dr. C. W. Caldwell, and Dr. G. A. Glass.

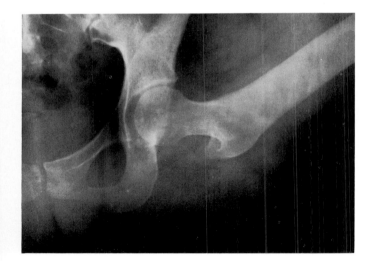

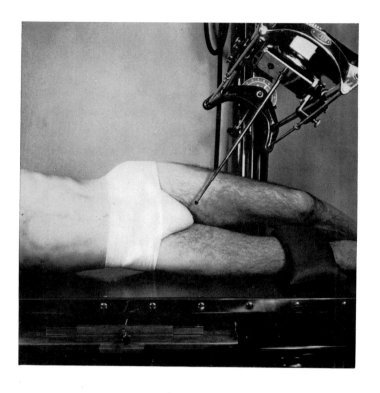

HIP
Inferosuperior projection
Friedman position

Film: $10'' \times 12''$ lengthwise.

Position of patient

Have the patient lie in the lateral recumbent position on the affected side. Center the midaxillary plane of the body to the midline of the table.

Position of part

Fully extend the affected extremity, adjust it in a true lateral position, and immobilize it with sandbags.

Have the patient grasp the side of the table to aid in stabilizing the position. Roll the upper side gently backward approximately 10 degrees, and place sandbags under the knee to support it at hip level. The affected femur will not change position if it is properly immobilized; the pelvis will rotate from the femoral head.

With the cassette in the Potter-Bucky tray, adjust its position so that the midpoint of the film will coincide with the central ray.

Central ray

Direct the central ray to the femoral neck at an angle of 35 degrees toward the head.

Kisch[1] recommends that the central ray be angled 15 or 20 degrees toward the head for this projection.

Structures shown

An axiolateral view of the head, neck, trochanters, and upper shaft of the femur.

[1]Kisch, Eugen: Eine neue Methode für röntgenologische Darstellung des Hüftgelenks in frontaler Ebene, Fortschr. Roentgenstr. **27:**309, 1920.

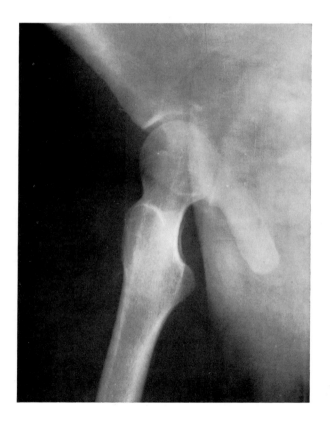

HIP JOINT
Lauenstein and Hickey projections
Lateral body position

These projections are used to demonstrate the hip joint and the relationship of the femoral head to the acetabulum. Because of the danger of fragment displacement or injury, this body position is not used in the presence of either an unhealed fracture or a destructive disease.

Film: $10'' \times 12''$ crosswise.

Position of patient

Following the anteroposterior projection, have the patient turn toward the affected side to a near lateral position and grasp the side of the table for support.

Position of part

Adjust the body so as to center the affected hip to the midline of the table. Ask the patient to flex the dependent knee and draw the thigh up to a near right-angle position. Extend the opposite thigh and support it at hip level on sandbags. Adjust the position of the pelvis so that the upper side is rotated backward just enough to prevent its superimposition on the affected hip.

Position the Potter-Bucky tray so that the midpoint of the film will coincide with the central ray.

Central ray

Direct the central ray through the hip joint, which is located at a point midway between the anterior superior iliac spine and the pubic symphysis, (1) vertically to obtain the Lauenstein projection, and (2) at a cranial angle of 20 to 25 degrees to obtain the Hickey projection.

Structures shown

A lateral projection of the hip, showing the acetabulum, the upper end of the femur, and the relationship of the femoral head to the acetabulum.

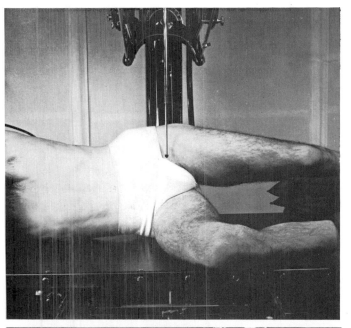

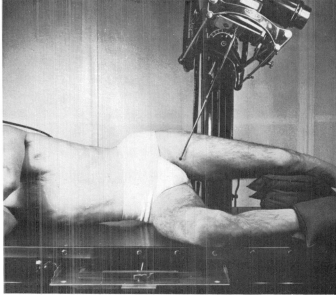

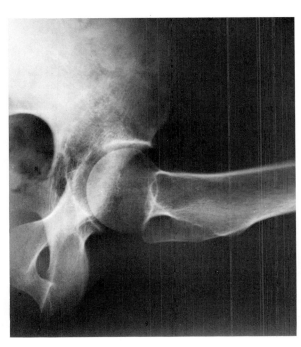

Lauenstein projection.

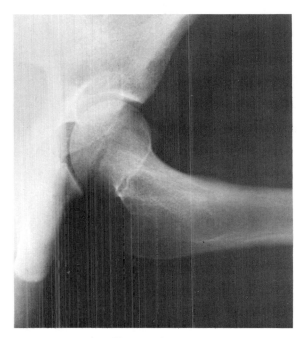

Hickey projection.

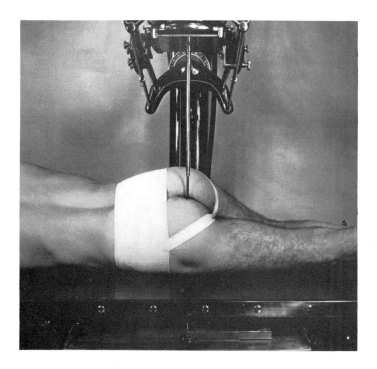

HIP
Posterior oblique projection
Hsieh position

Film: $10'' \times 12''$ lengthwise.

Position of patient

Place the patient in the semiprone position and center the affected hip to the midline of the table.

Position of part

Elevate the unaffected side approximately 40 to 45 degrees and have the patient support himself on the flexed knee and forearm of the elevated side.

Adjust the position of the body so as to place the posterior surface of the dependent iliac bone over the midline of the table.

With the cassette in the Potter-Bucky tray, adjust its position so that the center of the film will lie at the level of the superior border of the greater trochanter.

Central ray

Direct the central ray perpendicularly to the midpoint of the film; it should pass between the posterior surface of the iliac blade and the dislocated femoral head.

Structures shown

An oblique view of the ilium, the hip joint, and the upper end of the femur. Hsieh[1] recommended this position for demonstrating posterior dislocations of the femoral head in other than acute fracture dislocations.

NOTE: Urist[2] has recommended an anterior oblique position for the demonstration of the posterior rim of the acetabulum in acute fracture-dislocation injuries of the hip. The patient is adjusted from the supine position for this projection. Elevate the injured hip 60 degrees to place the posterior rim of the acetabulum in profile, and adjust the body so as to center the sagittal plane passing through the anterior superior iliac spine to the midline of the table. Center the film at the level of the upper border of the greater trochanter. Direct the central ray vertically to the midpoint of the film.

[1]Hsieh, C. K.: Posterior dislocation of the hip, Radiology **27**:450-455, 1936.
[2]Urist, Marshall R.: Fracture-dislocation of the hip joint, J. Bone Joint Surg. **30-A**:699-727, 1948.

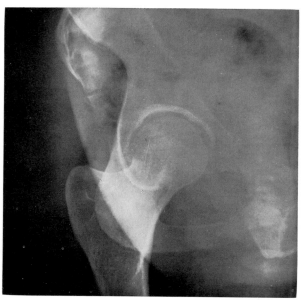

Hseih projection.

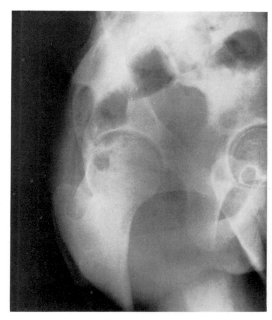

Urist projection.

HIP
Posterolateral projection
Lilienfeld position

Film: $10'' \times 12''$ lengthwise.

Position of patient

Have the patient lie in the lateral recumbent position on the affected side.

Position of part

Center the midaxillary plane of the body to the midline of the table. Fully extend the affected thigh, adjust it in a true lateral position, and immobilize it with sandbags.

Have the patient grasp the side of the table to aid in stabilizing the position. Roll the upper side gently forward approximately 15 degrees, or just enough to separate the two sides of the pelvis, and support the extremity at hip level on sandbags. If the affected side is well immobilized and the upper side is gently rolled forward, it will not change position; the pelvis will rotate from the femoral head.

With the cassette in the Potter-Bucky tray, adjust its position so that the center point of the film will lie at the level of the greater trochanter.

Central ray

Direct the central ray perpendicularly to the midpoint of the film.

Structures shown

A posterolateral projection of the ilium, the acetabulum, and the upper end of the femur.

NOTE: The Lilienfeld position is not used with patients who have an acute hip injury because of the danger of fragment displacement. These patients can be comfortably, safely, and satisfactorily examined in the position described by Colonna.[1] The patient is positioned for this projection in approximately the manner described for the Lilienfeld position, except that he is placed *on the unaffected side* and adjusted so as to center the uppermost hip to the midline of the table. Colonna recommended that the uppermost side, the affected side, be rotated about 17 degrees forward from the true lateral position. He stated that this degree of rotation separates the shadows of the hip joints and gives the optimum view of the slope of the acetabular roof and the depth of the socket.

[1]Colonna, Paul C.: A diagnostic roentgen view of the acetabulum, Surg. Clin. N. Amer. **33**:1565-1569, 1953.

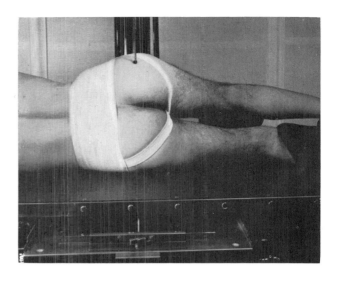

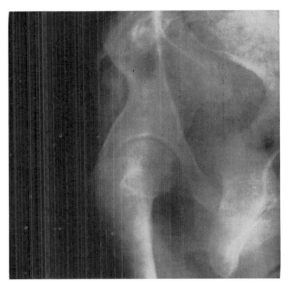

Lilienfeld projection.

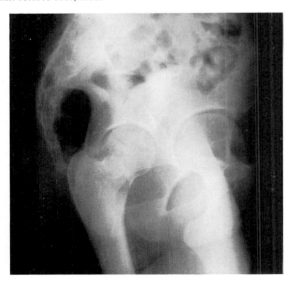

Colonna projection.

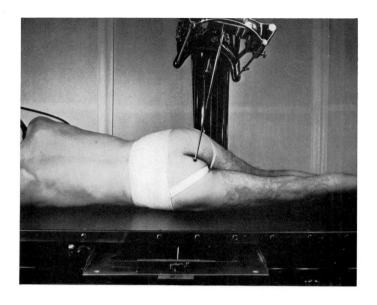

ACETABULUM
Posterior oblique projection
Teufel position

Film: 8″ × 10″ lengthwise.

Position of patient

Have the patient lie in a semiprone position on the affected side, and have him support himself on the forearm and flexed knee of the elevated side.

Position of part

Align the body so as to center the hip being examined to the midline of the table. Adjust the elevation of the unaffected side so that the anterior surface of the body will just touch the hypotenuse of a 38-degree cardboard triangle. Place sandbags under the flexed knee and the ankles to relieve pressure.

With the cassette in the Potter-Bucky tray, adjust its position so that the midpoint of the film will coincide with the central ray.

Central ray

Direct the central ray through the acetabulum at an angle of 12 degrees toward the head. The central ray enters the body about 2 inches above the gluteal fold and 2 inches lateral to the median sagittal plane.

Structures shown

Teufel[1] recommended this position for the demonstration of the fovea capitis, the acetabular incisura, and, particularly, the upper posterior wall of the acetabulum.

[1]Teufel, Siegfried: Eine gezielte Aufsichtsaufnahme der Hüftgelenkspfanne, Roentgenpraxis **10**:398-402, 1938.

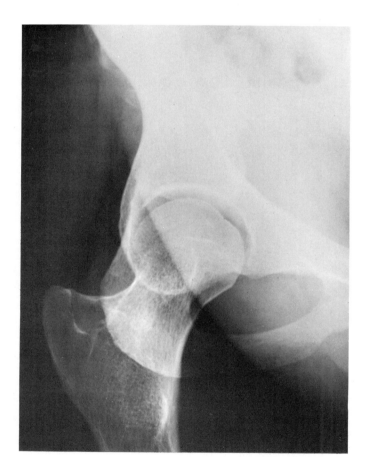

ACETABULA
Superoinferior projection
Dunlap, Swanson, and Penner position

Film

Select a $7'' \times 17''$ or $14'' \times 17''$ film and place it crosswise for bilateral projections of adults. An extension cylinder is used to restrict the radiation to the adjacent half of the film, which makes it unnecessary to mask the opposite half when examining adults.

Position of patient

The patient is placed in the seated-erect position on the side of the table.

Position of part

Ask the patient to move back far enough to place the posterior surface of his knees in contact with the edge of the table. When the patient is not tall enough for this position to center the midaxillary plane of the body to the midline of the table, both the x-ray tube and the film must be shifted forward. The transverse axis of the film can be centered to or near the midaxillary plane of the body by moving the cassette forward in the grid tray. To prevent the cassette from slipping when the grid is shifted for the second exposure, place a strip of wood of suitable width and thickness between it and the back locking device of the tray.

Center the midline of the longitudinal half of the film opposite to the side being examined to the median sagittal plane of the body. Mark the position of the grid so that it can be moved back to this position for the second exposure without disturbing the patient's position, and then center the opposite half of the film to the median sagittal plane of the body for the first exposure.

Ask the patient to sit erect with his thighs together, and have him cross his arms over his chest so that they will be well away from the iliac crests. Instruct him to maintain the exact position when the x-ray tube is shifted for the second exposure. Respiration need not be suspended for the exposures.

Central ray

Direct the central ray to the crest of the ilium at a medial angle of 30 degrees, first from one side and then from the other.

The originators[1] of this position stated that the plane of the acetabulum forms an angle of 35 degrees with the sagittal plane in the average adult, and 32 degrees in children, but they have found that a central ray angulation of 30 degrees results in the least superimposition of parts.

Structures shown

A profile view of the acetabula projected from a plane at right angles to the frontal view, and the relationship of the femoral heads to the acetabula. The femoral heads, necks, and trochanters are seen from a near frontal plane because there is little change in the position of the femora between the supine and the seated positions.

[1]Dunlap, K., Swanson, A. B., and Penner, R. S.: Studies of the hip joint by means of lateral acetabular roentgenograms, J. Bone Joint Surg. **38-A:**1218-1230, 1956.

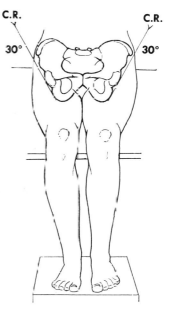

Drawing adapted from Dr. K. Dunlap, Dr. A. B. Swanson, and Dr. R. S. Penner

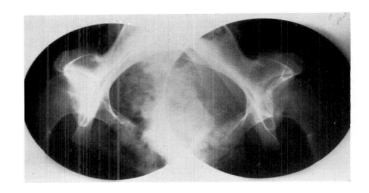

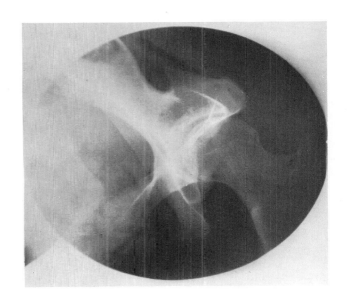

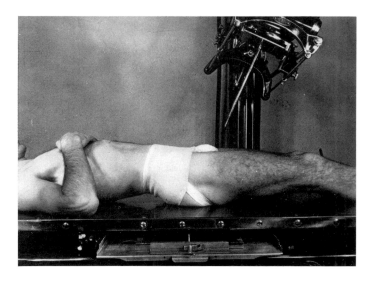

ANTERIOR PELVIC BONES
Semiaxial anteroposterior projection
Taylor position

Film: $10'' \times 12''$ crosswise.

Position of patient

Place the patient in the supine position and adjust a long sandbag under the knees to relieve strain.

Position of part

Center the median sagittal plane of the body to the midline of the table and then adjust it in a true anteroposterior position.

With the cassette in the Potter-Bucky tray, adjust its position so that the midpoint of the film will coincide with the central ray.

Central ray

Males. Direct the central ray approximately 25 degrees (20 to 35 degrees) toward the head and center to a point 2 inches distal to the upper border of the symphysis pubis.

Females. Direct the central ray approximately 40 degrees (30 to 45 degrees) toward the head and center to a point 2 inches distal to the upper border of the symphysis pubis.

The localization point may be established with sufficient accuracy from the most prominent lateral projection of the greater trochanter.

Structures shown

An inferosuperior view of the pubic and ischial rami, projected free of superimposition.

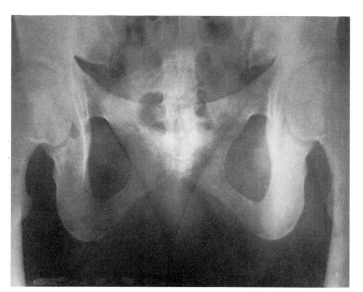

Male pelvis.

Female pelvis.

ANTERIOR PELVIC BONES
Posteroanterior projection

Film: 8″ × 10″ crosswise.

Position of patient

Place the patient in the prone position and center the median sagittal plane of the body to the midline of the table.

Position of part

Adjust the body in a true posteroanterior position. Place sandbags under the ankles so that the weight of the feet will not rest on the toes.

With the cassette in the Potter-Bucky tray, center at the level of the greater trochanters; this will center the film to the symphysis pubis.

Central ray

Direct the central ray perpendicularly to the midpoint of the film.

Structures shown

A posteroanterior projection of the pubic and ischial bones, the pubic symphysis, and the obturator foramina.

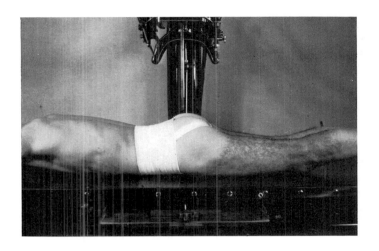

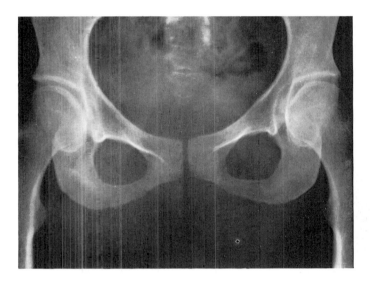

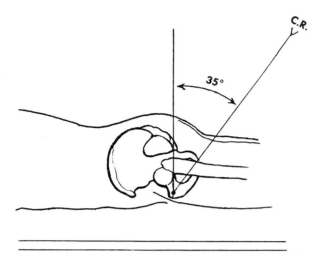

ANTERIOR PELVIC BONES
Semiaxial projection
Staunig position

Film: $8'' \times 10''$ crosswise.

Position of patient

Place the patient in the prone position. Support the ankles on sandbags so that the weight of the feet will not rest on the toes.

Position of part

Center the median sagittal plane of the body to the midline of the table. Adjust the body in a true postero-anterior position.

With the cassette in the Potter-Bucky tray, adjust its position so that the midpoint of the film will coincide with the central ray.

Central ray

With the central ray at an angle of 35 degrees toward the head, center to the symphysis pubis, which lies in the median sagittal plane at the level of the greater trochanters.

Structures shown

An inferosuperior projection of the pubic and ischial bones and of the symphysis pubis.

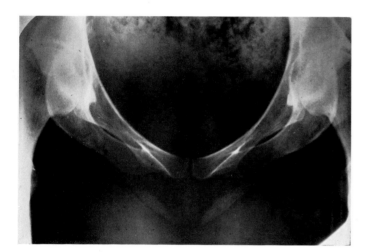

ANTERIOR PELVIC BONES
Axial projection
Lilienfeld position
Film: $8'' \times 10''$ crosswise.

Position of patient

Place the patient on the radiographic table in a seated-erect position.

Position of part

Center the median sagittal plane of the body to the midline of the table. In order to relieve strain, flex the knees slightly and support them on sandbags. If the travel of the cassette tray is great enough to permit centering near the end of the table, the patient will be more comfortable seated so that his legs can hang over and his feet can rest on a suitable support.

Have the patient extend his arms for support, lean backward 45 or 50 degrees, and then arch his back to place the pubic arch in a vertical position.

With the cassette in the Potter-Bucky tray, center at the level of the greater trochanters.

Central ray

Direct the central ray vertically to the midpoint of the film.

Structures shown

A superoinferior projection of the pubic and ischial bones and of the symphysis pubis.

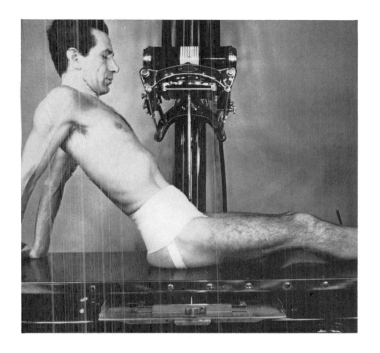

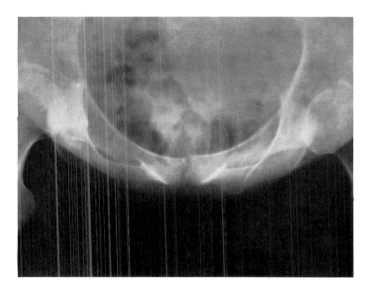

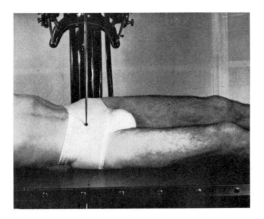

ILIUM
Anterior and posterior oblique projections

Film: $10'' \times 12''$ lengthwise.

Anterior oblique position
Posterior oblique view

Place the patient in the supine position and center the sagittal plane passing through the hip joint of the affected side to the midline of the table. Elevate the unaffected side approximately 40 degrees to place the broad surface of the wing of the dependent ilium parallel with the plane of the film. Support the elevated shoulder, hip, and knee on sandbags. Adjust the position of the uppermost extremity so as to place the anterior superior iliac spines in the same transverse plane.

Posterior oblique position
Anterior oblique view

Place the patient in the prone position and center the sagittal plane passing through the hip joint of the affected side to the midline of the table. Elevate the unaffected side about 40 degrees to place the dependent ilium at or near right angles to the plane of the film. Have the patient rest on the forearm and flexed knee of the elevated side. Adjust the position of the uppermost thigh so as to place the anterior superior iliac spines in the same transverse plane.

Center the film at the level of the transverse plane passing midway between the anterior superior iliac spines and the upper border of the greater trochanters.

Central ray

Direct the central ray perpendicularly to the midpoint of the film.

Structures shown

The anterior oblique projection shows an unobstructed view of the iliac wing and of the sciatic notches, and a profile view of the acetabulum.

The posterior oblique projection shows an oblique view of the ilium and of the upper end of the femur.

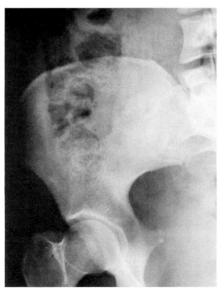

Anterior oblique projection.

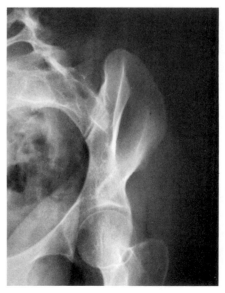

Posterior oblique projection.

Anatomy and positioning
of the
vertebral column

The vertebral column

The vertebral column, which forms the central axis of the skeleton, is situated in the median sagittal plane of the posterior part of the trunk. It encloses and protects the spinal cord, and acts as a support for the trunk; it supports the skull above, and affords attachment for the ribs laterally, through which it supports the upper extremities. The column is supported by the hipbones at the sacroiliac joints, which, through the hip joints, transmit the weight of the trunk to the lower extremities. The column is composed of small segments of bone with disks of fibrocartilage interposed between their bodies to act as cushions; the whole is held together by ligaments and is so jointed and so curved that it has considerable flexibility and resilience.

In early life the vertebral column normally consists of thirty-three small, irregular bones called vertebrae. The vertebrae are divided into five groups and named according to the regions they occupy. The upper seven vertebrae occupy the region of the neck and are termed cervical vertebrae; the succeeding twelve bones lie in the dorsal portion of the thorax and are called the thoracic vertebrae. The five vertebrae occupying the region of the loin, or lumbus, are termed lumbar vertebrae, the following five are termed sacral vertebrae, and the vertebrae in the terminal group, which vary from three to five in number, are called the coccygeal vertebrae. The twenty-four segments in the upper three regions remain distinct throughout life and are termed the true, or movable, vertebrae. The segments in the two lower regions are called false, or fixed, vertebrae because of the change they undergo in the adult; the sacral segments always fuse into one bone termed the sacrum, while the coccygeal segments, referred to as the coccyx, have a tendency to fuse into one bone.

Viewed from the side, the vertebral column presents four anteroposterior curves that arch forward and backward from the midaxillary line of the body. These curves are called cervical, thoracic, lumbar, and pelvic curves, for the regions they occupy. The cervical and lumbar curves are convex forward, while the thoracic and pelvic curves are concave forward. The upper curves merge smoothly, but the lumbar and pelvic curves are joined at an obtuse angle, the lumbosacral, or sacrovertebral, angle, which varies in different subjects. The thoracic and pelvic curves are called primary curves because they are present at birth. The cervical and lumbar curves are called secondary, or compensatory, curves because they are developed after birth. The cervical curve, which is the least pronounced of the curves, develops when the child begins to hold his head up at about 3 or 4 months of age, and when he begins to sit alone at about 8 or 9 months of age. The lumbar curve develops when the child begins to walk at about 1 to 1½ years of age. The lumbar and pelvic curves are more pronounced in the female, causing a more acute angle at the lumbosacral junction.

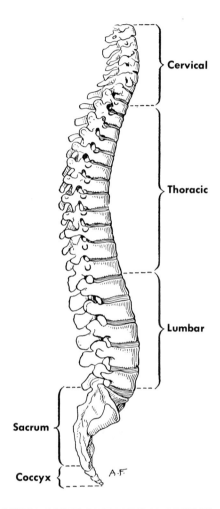

LATERAL ASPECT OF VERTEBRAL COLUMN

Viewed from the front, the vertebral column is seen to vary in width in the several regions. Generally, the width gradually increases from the second cervical vertebra to the upper part of the sacrum, from which level it decreases sharply. There is sometimes a slight lateral curvature in the upper thoracic region. The convexity of this curve is to the right in right-handed persons and to the left in left-handed persons; for this reason, it is believed to be the result of muscle action and to be influenced by occupation.

The vertebral articulations consist of two types of joints: (1) amphiarthrodial joints, which are between the bodies of the vertebrae and which permit only slight movement to individual vertebrae, and (2) diarthrodial joints, which are between the vertebral arches and which permit gliding movements. The movements permitted in the vertebral column by the combined action of the joints are flexion, extension, lateral, and rotary.

Typical vertebra. A typical vertebra is composed of two main parts—an anterior mass of bone called the body, and a posterior ringlike portion called the vertebral arch. The body and the vertebral arch enclose a space called the vertebral foramen. In the articulated column the vertebral foramina form the spinal, or neural, canal.

The body of the vertebra is composed largely of cancellous tissue covered by a layer of compact tissue. It is approximately cylindrical in shape. From above downward, its posterior surface is flattened and its anterior and lateral surfaces are concave. The superior and inferior surfaces of the bodies are flattened and are covered by a plate of articular cartilage. In the articulated column the bodies are separated by cartilaginous disks that consist of a central mass of soft, pulpy, semigelatinous material called the nucleus pulposus, surrounded by an outer, firm portion called the annulus fibrosus.

The vertebral arch is formed by two pedicles and two laminae that support four articular processes, two transverse processes, and one spinous process. The pedicles are short, thick processes that project backward, one from each side, from the upper lateral part of the posterior surface of the body. The upper and lower surfaces of the pedicles, or roots, are concave. These concavities are called vertebral notches, and by articulation with the vertebrae above and below, the notches form intervertebral foramina for the transmission of the spinal nerves and blood vessels. The laminae are broad and flat and are directed backward and medialward from the pedicles.

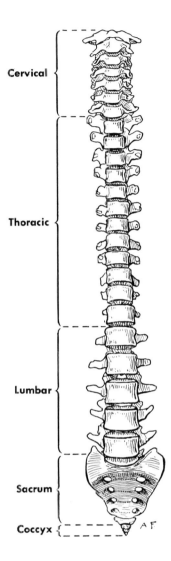

Cervical

Thoracic

Lumbar

Sacrum

Coccyx

ANTERIOR ASPECT OF VERTEBRAL COLUMN

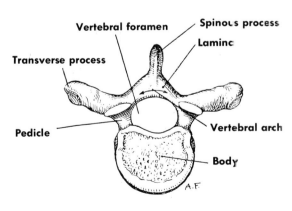

Transverse process

Vertebral foramen

Spinous process

Lamina

Pedicle

Vertebral arch

Body

SUPERIOR ASPECT OF TYPICAL VERTEBRA

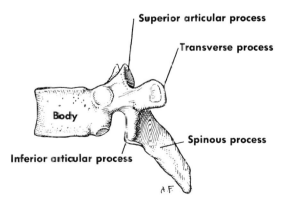

Superior articular process

Transverse process

Body

Inferior articular process

Spinous process

LATERAL ASPECT OF TYPICAL VERTEBRA

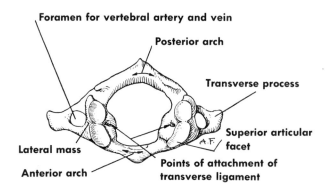

SUPERIOR ASPECT OF ATLAS

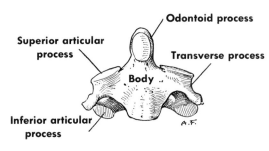

ANTERIOR ASPECT OF AXIS

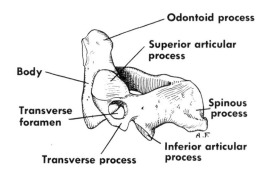

LATERAL ASPECT OF AXIS

The four articular processes (zygapophyses), two superior and two inferior, arise from the junction of the pedicles and laminae to articulate with the superjacent and subjacent vertebrae. Each superior zygapophysis presents an articular facet on its posterior surface, while the inferior processes present facets on their anterior surface. The planes of the facets vary in direction in the different regions and often in the same vertebra. The articulations between the vertebral arches are referred to as zygapophysial, or apophysial, joints to distinguish them from the articulations between the bodies of the vertebrae.

The transverse processes project lateralward and slightly backward from the junction of the pedicles and laminae. The spinous process projects backward and downward from the junction of the laminae in the posterior midline.

The movable vertebrae, with the exception of the first and second cervical, are similar in general structure; however, each group has certain distinguishing characteristics that must be considered in radiography of the vertebral column.

THE CERVICAL VERTEBRAE

The *atlas*, the first cervical vertebra, is a ringlike structure having no body and no spinous process. It consists of an anterior arch, a posterior arch, two lateral masses, and two transverse processes. The anterior and posterior arches extend between the lateral masses, and the ring formed by them is divided into anterior and posterior portions by a ligament called the transverse atlantal ligament. The anterior portion of the ring receives the odontoid process of the axis, and the posterior portion transmits the medulla oblongata.

The transverse processes are longer than those of the other cervical vertebrae, and they project lateralward and slightly downward from the lateral masses. Each lateral mass bears a superior and an inferior articular facet. The superior facets lie in a transverse plane, are large and deeply concave, and are shaped for the reception of the condyles of the occipital bone of the cranium. The articulations between the atlas and the occipital bone are diarthroses and are called the occipitocervical, or occipito-atlantal, articulations. The inferior facets are directed lateralward and slightly downward to articulate with the axis.

The *axis*, the second cervical vertebra, has a strong, conical process arising from the upper surface of its body, which is called the odontoid process, or the dens. The odontoid is received into the anterior portion of the atlantal ring to act as a pivot or body for the atlas. At each side of the odontoid, on the upper surface of the body, the transverse processes and the pedicles, are the superior articular facets, which are adapted to the inferior facets of the atlas. This pair of joints differs in both position and direction from the other cervical apophysial joints. The inferior articular processes of the axis have the same direction as those of the succeeding cervical vertebrae. The laminae of the axis are broad and thick. The spinous process is long and is horizontal in position.

The seventh cervical vertebra, which is termed the *vertebra prominens*, has a long, prominent spinous process that projects almost horizontally backward. The spinous process of the vertebra prominens is easily palpable at the base of the neck posteriorly. It is convenient to use this process as a guide in localizing other vertebrae.

The *typical cervical* vertebrae have small, transversely oblong bodies that have slightly prolonged anteroinferior borders, resulting in an anteroposterior overlapping of the bodies in the articulated column.

The transverse processes of the cervical vertebrae arise partially from the side of the body and partially from the vertebral arch, are short and wide, are perforated by the transverse foramen for the transmission of the vertebral artery and vein, and present a deep concavity on their upper surfaces for the passage of the spinal nerves.

The roots (pedicles) project laterally and posteriorly from the body, and their superior and inferior vertebral notches are nearly equal in depth. The laminae are narrow and thin. The spinous processes are short, have bifid tips, and are directed backward and slightly downward; their palpable tips lie at the level of the interspace below the body of the vertebra from which they spring.

The superior and inferior articular processes are situated behind the transverse process, where, arising at the junction of the pedicle and the lamina, they form a short column of bone that is usually referred to as the articular pillar. The superior and inferior articulating surfaces of the pillars are directed obliquely backward and downward so that the apophysial joints are not radiographically demonstrable in conventional frontal plane projections. The apophysial joints of the lower six cervical vertebrae are situated at right angles to the median sagittal plane of the body so that they are clearly demonstrated in a true lateral projection.

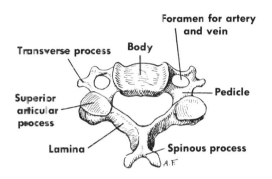

SUPERIOR ASPECT OF TYPICAL CERVICAL VERTEBRA

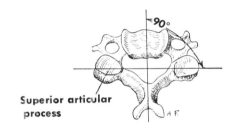

DIRECTION OF CERVICAL APOPHYSIAL JOINTS

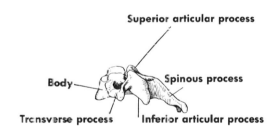

LATERAL ASPECT OF TYPICAL CERVICAL VERTEBRA

The *intervertebral foramina* of the cervical region lie at an angle of 45 degrees, open forward, to the median sagittal plane of the body, and at an angle of approximately 15 degrees, open downward, to the transverse plane of the body. Accurate roentgenographic demonstration of these foramina requires a longitudinal angulation of the central ray as well as medial rotation of the patient or a medial angulation of the central ray.

THE THORACIC VERTEBRAE

The bodies of the thoracic segments increase in size from above downward and vary in form from those resembling the cervical bodies in the upper part of the region to those resembling the lumbar bodies in the lower part of the region. The bodies of the typical thoracic vertebrae, from the third to the ninth, are approximately triangular in form. The thoracic bodies are deeper behind than in front, and their posterior surface is concave from side to side. On each side of the bodies, at both the upper and lower posterior borders, are demifacets that form, with the demifacet of the superjacent and subjacent vertebrae, the articular surfaces for the heads of the ribs. The body of the first thoracic vertebra presents a whole facet above for the first rib, and a demifacet below; the tenth, eleventh, and twelfth bodies present whole facets above and none below. The articulations between the ribs and the vertebral bodies are called costovertebral joints.

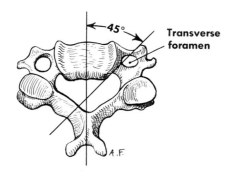

DIRECTION OF CERVICAL INTERVERTEBRAL FORAMINA

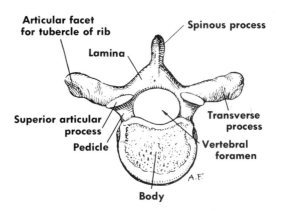

SUPERIOR ASPECT OF THORACIC VERTEBRA

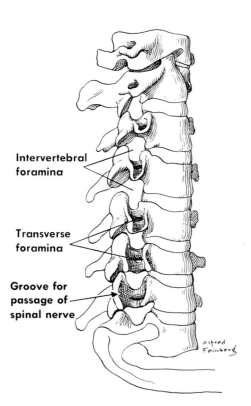

ANTEROLATERAL ASPECT OF CERVICAL VERTEBRAE SHOWING INTERVERTEBRAL AND TRANSVERSE FORAMINA

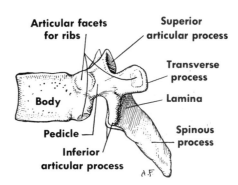

LATERAL ASPECT OF THORACIC VERTEBRA

The transverse processes of the thoracic vertebrae project obliquely lateralward and backward, and with the exception of the eleventh and twelfth pairs, each process has, on the anterior surface of its extremity, a small concave facet for articulation with the tubercle of a rib. The articulations between the ribs and the transverse processes of the thoracic vertebrae are termed the costotransverse joints. The laminae are broad and thick and overlap the subjacent lamina. The spinous processes are long. From the fifth to the ninth vertebrae, they project sharply downward and overlap each other but are less vertical in direction above and below this region. The palpable tips of the spinous processes of the fifth to the ninth vertebrae correspond in position with the body of the subjacent vertebra; the upper and lower processes correspond in position with the interspace below the body from which they spring.

The *apophysial joints* of the thoracic region, except the inferior processes of the twelfth vertebra, which are similar in direction to those of the lumbar region, angle forward approximately 15 to 20 degrees to form an angle of 70 to 75 degrees, open forward, to the median sagittal plane of the body. For the roentgenographic demonstration of the apophysial joints of the thoracic region, the body must be rotated 15 to 20 degrees from the lateral position, using forward rotation to demonstrate the joints nearer the film, and backward rotation to demonstrate those farther from the film.

The *intervertebral foramina* of the thoracic region are at right angles to the median sagittal plane of the body. They are clearly demonstrated radiographically in a true lateral position. The arms must be raised enough to elevate the ribs, which otherwise cross the intervertebral foramina.

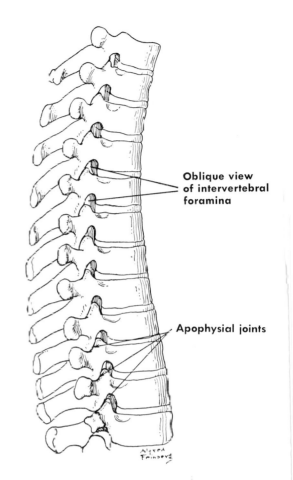

POSTEROLATERAL ASPECT OF THORACIC VERTEBRAE
SHOWING APOPHYSIAL JOINTS

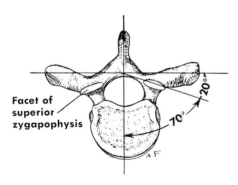

DIRECTION OF THORACIC APOPHYSIAL JOINTS

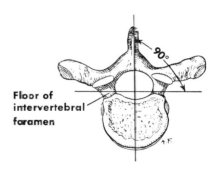

DIRECTION OF THORACIC INTERVERTEBRAL FORAMINA

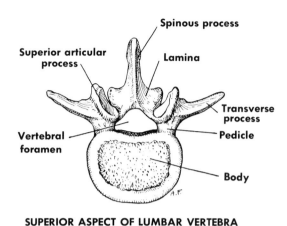

SUPERIOR ASPECT OF LUMBAR VERTEBRA

Spinous process

Superior articular process

Lamina

Transverse process

Vertebral foramen

Pedicle

Body

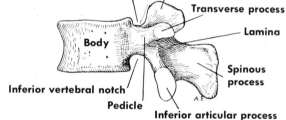

LATERAL ASPECT OF LUMBAR VERTEBRA

Superior articular process

Superior vertebral notch

Transverse process

Lamina

Body

Spinous process

Inferior vertebral notch

Pedicle

Inferior articular process

THE LUMBAR VERTEBRAE

The lumbar segments have large, bean-shaped bodies that increase in size from above downward. They are deeper in front than behind, and their superior and inferior surfaces are flattened or slightly concave. The lumbar body, at its posterior surface, is flattened from above downward and is transversely concave. Its anterior and lateral surfaces are concave from above downward.

The transverse processes are smaller than those of the thoracic region. The upper three pairs are directed almost exactly lateralward, while the lower two pairs are inclined slightly upward. The spinous processes are large, thick, and blunt, and project almost horizontally backward; their palpable tips correspond in position with the interspace below the vertebra from which they spring.

The body of the fifth lumbar segment is considerably deeper in front than behind, which gives it a wedge shape that adapts it for articulation with the sacrum. The articular disk of this joint is also more wedge-shaped than are those in the interspaces above. The spinous process of the fifth lumbar vertebra is smaller and shorter, and the transverse processes are much thicker, than are those of the upper lumbar vertebrae.

The *apophysial joints* of the lumbar region are inclined backward from the coronal plane, forming an angle, open backward, of 30 to 50 degrees to the median sagittal plane of the body. These joints can be demonstrated radiographically by rotating the body from either the anteroposterior or the posteroanterior position.

The *intervertebral foramina* of the lumbar region are situated at right angles to the median sagittal plane of the body, except the fifth, which turns slightly forward. The upper four pairs of foramina are demonstrated in a true lateral projection; the last pair requires a slight obliquity of the body.

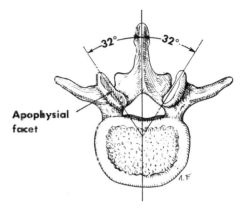

DIRECTION OF LUMBAR APOPHYSIAL JOINTS

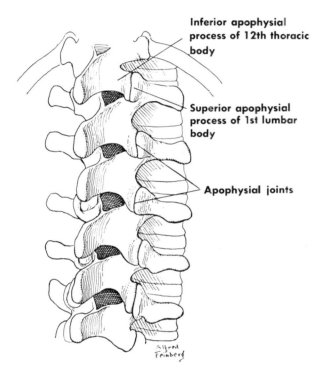

POSTEROLATERAL ASPECT OF LUMBAR VERTEBRAE
SHOWING APOPHYSIAL JOINTS

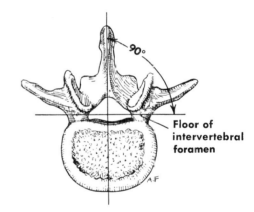

DIRECTION OF LUMBAR INTERVERTEBRAL FORAMINA

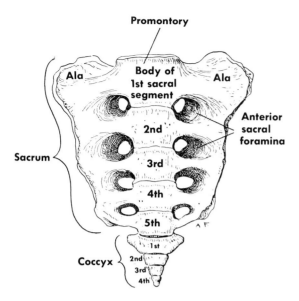

ANTERIOR ASPECT OF SACRUM AND COCCYX

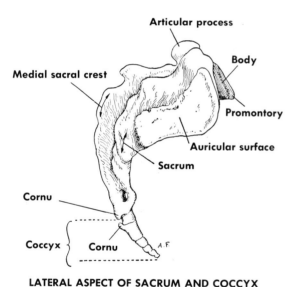

LATERAL ASPECT OF SACRUM AND COCCYX

THE SACRUM AND THE COCCYX

The *sacrum* is formed by the fusion of the five sacral segments into a curved, triangular bone. The sacrum is wedged between the iliac bones of the hips, its broad base directed obliquely upward and forward, and its apex directed backward and downward. While there is a considerable variation in the size and in the degree of curvature of the sacrum in different subjects, the bone is normally longer, narrower, more evenly curved, and more vertical in position in the male than in the female. In the female, the sacrum is more acutely curved on itself, the greatest curvature being in the lower half of the bone, and it lies in a more oblique plane, which results in a sharper angle at the junction of the lumbar and pelvic curves.

The upper portion of the first sacral segment remains distinct and resembles the vertebrae of the lumbar region. The superior surface of the body of the sacrum corresponds in size and shape to the inferior surface of the last lumbar segment, with which it articulates to form the sacrovertebral, or lumbosacral, junction. The concavities on the upper surface of the pedicles of the first sacral segment, with the corresponding concavities on the lower surface of the pedicles of the last lumbar segment, form the last pair of intervertebral foramina. The superior articular processes of the first sacral segment articulate with the inferior articular processes of the last lumbar vertebra to form the last pair of apophysial joints.

The body of the sacrum has a prominent ridge at its upper anterior margin that is termed the sacral promontory. Directly behind the body is the sacral canal, the continuation of the spinal canal, which is contained within the bone and transmits the sacral nerves. The anterior and posterior walls of the sacral canal are each perforated by four pairs of foramina for the passage of the sacral nerves and blood vessels.

On each side of the sacral body is a large, winglike lateral mass, or ala. At the upper anterior part of the lateral surface of each ala is a large articular process, the auricular surface, for articulation with similarly shaped processes on the iliac bones of the hips. The articulations between the sacrum and the ilia, the sacroiliac joints, slant obliquely backward and medialward at an angle of 25 to 30 degrees, open forward, to the median sagittal plane of the body. These joints are amphiarthroses.

The inferior surface of the apex of the sacrum has an oval facet for articulation with the coccyx, and two processes, the sacral cornua, which project downward from the posterolateral aspect of the last sacral segment to join the cornua of the coccyx.

The *coccyx* is composed of three to five (usually four) rudimentary vertebrae that have a tendency to fuse into one bone in the adult. The coccyx diminishes in size from its base downward to its apex. From its articulation with the sacrum, it curves downward and forward, often deviating from the median sagittal plane of the body. There are two processes, the coccygeal cornua, which project upward from the posterolateral aspect of the first coccygeal segment to join the sacral cornua.

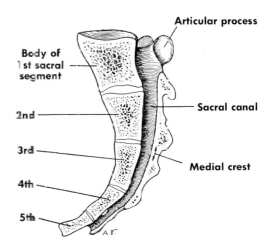

SAGITTAL SECTION OF SACRUM

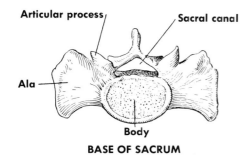

BASE OF SACRUM

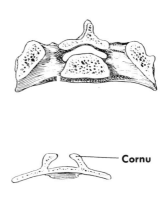

TRANSVERSE SECTIONS OF SACRUM

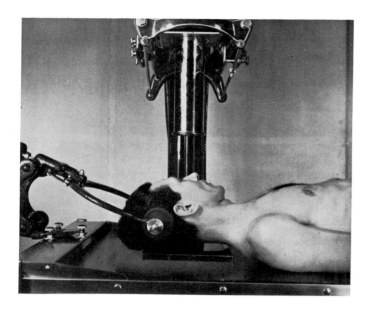

OCCIPITOCERVICAL ARTICULATIONS
Oblique anteroposterior projection
Oblique posteroanterior view

Film: $8'' \times 10''$ crosswise for two exposures on one film.

Position of patient

Place the patient in the supine position. Center the median sagittal plane of the body to the midline of the table and adjust the shoulders to lie in the same transverse plane.

Position of part

Place the cassette under the patient's head and adjust it so that the midpoint of the unmasked half is about 1 inch lateral to the median sagittal plane of the head at the level of the external auditory meatuses.

Rotate the head away from the side being examined enough to place the midpoint of the orbit perpendicular to the film. Adjust the flexion of the head to place the infraorbitomeatal line perpendicular to the film.

Use a head clamp or place sandbags against the head for immobilization. Respiration is suspended for the exposure.

Central ray

Direct the central ray vertically to the midpoint of the film; it enters the outer margin of the orbit and emerges at the occipitoatlantal articulation.

Structures shown

A slightly oblique anteroposterior projection of the occipitoatlantal articulation, the joint being projected between the orbit and the vertical ramus of the mandible. Both sides are examined for comparison.

The odontoid process of the axis is also well demonstrated in this projection so that it can be used for this purpose when a patient cannot be adjusted in the open-mouth position.

NOTE: Buetti[1] recommends a position for the occipitocervical articulations wherein the head is turned 45 to 50 degrees to one side and, with the mouth wide open, the chin is drawn down as much as the open mouth will allow. The central ray is then directed vertically through the open mouth to the dependent mastoid tip.

[1]Buetti, C.: Zur Darstellung der Atlanto-epistropheal-Gelenke bzw. der Procc. transversi atlantis und esistrophei, Radiol. Clin. **20:**168-172, 1951.

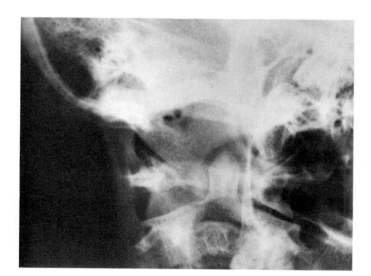

OCCIPITOCERVICAL ARTICULATIONS
Bilateral posteroanterior projection
Anteroposterior view

Film: $8'' \times 10''$ crosswise.

Position of patient

With the patient in the prone position, center the median sagittal plane of the body to the midline of the table. If the patient is thin, place a small, firm pillow under the chest to relieve strain in holding the position. Flex the patient's elbows, place the arms in a comfortable position, and adjust the shoulders to lie in the same transverse plane. Place sandbags under the ankles to prevent the weight of the feet from resting on the toes.

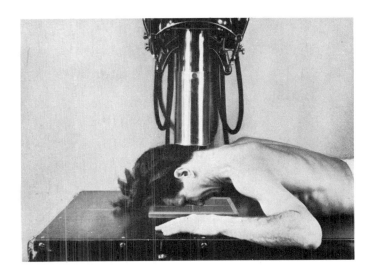

Position of part

Rest the patient's head on his forehead and nose and adjust it so that its median sagittal plane is perpendicular to the midline of the table or cassette.

Adjust the flexion of the head to place the orbitomeatal line vertical, and if using non-Bucky technique, center the film at or slightly below the level of the infraorbital margins.

Immobilize the head with a head clamp or with a weighted band. Respiration is suspended for the exposure.

Central ray

Direct the central ray perpendicularly to the midpoint of the film; it enters the nape of the neck at the level of the infraorbital margins.

Structures shown

An anterior view (posteroanterior projection) of the occipitocervical joints projected through the antra.

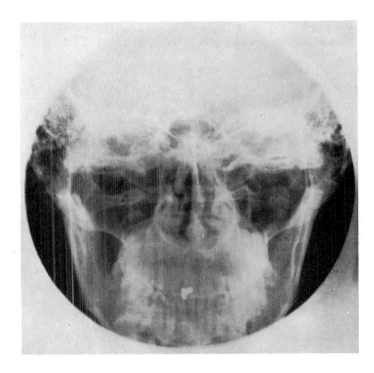

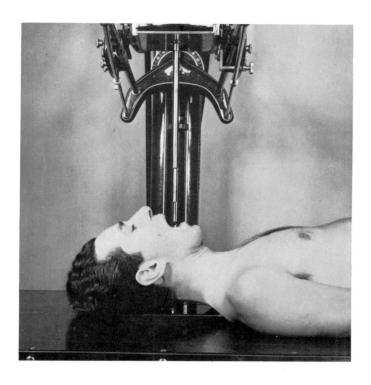

ATLAS AND AXIS
Anteroposterior projection
Posteroanterior view
Open-mouth position

This position was described by Albers-Schönberg[1] in 1910, and by George[2] in 1919.

Film: $5'' \times 7''$ crosswise.

Position of patient

With the patient in the supine position, center the median sagittal plane of the body to the midline of the table. Place the patient's arms along the sides of his body, and adjust the shoulders to lie in the same transverse plane.

Position of part

Place the cassette under the patient's neck and center it to the median sagittal plane at the level of the second cervical segment. Place a folded towel or other pad under the head so that it overlaps the upper border of the cassette; this prevents the cassette from slipping and is more comfortable for the patient.

Set the machine for the exposure, and move the x-ray tube into position so that any minor change can be made quickly after the final adjustment of the patient's head. This position is not an easy one to hold; however, the patient is usually able to cooperate fully unless he is kept in the final, strained position too long.

Have the patient open his mouth as wide as possible, and then adjust the head so that a line from the lower edge of the upper incisors to the tip of the mastoid process is perpendicular to the film. Immobilize the head with a head clamp or with sandbags placed against the sides of the head.

Instruct the patient to keep his mouth wide open and to softly phonate "ah" during the exposure. This will fix the tongue in the floor of the mouth so that its shadow will not be projected on that of the atlas and axis, and will prevent movement of the jaw.

Central ray

Direct the central ray vertically to the midpoint of the open mouth.

Structures shown

An anteroposterior projection of the atlas and axis through the open mouth.

If the patient has a deep head or a long upper jaw, the entire atlas will not be demonstrated. When the exactly superimposed shadows of the inferior margins of the upper teeth and the base of the skull are in line with those of the tips of the mastoid processes, the position cannot be improved.

[1]Albers-Schönberg, H. E.: Die Röntgentechnik, Hamburg, 1910.
[2]George, A. W.: Method for more accurate study of injuries to the atlas and axis, Boston Med. Surg. J. **181**:395-398, 1919.

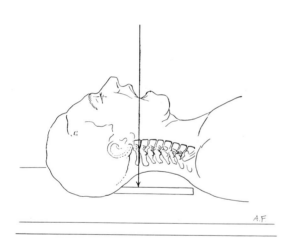

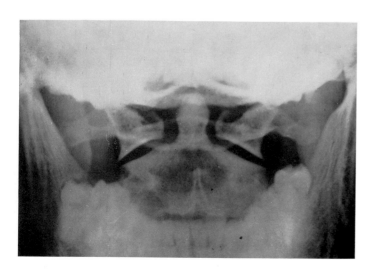

ODONTOID PROCESS
Anteroposterior projection
Posteroanterior view
Fuchs position

Film: $5'' \times 7''$ or $8'' \times 10''$ crosswise.

Position of patient

With the patient in the supine position, center the median sagittal plane of the body to the midline of the table. Place the arms along the sides of the body and adjust the shoulders to lie in the same transverse plane.

Position of part

For non-Bucky technique, place the cassette under the patient's upper neck and center it to the median sagittal plane at the level of the tips of the mastoid processes. In order to prevent the cassette from slipping when the head is adjusted, and to make the patient more comfortable, place a folded towel under the head so that it overlaps the upper edge of the cassette.

Tip the head backward until a line passing through the tip of the chin and the tip of the mastoid process is vertical. Adjust the head so that its median sagittal plane is vertical.

Immobilize the head with a head clamp or by placing sandbags against the sides of the head. Respiration is suspended for the exposure.

Central ray

Direct the central ray vertically to the midpoint of the film; it enters the neck just distal to the tip of the chin.

Structures shown

An anteroposterior projection of the odontoid process lying within the shadow of the foramen magnum.

Fuchs[1] recommended this position for the demonstration of the dens when its upper half is not clearly shown in the open-mouth position. He stated, however, that the position should not be attempted by the technologist if there is a fracture or a degenerating disease of the upper cervical region.

[1]Fuchs, Arthur W.: Cervical vertebrae (part 1), Radiogr. Clin. Photogr. **16:**2-17, 1940.

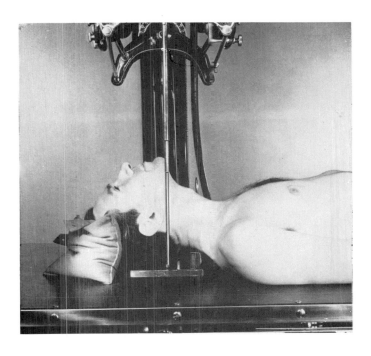

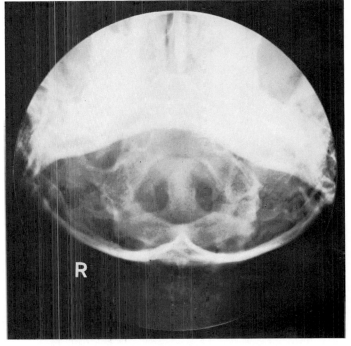

Courtesy Arthur W. Fuchs.

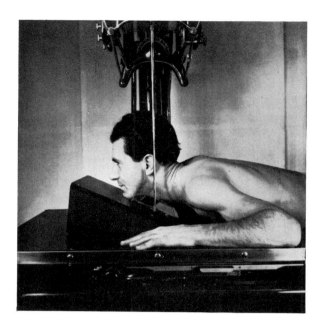

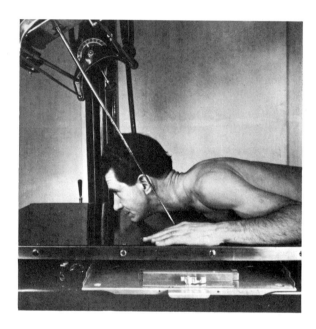

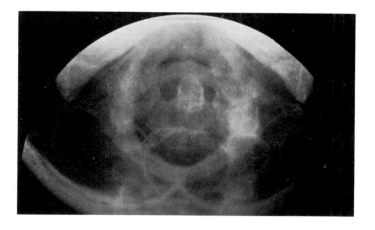

ATLAS AND ODONTOID PROCESS
Semiaxial projection
Jackson position[1]
Film: $5'' \times 7''$ or $8'' \times 10''$ crosswise.

Position of patient

With the patient in the prone position, center the median sagittal plane of the body to the midline of the table. Flex the elbows, place the arms in a comfortable position, and adjust the shoulders to lie in the same transverse plane.

Position of part

Place the cassette on a 23-degree angle block inclined toward the feet, slide it into position, and have the patient extend his chin and rest it on the upper border of the cassette. Immobilize the angle block with sandbags to prevent it from slipping.

Center the film to the median sagittal plane of the throat at the level of the upper border of the thyroid cartilage (approximately $1\frac{1}{2}$ inches distal to the tip of the mastoid process) to allow for the angulation displacement of the part. Adjust the head so that its median sagittal plane is vertical. Respiration is suspended for the exposure.

Central ray

Direct the central ray vertically to the midpoint of the film; it enters the head midway between the tips of the mastoid processes.

Structures shown

A semiaxial view of the atlas and an anterior view of the odontoid process projected into the shadow of the foramen magnum.

Variation

When Potter-Bucky technique is preferred, Davis[2] recommends the following position for obtaining a view similar to the one described above: rest the head on the fully extended chin and adjust it so that the median sagittal plane is vertical and centered to the midline of the table; direct the central ray through the odontoid process (midway between the mastoid tips) at an angle that is parallel with the localization plane of the face.

NOTE: Neither of these positions is recommended for use with the patient who has a suspected fracture, nor with the patient who has a destructive disease of the upper cervical region.

[1]As accredited to Jackson in Pancoast, H. K., Pendergrass, E. P., and Schaeffer, J. P.: The head and neck in roentgen diagnosis, Springfield, Ill., 1940, Charles C Thomas, Publisher, p. 148.
[2]Davis, Dorothy W.: Personal communication.

ATLAS AND ODONTOID PROCESS
Posteroanterior projection
Anteroposterior view
Judd position

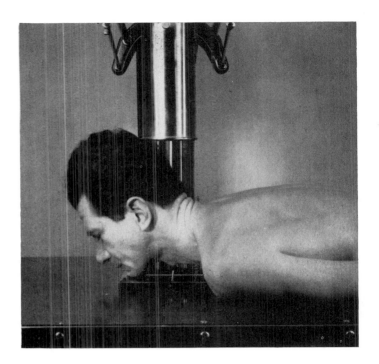

Film: $5'' \times 7''$ crosswise.

Position of patient

With the patient in the prone position, center the median sagittal plane of the body to the midline of the table. Flex the patient's elbows, place the arms in a comfortable position, and adjust the shoulders to lie in the same transverse plane. Place sandbags under the ankles to prevent the weight of the feet from resting on the toes.

Position of part

Have the patient extend his chin and rest it on the upper border of the transversely placed film. Adjust the film so that its midpoint is centered to the throat at the level of the upper margin of the thyroid cartilage.

Adjust the head so that the tip of the nose is about 1 inch from the tabletop, and so that the median sagittal plane is vertical.

Use a head clamp or a weighted band for immobilization. Respiration is suspended for the exposure.

Central ray

Direct the central ray vertically to the midpoint of the film; it enters the occiput just posterior to the mastoid tips.

Structures shown

An anterior view of the odontoid process projected into the shadow of the foramen magnum.

The technologist should not attempt this position with the patient who has an unhealed fracture, nor with the patient who has a destructive disease of the upper cervical region.

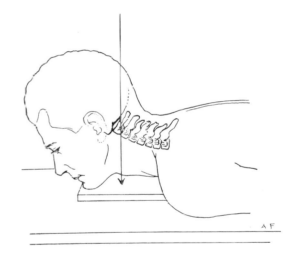

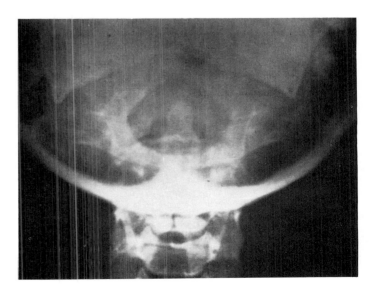

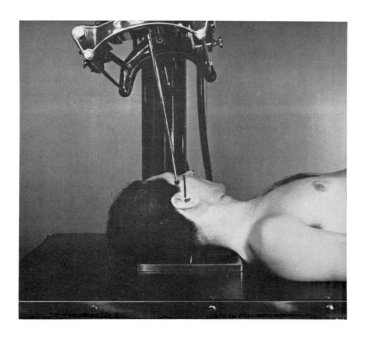

ODONTOID PROCESS
Anterior oblique projection
Posterior oblique view
Kasabach position

Film: $8'' \times 10''$ crosswise for two exposures.

Position of patient

With the patient in the supine position, center the median sagittal plane of the body to the midline of the table. Place the arms along the sides of the body and adjust the shoulders to lie in the same transverse plane.

Position of part

For non-Bucky technique, place the film under the upper neck and center the unmasked half to the median sagittal plane at the level of the mastoid tip.

Rotate the head approximately 40 to 45 degrees away from the side being examined and adjust the head so that the infraorbitomeatal line is vertical. Immobilize the head with a head clamp or by placing a sandbag against the vertex. Respiration is suspended for the exposure.

For right-angle views of the odontoid, make one exposure with the head turned to the right and one with it turned to the left.

Central ray

With the central ray angulated 10 to 15 degrees toward the feet, center to a point midway between the outer canthus and the external auditory meatus.

Structures shown

An oblique view of the odontoid process, which Kasabach[1] recommended for use in conjunction with the antero-posterior and lateral views.

The head of a patient who has a possible fracture or destructive disease must not be rotated. Kasabach[1] recommended that the entire body, rather than only the head, be rotated.

NOTE: Herrmann and St. Stender[2] described a position for the demonstration of the occipitoatlantal-odontoid relationship, wherein the head is adjusted as for the Kasabach position. The central ray is then directed vertically midway between the mastoid processes at the level of the occipitocervical joints.

[1]Kasabach, H. H.: A roentgenographic method for the study of the second cervical vertebra, Amer. J. Roentgen. **42**:782-785, 1939.
[2]Herrmann, E., and St. Stender, H.: Ein einfache Aufnahmetechnik zur Darstellung der Dens axis, Fortschr. Roentgenstr. **96**:115-119, 1962.

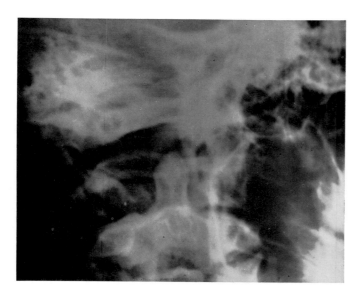

ATLAS AND AXIS
Lateral projection

Film: $5'' \times 7''$ crosswise.

Position of patient

With the patient supine, adjust the body in a true anteroposterior position. Place the arms along the sides of the body and adjust the shoulders to lie in the same transverse plane.

Position of part

With the cassette in the vertical position and in contact with the upper neck, center at the level of the atlanto-axial articulation (1 inch distal to the tip of the mastoid process). Adjust the cassette so that it is parallel with the median sagittal plane of the neck and then support it in position with sandbags.

Extend the head slightly so that the shadow of the mandibular rami will not overlap that of the spine. Adjust the head so that its median sagittal plane is vertical.

Immobilize the head with a head clamp or by placing sandbags against the parietal regions of the skull. Respiration is suspended for the exposure.

Central ray

Direct the central ray horizontally to a point 1 inch distal to the adjacent mastoid tip.

Structures shown

A lateral view of the atlas and axis. The occipitocervical articulations are also demonstrated. Because of the short part-film distance, better detail is obtained with this method than with the customary method of performing the lateral examination of the cervical vertebrae. A small cone should be used and, if possible, a grid-front cassette or a wafer grid, in order to minimize secondary radiation.

Pancoast, Pendergrass, and Schaeffer[1] recommend that the head be rotated slightly to prevent superimposition of the laminae of the atlas. They recommend a slight transverse tilt of the head for the demonstration of the arches of the atlas.

[1]Pancoast, H. K., Pendergrass, E. P., and Schaeffer, J. P.: The head and neck in roentgen diagnosis, Springfield, Ill., 1940, Charles C Thomas, Publisher.

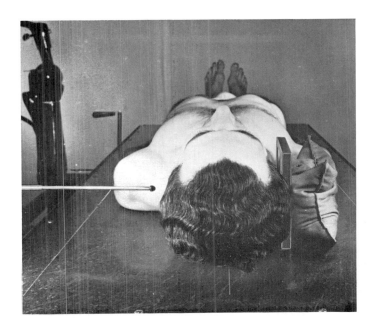

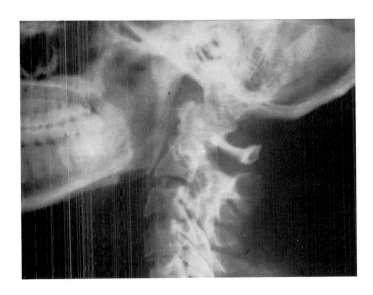

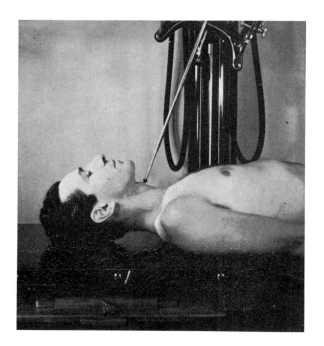

LOWER CERVICAL VERTEBRAE
Anteroposterior projection
Posteroanterior view

Film: $8'' \times 10''$ lengthwise.

Position of patient

The patient is placed in the anteroposterior position, either recumbent or erect.

Position of part

Center the median sagittal plane of the patient's body to the midline of the table or vertical Potter-Bucky stand. Adjust the shoulders to lie in the same transverse plane to prevent rotation.

Extend the head enough to place the occlusal plane and the mastoid tips in the same transverse plane in order to prevent superimposition of the mandible and the midcervical vertebrae.

Adjust the position of the cassette so that the center point of the film will coincide with the central ray.

Immobilization can usually be obtained by having the patient softly phonate an m-m-m sound during the exposure of the film.

Central ray

Direct the central ray through the fourth cervical body at an angle of 15 to 20 degrees toward the head; it enters at the most prominent point of the thyroid cartilage.

Structures shown

A frontal view of the lower five cervical bodies and the upper two or three thoracic bodies, the interpediculate spaces, the superimposed transverse and articular processes, and, when the central ray is angulated 15 to 20 degrees toward the head, the intervertebral disk spaces.

This position is also used to demonstrate the presence or absence of cervical ribs.

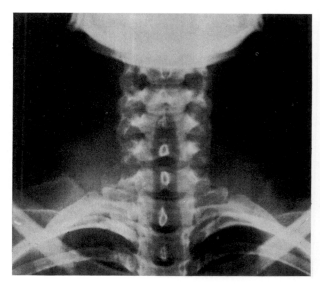

Central ray 20 degrees toward head.

Central ray perpendicular, opposite patient.

CERVICAL VERTEBRAE
Anteroposterior projection
Posteroanterior view
Ottonello method

With the Ottonello method, the mandibular shadow is blurred if not obliterated by utilizing even, rhythmical motion of the mandible during the exposure. Needless to say, the head must be rigidly immobilized to prevent movement of the vertebrae. The exposure time must be long enough, preferably ten seconds, to cover several complete excursions of the mandible.

Film: 8″ × 10″ lengthwise.

Position of patient

With the patient in the supine position, center the median sagittal plane of the body to the midline of the table. Place the arms along the sides of the body and adjust the shoulders to lie in the same transverse plane. Place a long sandbag under the ankles for the patient's comfort.

Position of part

Place a thin, radioparent pad under the patient's head to prevent slipping during mandibular movement. Adjust the head so that its median sagittal plane is vertical. Elevate the chin enough to place the edges of the upper incisors and the mastoid tips in the same transverse plane. Immobilize the head with a head clamp and then have the patient practice opening and closing his mouth until he can move the mandible smoothly and fairly rapidly without striking the teeth together.

With the cassette in the Potter-Bucky tray, center it at the level of the fourth cervical vertebra.

Central ray

Direct the central ray vertically to the midpoint of the film.

Structures shown

An anteroposterior projection of the entire cervical column, the shadow of the mandible being blurred if not obliterated.

NOTE: Jacobs[1] recommends that a pure gum-rubber bag filled two-thirds full of water be placed under the lower cervical and shoulder regions to act as a filter in preventing overexposure of the lower vertebrae. The bag must be placed so that it will not overlap the area covered by the excursion of the mandible in order to prevent underexposure of that region.

[1]Jacobs, Lewis: Roentgenography of the cervical second vertebra by Ottonello's method, Radiology **31**:412-413, 1938.

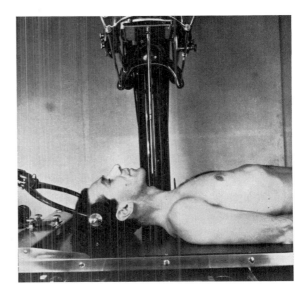

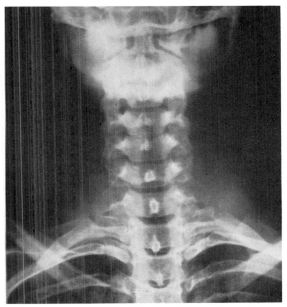

Ottonello projection.

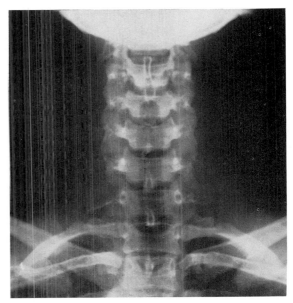

Conventional projection.

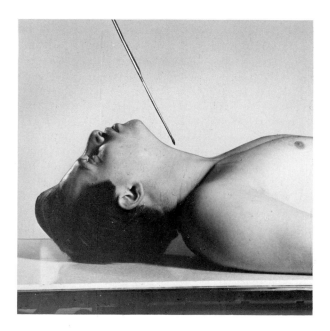

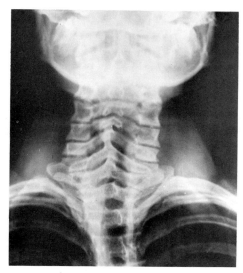

Central ray coincident with plateau of the articular facets.

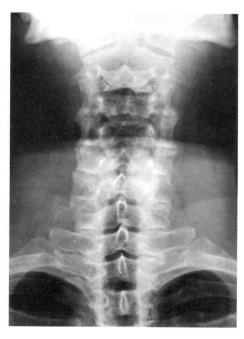

Head fully extended but central ray angulation inadequate.

CERVICAL AND UPPER THORACIC VERTEBRAE

Vertebral arch projections[1,2]

The vertebral arch projections, sometimes referred to as *pillar* projections, are employed for the demonstration of the posterior elements of the cervical and upper three or four thoracic vertebrae, the articular processes and their facets, the laminae, and the spinous processes. The central ray angulations employed project the vertebral arch elements free of the shadows of the anteriorly situated vertebral bodies and transverse processes so that, when the central ray angulation is correct, the resultant film resembles a hemisection of the vertebrae. In addition to frontal plane delineation of the articular pillars and facets, these projections are especially useful for the demonstration of the cervicothoracic spinous processes in patients with a whiplash injury.[3]

Film: According to the area to be included, 8″ × 10″ or 10″ × 12″ lengthwise.

Anteroposterior projection

Position of patient

The patient is adjusted in the supine position, with the median sagittal plane of the body centered to the midline of the table. Depress his shoulders and adjust them to lie in the same transverse plane; if necessary, place a long strip of bandage around the patient's feet and, with his knees slightly flexed, have him grasp the ends of the bandage and then extend his knees to hold the shoulders in position.

Position of part

With the median sagittal plane of the head vertical, *hyperextend* the head; the success of the direct anteroposterior projection depends upon the hyperextension. When the patient cannot tolerate hyperextension without undue discomfort, use the oblique projections instead.

Adjust the position of the cassette so that the upper edge of the film is at the level of the external auditory meatuses.

Central ray

Direct the central ray to the seventh cervical vertebra at an average angle of 25 (20 to 30) degrees toward the feet; it enters the neck in the region of the thyroid cartilage.

The degree of central ray angulation is determined by the cervical lordosis. The aim is to have the central ray coincide with the plane of the articular facets, so that a greater angle is required when the cervical curve is accentuated, and a lesser angle is required when the curve is diminished. The originators[2] suggested that, in order to reduce an accentuated cervical curve and thus place the third to seventh cervical vertebrae in the same plane as the first to fourth thoracic vertebrae, a radioparent wedge be placed under the neck and shoulders, with the head extended somewhat over the edge of the wedge.

[1] Dorland, P., and Frémont, J.: Aspect radiologique normal du rachis postérieur cervicodorsal (vue postérieure ascendante), Semaine Hôp. pp. 1457-1464, 1957.

[2] Dorland, P., Frémont, J., Parer, and Perez: Techniques d'examen radiologique de l'arc postérieur des vertebres cervicodorsales, J. Radiol. Electr. 39:509-519, 1958.

[3] Abel, Martin S.: Moderately severe whiplash injuries of the cervical spine and their roentgenologic diagnosis, Clin. Orthop. 12:189-208, 1958.

CERVICAL AND UPPER THORACIC VERTEBRAE
Vertebral arch projections—cont'd
Oblique anteroposterior projection

Position of part

With the patient adjusted in the supine position, as for the direct anteroposterior projection, rotate the head 45 to 50 degrees to one side (both sides are examined for comparison). A 45- to 50-degree rotation of the head usually demonstrates the articular facets of the second to seventh cervical vertebrae and of the first thoracic vertebra, but a rotation of as much as 60 to 70 degrees is sometimes required for the demonstration of the facets of the sixth and seventh cervical vertebrae and of the first to fourth thoracic vertebrae.

Central ray

The central ray is directed to the seventh cervical vertebra at an average angle of 35 (30 to 40) degrees toward the feet.

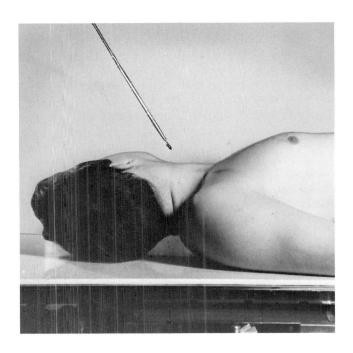

Oblique posteroanterior projection
Position of patient

The patient is adjusted in the prone position, which seems to be more comfortable for injured patients than the supine position. Center the median sagittal plane of the body to the midline of the table. When examining a thin patient, place a pillow under his chest to obviate accentuation of the cervical curve. Depress the shoulders and adjust them to lie in the same transverse plane.

Position of part

Rest the patient's head on one cheek (both sides are examined for comparison) and adjust the head so that its median sagittal plane is at an angle of 45 degrees.

For the demonstration of the second to fifth cervical vertebrae, flex the head somewhat to reduce the cervical curve; for the demonstration of the fifth to seventh cervical vertebrae and the first to fourth thoracic vertebrae, adjust the head in moderate extension.

Position the cassette so that the distal edge of the film is at the level of the tip of the seventh cervical spinous process.

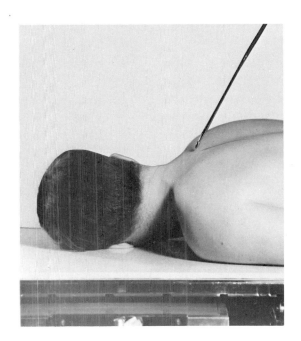

Central ray

Direct the central ray to the seventh cervical vertebra at an average angle of 35 (30 to 40) degrees toward the head; it exits at the level of the mandibular symphysis.

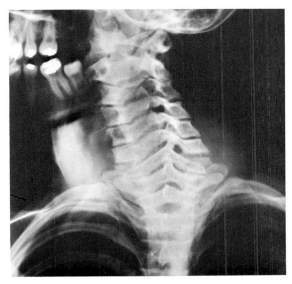

Oblique anteroposterior projection.

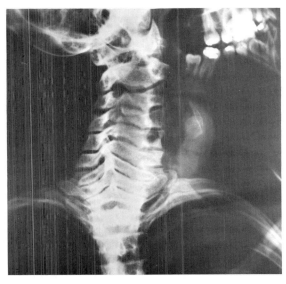

Oblique posteroanterior projection.

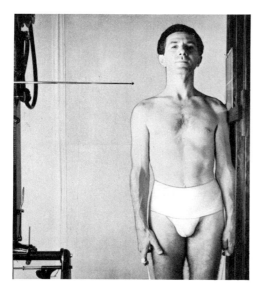

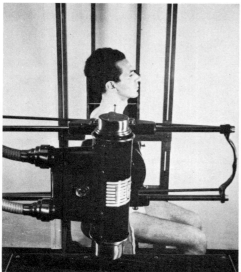

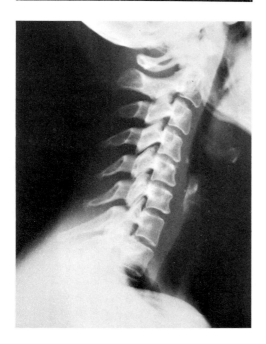

CERVICAL VERTEBRAE
Lateral projection
Grandy method
Film: $8'' \times 10''$ lengthwise.

Position of patient

Place the patient in a lateral position, either seated or standing, before a vertical cassette stand. Have him sit or stand straight, and then adjust the height of the film so that it is centered at the level of the fourth cervical segment.

Position of part

Center the coronal plane that passes through the tips of the mastoid processes to the midline of the film. Move the patient close enought to the stand to permit him to rest the adjacent shoulder against it for support.

Rotate the shoulders forward or backward, according to the natural kyphosis of the back: if the subject is round-shouldered, rotate them forward; otherwise, rotate them backward. Adjust the shoulders to lie in the same transverse plane, depress them as much as possible, and immobilize them by having the patient hold, one in each hand, two small sandbags of equal weight. Another method that is sometimes more suitable is to place a long strip of gauze bandage under the patient's feet or, if he is seated, under the rungs of the chair, and have him grasp one end of the gauze in each hand and pull. In this way, by the placement of the gauze strip, the shoulders can be depressed forward or backward, according to the needs of the particular patient.

Adjust the body in a true lateral position, with the long axis of the cervical vertebrae parallel with the plane of the film. Elevate the chin slightly to prevent superimposition of the mandibular rami and the spine, and with the median sagittal plane of the head vertical, ask the patient to look steadily at one spot on the wall to aid in maintaining the position of his head. The fraction of a second (two-tenths or less) needed for the exposure time of this projection makes elaborate immobilization measures unnecessary in a majority of cases.

Respiration is suspended at the end of full exhalation in order to obtain maximum depression of the shoulders.

NOTE: This method of obtaining the lateral view of the cervical spine was described by Grandy[1] in 1925. Prior to that time, the patient was examined in the recumbent position, with the cassette in contact with the neck.

[1]Grandy, C. C.: A new method for making radiographs of the cervical vertebrae in the lateral position, Radiology 4:128-129, 1925.

CERVICAL VERTEBRAE

Lateral projections

Central ray

Direct the central ray horizontally to the midpoint of the film.

Taylor[1] recommends centering at the level of the external auditory meatuses for the purpose of projecting the magnified shadow of the shoulder remote from the film below those of the lower cervical segments.

Because of the great part-film distance, the focal-film distance should be 72 inches in order to obtain the finest detail possible.

Structures shown

A lateral view of the cervical bodies and their interspaces, the articular pillars, the lower five articular facets, and the spinous processes. Depending upon how well the shoulders can be depressed and rotated, the seventh cervical vertebrae, and sometimes the upper one or two thoracic vertebrae.

Flexion-extension studies

As for the neutral, lateral view of the cervical vertebrae, the patient is adjusted in an exact lateral position and instructed to sit or stand erect.

While keeping the median sagittal plane of his head and neck parallel with the plane of the film:

1. Ask the patient to drop his head forward and then to draw his chin as close as possible to his chest in order to place the cervical vertebrae in a position of extreme flexion for the first exposure.

2. Ask the patient to elevate his chin as much as possible so as to place the cervical vertebrae in a position of extreme extension for the second exposure.

Functional studies of the cervical vertebrae in the lateral position are made for the purpose of demonstrating normal forward-backward movement or, as a result of trauma or disease, an absence of movement. The spinous processes are elevated and widely separated in the flexion position and are depressed in close approximation in the extension position.

Spinous processes

The demonstration of the cervicothoracic spinous processes is frequently requested for patients who have sustained an injury of either a direct or a whiplash type. When the patient has reasonably flexible shoulders, he can be adjusted in a direct lateral position, as described below. When, because of pain, bodily habitus, or obesity, the patient cannot be so positioned, the spinous processes can be demonstrated quite satisfactorily with the anterior oblique (backward rotation) apophysial joint position, described on pages 244 and 245.

Seat the patient in a lateral position before a Potter-Bucky grid. Center the film and the central ray at the level of the second or third thoracic vertebra. Rotate the shoulders well forward and downward, and have the patient hold them in position by grasping his knees, or by crossing his forearms and grasping his upper arms. Readjust the body position so as to center the cervicothoracic vertebrae to the midline of the grid. Instruct the patient to drop his head forward and pull his chin down as much as possible in order to elevate the spinous processes into a position of prominence. Respiration is suspended for the exposure.

The use of the lateral thoracic technique (less approximately one-third the milliampere-second factor) produces a satisfactory view of the spinous processes of the thoracic region. The cervical processes must usually be viewed by a spotlight.

[1]Taylor, Henry K.: Personal communication.

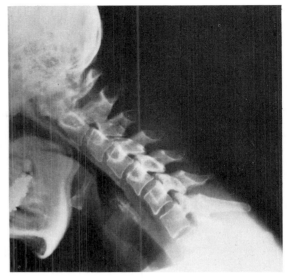

Flexion.

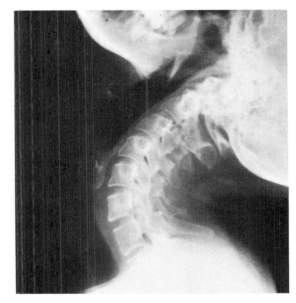

Extension.

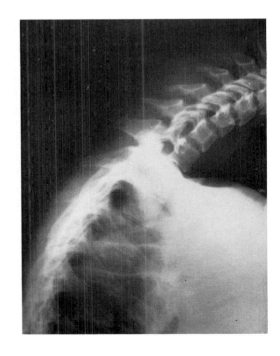

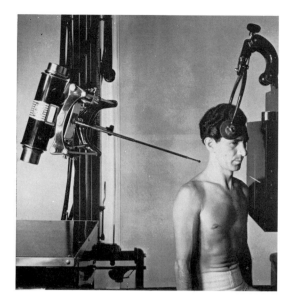

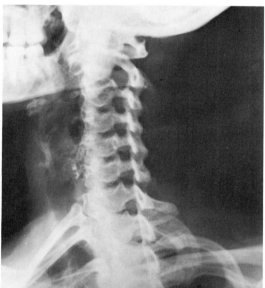

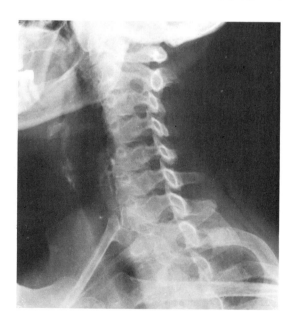

CERVICAL INTERVERTEBRAL FORAMINA
Oblique posteroanterior projection
Oblique anteroposterior view

Oblique projections for the demonstration of the cervical intervertebral foramina were first described by Barsony and Koppenstein.[1,2]

Film: $8'' \times 10''$ lengthwise.

Position of patient

The patient is placed in the posteroanterior position. For the patient's comfort and to facilitate accurate adjustment of the part, the standing or seated erect position is preferable for oblique studies of the cervical spine. The part-film distance here is such that secondary radiation is largely filtered out into the air so that these studies may, with the equivalent of a 6-kilovolt reduction in exposure, be made with the same nongrid, 72-inch focal-film distance technique used for the lateral projection. When a patient must be examined in the semiprone position, a grid technique should be used to eliminate secondary radiation, which would otherwise reach the film because of the decrease in part-film distance.

Position of part

Keeping one shoulder adjacent to the film (both sides are examined for comparison), rotate the patient's *entire body* to approximately the 45-degree angle required to place the foramina parallel with the film, and then center the cervical spine to the midline of the vertical stand or table.

In order to allow for the caudal angulation of the central ray, the film is centered at the level of the fifth cervical segment (1 inch distal to the most prominent point of the thyroid cartilage).

Erect position. Ask the patient to sit or stand straight without strain and, with the arm hanging free, to rest the adjacent shoulder against the stand. Adjust the degree of body rotation with the use of a protractor or with a 45-degree cardboard triangle.

With the median sagittal plane of the head coextensive with that of the spine, elevate the chin slightly to prevent superimposition of the shadows of the mandibular rami and the foramina; if preferred, the head may be turned slightly, but care must be exercised to avoid rotation of the upper cervical segments.

Immobilize by having the patient grasp the side of the stand with the hand of the side remote from the film, and by having him softly phonate an m-m-m sound during the exposure.

[1]Barsony, T., und Koppenstein, E.: Eine neue Method zur Röntgenuntersuchung der Halswirbelsäule, Fortschr. Roentgenstr. **35**:593-594, 1926.
[2]Barsony, T., and Koppenstein, E.: Beitrag zur Aufnahmetechnik der Halswirbelsäule; Darstellung der Foramina intervertebralia, Roentgenpraxis **1**:245-249, 1929.

CERVICAL INTERVERTEBRAL FORAMINA
Oblique posteroanterior projection
Oblique anteroposterior view
Position of part—cont'd

Semiprone position. With the patient's body at an angle of about 45 degrees and the cervical spine centered to the midline of the table, have the patient support himself on the forearm and flexed knee of the elevated side. Place sandbags under the ankles and the flexed knee. Adjust a suitable support under the head to place the long axis of the cervical column parallel with the film.

Check and adjust the degree of body rotation with a protractor or with a 45-degree cardboard triangle.

Adjust the position of the patient's head so that its median sagittal plane is coextensive with that of the spine, and extend the head just enough to prevent superimposition of the shadows of the mandibular rami and the intervertebral foramina.

When necessary, use a head clamp or a suitably backed strip of adhesive tape for immobilization; otherwise, have the patient softly phonate an m-m-m sound during the exposure.

Central ray

Direct the central ray to the fourth cervical vertebra at an angle of 15 to 20 degrees toward the feet so that it will coincide with the angle of the foramina.

Structures shown

A profile view of the intervertebral foramina and pedicles adjacent to the film, and an oblique view of the bodies and other parts of the cervical column.

Oblique flexion-extension projections

Bolyston[1] has suggested functional studies of the cervical vertebrae in the oblique position for the demonstration of fractures of the articular processes, and of obscure dislocations and subluxations, the manipulation of the patient's head to be performed by a physician when an acute injury has been sustained.

The patient is placed in a direct posteroanterior position, seated or standing erect, with his shoulders held firmly against the Potter-Bucky diaphragm. The head is then rotated maximally to one side and kept so, while the neck is flexed for the first exposure, and extended for the second exposure. Both sides are examined.

[1]Bolyston, B. F.: Oblique roentgenographic views of the cervical spine in flexion and extension; an aid in the diagnosis of cervical subluxations and obscure dislocations, J. Bone Joint Surg. 39-A:1302-1308, 1957.

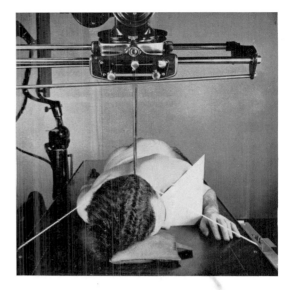

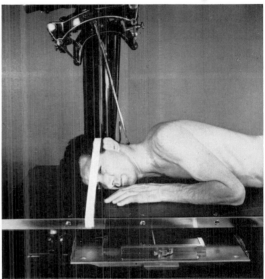

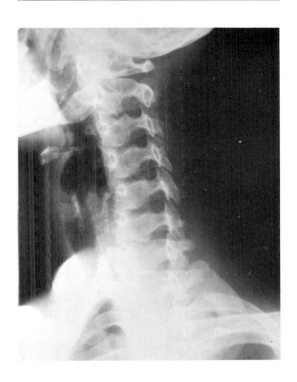

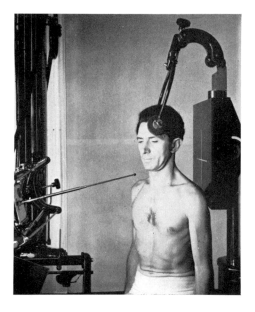

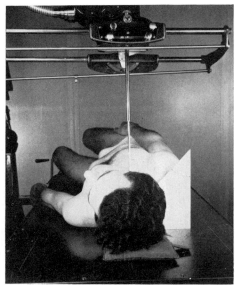

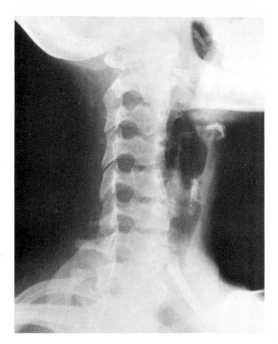

CERVICAL INTERVERTEBRAL FORAMINA
Oblique anteroposterior projection
Oblique posteroanterior view
Film: $8'' \times 10''$ lengthwise.

Position of patient

The patient is placed in the anteroposterior position. The erect position, standing or seated, is preferable for the patient's comfort and for greater ease of adjustment. The reader is referred to the comments made in the first paragraph on page 232.

Position of part

Adjust the body at approximately the 45-degree angle required to profile the foramina, and then center the cervical spine to the midline of the vertically placed cassette or the table.

To compensate for the cranial angulation of the central ray, center the film to the third cervical body (1 inch proximal to the most prominent point of the thyroid cartilage).

Erect position. Ask the patient to sit or stand straight without strain and to rest the adjacent shoulder firmly against the stand for support. Check and adjust the degree of body rotation with a protractor or with a 45-degree cardboard triangle. Being careful not to rotate the cervical spine, turn the head away from the side being examined (the side remote from the film) just enough to prevent superimposition of the shadows of the mandibular rami and the foramina.

When necessary, immobilize patient's head with a head clamp or by placing a cardboard box or other suitable support between the head and the cassette. Having the patient softly phonate an m-m-m sound during the exposure usually gives sufficient immobilization.

Semisupine position. With the patient's body rotated approximately 45 degrees and the cervical spine centered to the midline of the table, place suitable supports under the lower thorax and the elevated hip. Place a support under the head and adjust it so that the cervical column is horizontal.

Using a protractor or a 45-degree cardboard triangle, check and adjust the degree of body rotation. Turn the head just enough to prevent superimposition of the shadows of the mandibular rami and the foramina, being careful to avoid rotation of the cervical spine.

Central ray

Direct the central ray to the fourth cervical vertebra at an angle of 15 to 20 degrees toward the head, so that the beam coincides with the angle of the foramina.

Structures shown

A profile view of the intervertebral foramina and pedicles remote from the film, and an oblique view of the bodies and other parts of the cervical vertebrae.

CERVICAL VERTEBRAE
Intervertebral foramina
Oppenheimer method

This method of examining the intervertebral foramina requires a device consisting of two cassette tunnels standing at right angles to each other, each forming an angle of 45 degrees to the horizontal.

Film: 8″ × 10″ lengthwise.

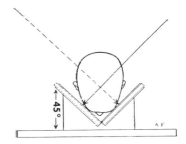

Position of patient

Place the patient in the prone position and center the median sagittal plane of the body to the midline of the table. If the patient is thin, place a pillow under the chest so that the long axis of the neck can be adjusted to lie parallel to the table without strain. Flex the elbows, place the arms in a comfortable position, and adjust the shoulders to lie in the same transverse plane.

Position of part

Place the cassette tunnel under the head and neck and center it to the midline of the table at the level of the fourth cervical vertebra.

Rest the patient's head on the forehead and nose within the tunnel device. When a head rest is not incorporated into the device, place a folded towel under the forehead and nose and adjust it so that the orbitomeatal line is vertical. Adjust the head so that its median sagittal plane is vertical.

The tunnel device usually affords sufficient support for the head. Respiration is suspended for the exposures.

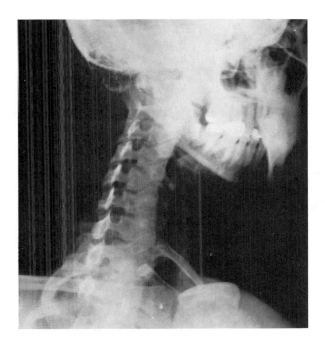

Central ray

The central ray is directed perpendicularly to the midpoint of the film, from the right side to project the left foramina, and from the left side to project the right foramina.

The focal-film distance should be at least 36 inches because of the comparatively great part-film distance.

Structures shown

An oblique view of the cervical vertebrae, demonstrating the intervertebral foramina. Both sides are examined for comparison.

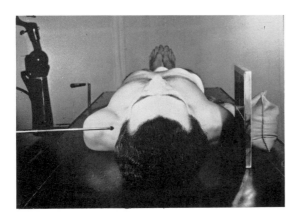

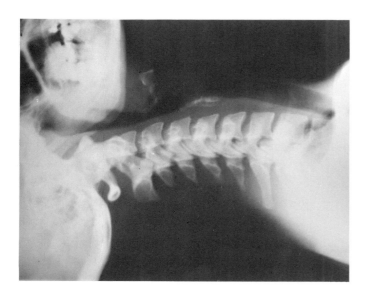

CERVICAL VERTEBRAE
Adaptation of positions to the severely injured patient

When a patient who has sustained a severe injury of the cervical spine arrives by stretcher or bed, he is not transferred to the radiographic table, and he must not be rotated. In order to obviate the possibility of damaging the spinal cord by the sharp edge of a bone fragment or by a subluxated vertebra as a result of movement, any necessary manipulation of the patient's head must be performed by a physician.

If there is no specially equipped emergency room, the initial examination is performed with a mobile unit or in an examining room that is large enough to accommodate the placement of a stretcher or bed where the x-ray tube can be brought into position for the required views.

Grid-front cassettes or a stationary grid should be used for the anteroposterior and oblique projections.

Lateral projection

The lateral view, taken by horizontal ray projection, presents no problem because it requires little or no adjustment of the patient's head and neck.

The cassette is placed in the vertical position, with its lower portion in contact with the shoulder, centered to the fourth cervical vertebra, and then immobilized with sandbags. The central ray is directed horizontally to the fourth cervical vertebra.

For the demonstration of the seventh cervical vertebra, the shoulders must be fully depressed. Depending upon the patient's condition, this can be done by looping a long strip of bandage around his feet and, with his knees slightly flexed, having him grasp the ends of the bandage and then extend his knees to pull the shoulders down. Otherwise, an assistant can depress the shoulders by applying symmetrical traction on the arms.

CERVICAL VERTEBRAE

Adaptation of positions to the severely injured patient—cont'd

Anteroposterior projections

For anteroposterior projections, the bottom sheet must be drawn tight and, with the patient's head held to prevent it from turning, lifted enough for the cassette to be slipped into position without appreciable movement of the patient's head and neck.

Two anteroposterior projections may be made: (1) a 15- to 20-degree cranial angulation of the central ray for the demonstration of the vertebral bodies and their interspaces, and (2) a 20- to 30-degree caudal angulation of the central ray for the demonstration of the posterior vertebral elements, the articular pillars and facets, the laminae, and the spinous processes. The latter study should be made on a 10″ × 12″ film in order to include the upper three or four thoracic vertebrae.

Oblique anteroposterior projection

For the demonstration of the pedicles and the intervertebral foramina, the film must be positioned near the side opposite the one being examined so that its midpoint will coincide with the 45-degree lateromedial angulation of the central ray.

Have the patient's head lifted slightly with the tightly drawn sheet, and with the cassette held so that its midpoint is at the level of the third cervical body, gently slide it under the head just far enough to center it under the adjacent mastoid process. This centering places the midline of the film approximately 3 inches lateral to the median sagittal plane of the neck.

From the opposite side—the side being projected—the central ray is directed to the fourth cervical vertebra at an eccentric angle of 45 degrees toward the median sagittal plane and 15 to 20 degrees toward the head.

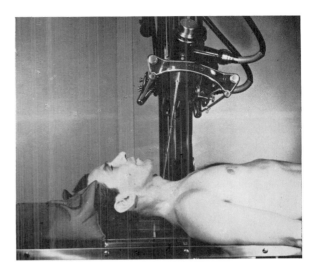

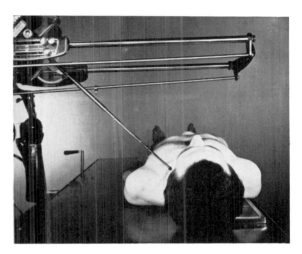

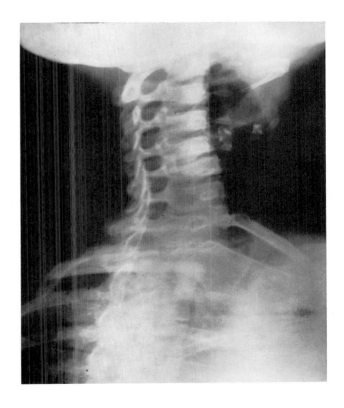

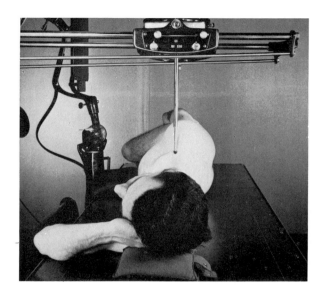

CERVICOTHORACIC REGION
Lateral projection
Pawlow position
Film: $10'' \times 12''$ lengthwise.

Position of patient

Place the patient in a lateral recumbent position with his head elevated on sandbags or small, firm pillows.

Position of part

Center the midaxillary line of the body to the midline of the table. Extend the patient's dependent arm and adjust it so as to place the humeral head either behind or in front of the vertebrae, the uppermost arm to be adjusted in the opposite direction. Adjust the support under the head, and place a folded sheet or loofah sponges under the lower thorax so that the long axis of the cervicothoracic vertebrae is horizontal.

Depress the upper shoulder, adjust it to separate the shoulder shadows, and immobilize it by having the patient grasp the dorsal surface of his thigh. Adjust the body in an exact lateral position.

Center the film at the level of the second or third thoracic vertebra.

Central ray

Direct the central ray to the midpoint of the film at an angle of 3 to 5 degrees toward the feet.

Structures shown

A lateral view of the cervicothoracic vertebrae projected between the shadows of the shoulders.

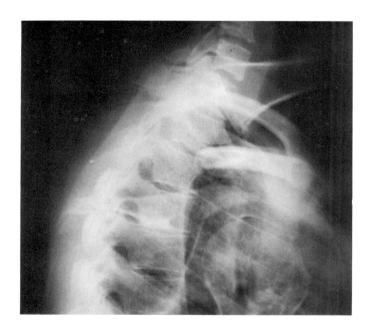

CERVICOTHORACIC REGION
Lateral projection
Twining position
Film: $10'' \times 12''$ lengthwise.

Position of patient

Place the patient in a lateral position, either seated or standing, before a vertical Potter-Bucky diaphragm. Have the patient sit or stand straight, and adjust the height of the cassette so that the film is centered at the level of the second thoracic vertebra.

Position of part

Center the mid-axillary line of the body to the midline of the film. Elevate the arm that is adjacent to the stand to a vertical position, flex the elbow, and rest the forearm on the patient's head.

Rotate the shoulder either backward or forward, according to what seems better for the individual patient; the opposite shoulder is rotated in the opposite direction. Move the patient close enough to the stand so that he can rest his shoulder firmly against it for support. Adjust the head so that its median sagittal plane is vertical.

Adjust the body in a true lateral position, with its median sagittal plane parallel with the plane of the film. Depress the shoulder that is remote from the film as much as possible, rotate it according to the placement of the opposite side, and immobilize it by having the patient hold a sandbag or an anchored strip of gauze. The goal is to have one shoulder rotated forward and the other backward just enough to prevent their superimposition on the shadow of the vertebrae. Respiration is suspended for the exposure.

Central ray

Direct the central ray to the midpoint of the film (1) perpendicularly if the shoulder is well depressed, or (2) at a caudal angle of 5 degrees when the shoulder cannot be well depressed.

Structures shown

A lateral view of the lower cervical and upper thoracic vertebrae, projected between the shadows of the shoulders.

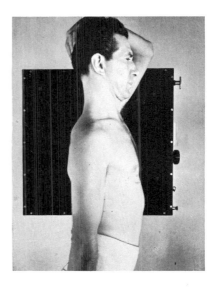

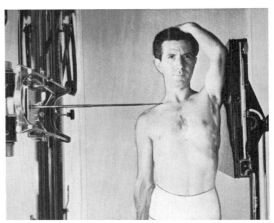

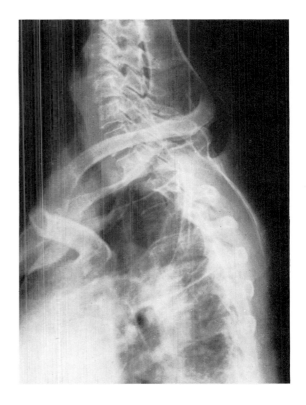

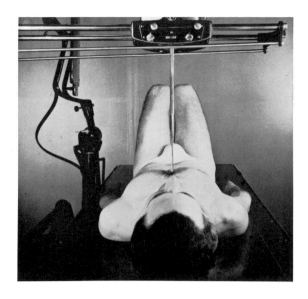

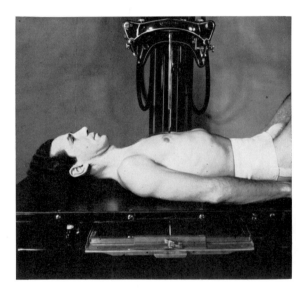

THORACIC VERTEBRAE
Anteroposterior projection
Posteroanterior view
Film: $14'' \times 17''$ lengthwise.

Position of patient

Place the patient in the anteroposterior position, either recumbent or erect. If the patient is supine, let the head rest directly on the table or on a thin pillow in order to avoid accentuating the dorsal kyphosis.

Position of part

Center the median sagittal plane of the body to the midline of the table or vertical Potter-Bucky diaphragm. Place the patient's arms along the sides of the body and adjust the shoulders to lie in the same transverse plane.

If the supine position is being used, further reduce the dorsal kyphosis by flexing the hips and knees enough to place the back in contact with the table. Adjust the thighs in a vertical position and immobilize the feet with sandbags. If the extremities cannot be flexed, support the knees on a long sandbag to relieve strain. Place another long sandbag under the ankles, invert the feet slightly, and immobilize them with sandbags.

When the erect position is used, have the patient stand so that his weight is equally distributed on the feet to prevent rotation of the vertebral column. If the lower extremities are of unequal length, place a support of correct height under the foot of the shorter side.

The patient may be allowed to breathe normally during the exposure unless his breathing is labored. In this case, respiration is suspended at the end of full exhalation in order to obtain a more uniform density. If compression is employed, the band should be applied at the level of the diaphragm.

The film is centered at the level of the sixth thoracic vertebra. Depending upon the stature of the patient, the anterior localization point will lie 3 to 4 inches distal to the manubrial notch; as a quick check, the upper edge of the film should lie 1½ to 2 inches above the upper border of the shoulders.

THORACIC VERTEBRAE
Anteroposterior projection
Posteroanterior view—cont'd
Central ray

Direct the central ray perpendicularly to the midpoint of the film.

As suggested by Fuchs,[1] a more uniform density of the thoracic vertebrae will be obtained if the "heel effect" of the tube is utilized. This is done by positioning the tube so that its long axis coincides with the median sagittal plane of the body, with the anode at the head end of the body, that is, with the anode facing caudally. With the tube in this position, the greatest concentration of the beam of radiation is projected toward the thickest region of the thoracic vertebrae, that is, toward the vertebrae situated behind the sternum and mediastinal structures and toward those below the diaphragm. Compare the radiographs.

Structures shown

An anteroposterior projection of the thoracic bodies, their interpediculate spaces, and the surrounding structures.

The intervertebral spaces are not well demonstrated unless the focal-film distance is adjusted to the center of the radius of the thoracic curve in order to place the spaces parallel with the divergent rays. This is not desirable as a routine procedure since, because it necessitates changing the focal-film distance for different patients, it results in varying degrees of magnification. It should be employed only when an anteroposterior projection of the spaces is indicated, and in conjunction with a roentgenogram made at the routine focal-film distance. A more practical method of demonstrating the disk spaces of a localized area is to angulate the central ray so that it forms a right angle to the long axis of the particular vertebral area. The degree of central ray angulation required can be estimated with reasonable accuracy by noting the angle of the dorsal curve at the area under investigation. Abnormal accentuation of the dorsal kyphosis requires that the patient be placed in the seated erect or decubitus position before a vertical Potter-Bucky diaphragm so that, by body adjustment, localized areas can be placed as nearly parallel with the film as possible.

[1]Fuchs, Arthur W.: Thoracic vertebrae, Radiogr. Clin. Photogr. **17**:2-13, 1941.

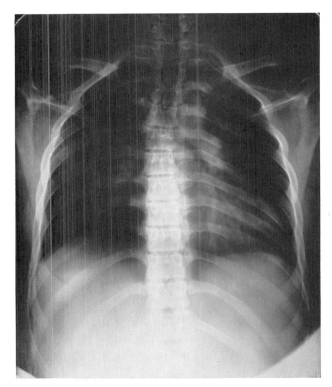

Anode facing cranially.

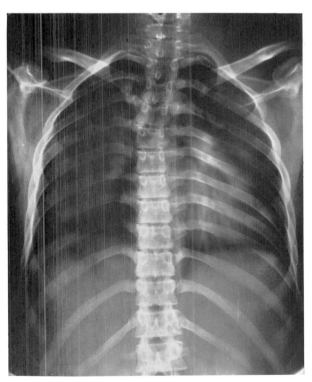

Anode facing caudally.

Radiographs courtesy Arthur W. Fuchs.

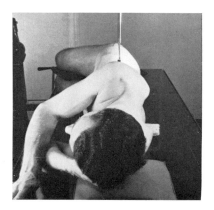

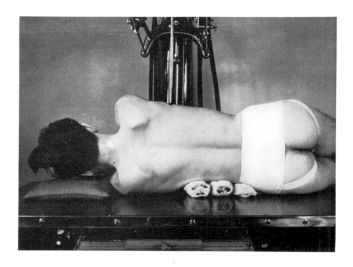

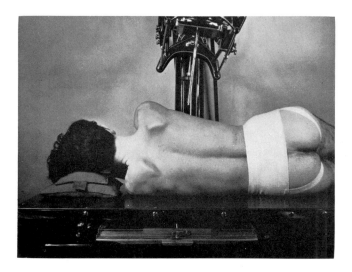

THORACIC VERTEBRAE
Lateral projection

Film: $14'' \times 17''$ lengthwise.

Position of patient

Place the patient in a lateral position, either recumbent or erect. If possible, the left lateral position should be used to place the heart closer to the film and thus minimize its shadow.

Oppenheimer[1] recommends the use of the orthostatic (erect) position to reproduce the physiologic conditions, and he says that the subject should be allowed to stand in a normal position—no attempt should be made to force him into an unwonted position, especially straightening of the vertebral column.

The patient should be dressed in an open-backed gown so that the vertebral column can be exposed for the adjustment of the position.

Recumbent position

Place a firm pillow or sandbags under the patient's head to elevate its median sagittal plane to the level of the long axis of the vertebral column. Flex the hips and knees to a comfortable position. Center the midaxillary line of the body to the midline of the table. Elevate the lower knee to hip level, support it on sandbags, and with the knees exactly superimposed to prevent rotation of the pelvis, place a small sandbag between them. Place sandbags under and between the ankles.

Adjust the arms at right angles to the long axis of the body to elevate the ribs enough to clear the intervertebral foramina. This placement of the arms gives a clear view of the vertebrae distal to the level of the glenohumeral joints. Drawing the arms forward or extending them to more than a right-angle position carries the scapulae forward where their shadows superimpose those of the upper thoracic vertebrae. Place the lower hand under the head or rest it on a sandbag beside the head. Have the patient grasp the side of the table with his upper hand and adjust its location so that the scapulae are in the same vertical plane.

Unless central ray angulation is to be used, place a folded sheet or loofah sponges under the lower thoracic region and adjust the position of the support so that the long axis of the vertebral column is horizontal.

Stand with your eyes in the vertical plane that passes down the posterior surface of the patient's back, and adjust the body in a true lateral position.

When necessary, apply a compression band across the trochanteric area of the pelvis. This does not interfere with the alignment of the body, as does a band placed higher. Respiration is suspended at the end of exhalation unless the exposure is to be made during quiet breathing.

[1]Oppenheimer, Albert: The apophyseal intervertebral articulations roentgenographically considered, Radiology **30**:724-740, 1938.

THORACIC VERTEBRAE
Lateral projection—cont'd

Erect position

Have the patient stand straight without strain, and then adjust the height of the Potter-Bucky diaphragm so that the midpoint of the film is at the level of the sixth thoracic vertebra. Center the midaxillary line of the body to the midline of the grid, and move the patient close enough to the stand to allow him to rest the adjacent shoulder firmly against the grid front for support.

The weight of the body must be equally distributed on the feet. If the extremities are of unequal length, place a support of correct height under the foot of the shorter side. Adjust the body so that the long axis of the vertebral column is parallel with the plane of the film.

In order to elevate the ribs, raise the arms to a position at right angles to the long axis of the body and support them in this position. An enema standard is very useful for this purpose; place it in front of the patient, immobilize it with sandbags, and, placing one of the patient's hands on the other for correct alignment of the arms, have him grasp the standard at the correct height.

The support of the upper extremities usually furnishes sufficient immobilization.

Breathing. In order to obliterate, or at least diffuse, overlapping shadows of the vascular markings and ribs, it is desirable to make the exposure during quiet breathing. This necessitates converting the basic milliampere-second factor to a low current–long time combination, a conversion allowing a time factor long enough to cover three or four phases of respiration. Heart action alone will usually satisfactorily diffuse vascular markings during an exposure of six or seven seconds, made on suspended respiration.

Central ray

Direct the central ray perpendicularly to the midpoint of the film.

If the vertebral column is not elevated to a horizontal plane when the patient is in a recumbent position, the tube should be tilted to direct the central ray at right angles to the long axis of the thoracic column, and then centered at the level of the sixth thoracic vertebra. An average angle of 10 degrees toward the head on female patients and, because of greater shoulder width, an average angle of 15 degrees on male patients is satisfactory for a majority of patients.

Structures shown

A lateral view of the thoracic bodies and their interspaces, the intervertebral foramina, and the lower spinous processes. Due to the overlapping shadows of the shoulders, the upper three or four segments are not demonstrated in this position.

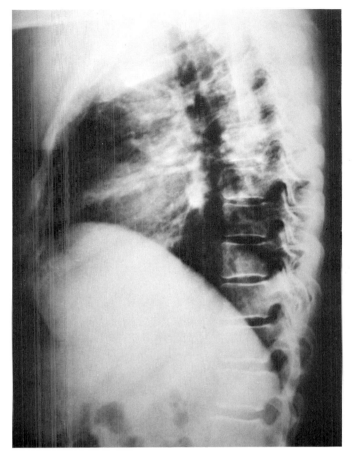

Suspended respiration for an exposure of ¾ second.

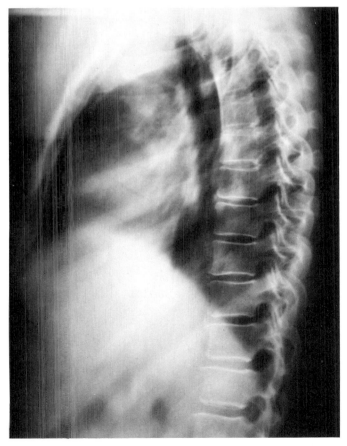

Suspended respiration for an exposure of 7½ seconds on above patient.

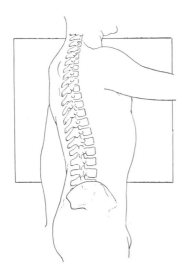

THORACIC VERTEBRAE
Apophysial articulations
Oblique projection

The thoracic apophysial joints may be examined by forward rotation of the body, as recommended by Oppenheimer,[1] or by backward rotation of the body, as recommended by Fuchs.[2] The joints are well demonstrated with either position, those of the side nearer the film with forward rotation, and those of the side farther from the film with backward rotation. While the difference in part-film distance between the two positions is not great, the same method of rotation should be used bilaterally in each case.

Film: $14'' \times 17''$ lengthwise.

Erect position

Position of patient

Place the patient in a lateral position before a vertical Potter-Bucky diaphragm. Adjust the height of the grid to center the film to the sixth thoracic vertebra.

Position of part

Rotate the body slightly, either forward or backward, so that the coronal plane forms an angle of 70 degrees with the plane of the film (the median sagittal plane forming an angle of 20 degrees with the film). Center the vertebral column to the midline of the Potter-Bucky diaphragm, and have the patient rest the adjacent shoulder firmly against it for support.

Flex the elbow of the arm adjacent to the stand and rest the hand on the hip. If the patient is rotated forward, have him grasp the side of the stand for support; if he is rotated backward, place his hand on his hip. Adjust the shoulders to lie in the same transverse plane.

Have the patient stand straight to place the long axis of the vertebral column parallel with the film. The weight of the body must be equally distributed on the feet, and the head must not be turned laterally.

Adjust the rotation of the body so that, according to the method of rotation, either the anterior or the posterior surface of the thorax will just touch the hypotenuse of a 20-degree cardboard triangle.

Having the shoulder rest against the Potter-Bucky stand usually furnishes sufficient support. Respiration is suspended at the end of exhalation.

[1]Oppenheimer, Albert: The apophyseal intervertebral articulations roentgenologically considered, Radiology **30**:724-740, 1938.
[2]Fuchs, A. W.: Thoracic vertebrae (part 2), Radiogr. Clin. Photogr. **17**:42-51, 1941.

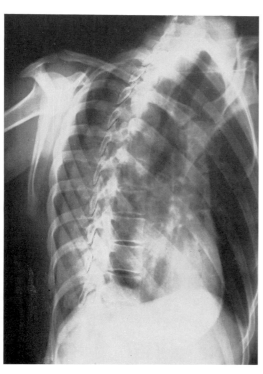

Forward rotation.

THORACIC VERTEBRAE
Apophysial articulations
Oblique projection—cont'd
Recumbent position

Position of patient

Place the patient in a lateral recumbent position. Elevate the head on sandbags or a firm pillow so that its median sagittal plane is continuous with that of the vertebral column. Flex the patient's hips and knees to a comfortable position.

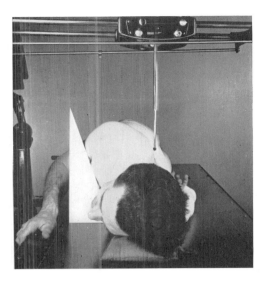

Position of part

For forward rotation, place the dependent arm behind the back. Have the patient grasp the side of the table with the opposite hand to aid in maintaining the position.

For backward rotation, adjust the dependent arm at right angles to the long axis of the body, flex the elbow, and place the hand under or beside the head. After the body has been adjusted, draw the opposite arm backward and support it on sandbags.

Rotate the body slightly, either forward or backward as preferred, so that the coronal plane forms an angle of 70 degrees with the horizontal (20 degrees with the vertical). Center the vertebral column to the midline of the table and then check and adjust the body rotation. This is done by placing the hypotenuse of a 20-degree cardboard triangle in contact with the thorax—at its anterior surface for forward rotation, or at its posterior surface for backward rotation—and then adjusting the body so that the chest or back will just touch the edge of the triangle.

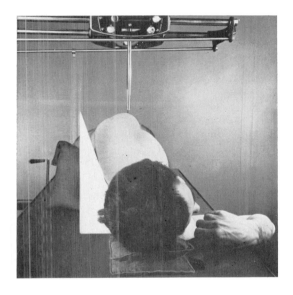

A compression band may be applied across the hips, but care must be used not to change the position. Respiration is suspended for the exposure.

With the cassette in the Potter-Bucky tray, center at the level of the sixth thoracic vertebra.

Central ray

Direct the central ray perpendicularly to the midpoint of the film.

Structures shown

An oblique view of the thoracic vertebrae, demonstrating the apophysial articulations. The number of joints shown depends upon the dorsal curve. A greater degree of rotation from the lateral position is required to show the joints at the proximal and distal ends of the region on patients having an accentuated dorsal kyphosis. The inferior facets of the twelfth thoracic vertebra, having an inclination of about 45 degrees, are not shown in this position.

NOTE: The backward rotation position gives an excellent demonstration of the cervicothoracic spinous processes and is used for this purpose when the patient cannot be satisfactorily positioned for a direct lateral projection.

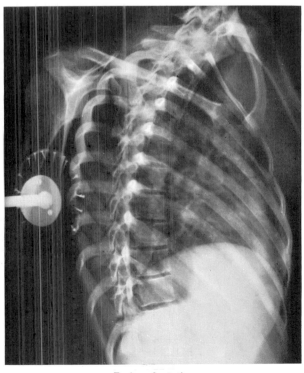

Backward rotation.

Courtesy Arthur W. Fuchs.

LUMBAR-LUMBOSACRAL VERTEBRAE

Frontal projections

It is desirable to have the intestinal tract free of gas and fecal material for examinations of the bones lying within the abdominal and pelvic regions. When bowel action is costive and it is possible to prepare the patient, he should be given either a nongas-forming cathartic or a saline enema, or both. The urinary bladder should be emptied just before the examination to eliminate the shadow cast by, and the secondary radiation set up within, the filled bladder; this is especially important in examinations of older male subjects, in whom it is frequently possible to detect prostatic enlargement, as shown by urinary retention.

Film: $14'' \times 17''$ for general survey examinations.

Position of patient

The frontal projection of the lumbar-lumbosacral spine may be taken from either the anteroposterior or the posteroanterior direction, and with the patient either recumbent or erect. Acute back disorders are excruciatingly painful. The technologist can spare the ambulatory patient much distress by radiographing him in the erect position whenever possible. When the patient cannot maintain the erect position without movement, he should be placed and positioned on the footboard of the elevated tilt table for each change in position and then returned to the horizontal position. This procedure takes a few minutes, but it nets a most grateful patient.

Because the posteroanterior position presents the concave side of the lordotic curve to the x-ray tube, it places the intervertebral disk spaces at an angle closely paralleling the divergence of the beam of radiation. For this reason, the posteroanterior position is used for erect studies of the lumbar-lumbosacral spine. The position does not increase the part-film distance, except with subjects who have an excessively large abdomen. When used in the recumbent position, it has the advantage of being more comfortable for the patient with a painful back and is especially more comfortable for the emaciated patient.

The anteroposterior position is generally used for recumbent examinations and, unfortunately, generally with the back fully arched by extension of the lower extremities. The extended position accentuates the lordotic curve, which in turn increases the angle between the vertebral bodies and the divergent rays, with resultant distortion of the bodies as well as poor delineation of the intervertebral disk spaces. The lordotic curve can be reduced and the intervertebral disk spaces clearly delineated in the anteroposterior direction simply by flexing the hips and knees enough to place the back in firm contact with the table.

Comparison of the films below shows that when the patient is correctly adjusted in the supine position, there is little difference between the anteroposterior and posteroanterior projections. This leaves only the patient's comfort to be considered.

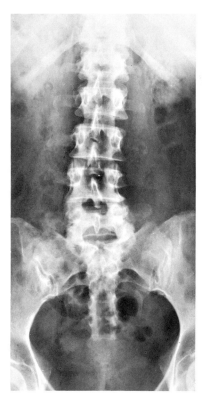

Anteroposterior projection, the extremities extended.

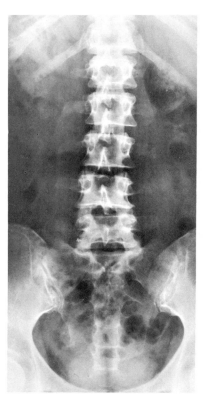

Anteroposterior projection, the extremities flexed.

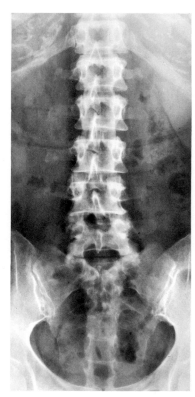

Posteroanterior projection. All projections are of the same patient.

LUMBAR-LUMBOSACRAL VERTEBRAE
Frontal projections—cont'd
Position of part

Supine position. Center the median sagittal plane of the body to the midline of the table. In order to prevent rotation of the spine, adjust the shoulders to lie in the same transverse plane and adjust the head so that its median sagittal plane is coextensive with that of the spine. So that the forearms will not lie within the exposure field, flex the patient's elbows and place his hands on the upper chest. When a soft tissue abnormality (atrophy or swelling) is causing rotation of the pelvis, adjust a radioparent support under the lower side.

In order to delineate the intervertebral disk spaces, it is necessary to adjust them at an angle closely paralleling that of the divergent beam of radiation. This requires that the lumbar lordosis be reduced by flexing the hips and knees enough to place the back in firm contact with the table. Have the patient lean his knees together for support, and then immobilize the feet with sandbags.

When the knees cannot be flexed and the patient cannot be turned for a posteroanterior projection, place supports under the knees to relieve strain. Place a sandbag under the ankles, grasp the heels and invert the feet 15 to 20 degrees, and immobilize them with sandbags.

Prone position. Center the median sagittal plane of the body to the midline of the table. Place a long sandbag under the ankles and adjust it to relieve pressure on the toes.

With the elbows flexed, adjust the arms and forearms in a comfortable, bilaterally symmetrical position. Adjust the shoulders to lie in the same transverse plane, and have the patient rest his head on the chin to prevent rotation of the spine.

Film centering

The 14" × 17" film is centered at the level of the iliac crests. Care must be used to palpate for the crest of the bone in order to avoid being misled by the contour of the heavy muscles and fatty tissue lying above it.

When two 10" × 12" films are used, the first is centered to the third lumbar body (at the level of the inferior mid-axillary costal margin), and the central ray is directed vertically. The second film is centered to coincide with the cranially or caudally angulated central ray, which is directed through the lumbosacral joint.

Central ray

Direct the central ray vertically to the midpoint of the film for the general survey study.

Structures shown

A frontal view (anteroposterior or posteroanterior) of the lumbar bodies and their intervening disk spaces, the interpediculate spaces, the laminae, and the spinous and transverse processes. When the larger film is used, one or two of the lower thoracic vertebrae, the sacrum and coccyx, the pelvic bones, and the hip joints are included. Because of the angle at which the last lumbar segment joins the sacrum, the lumbosacral disk space is not well shown in direct frontal projections. The positions used for this purpose are described on the two following pages.

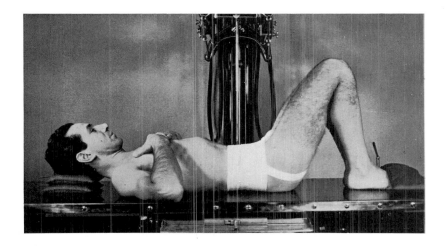

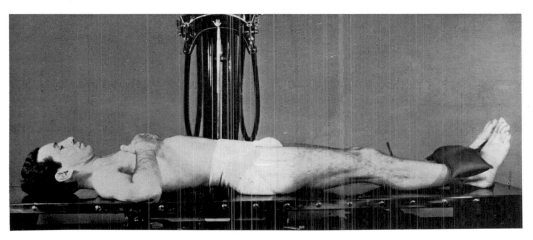

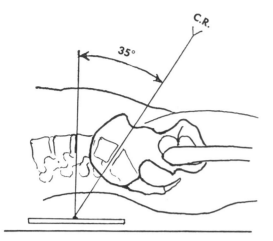

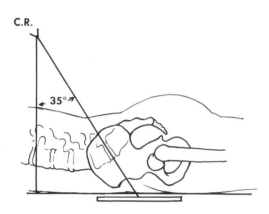

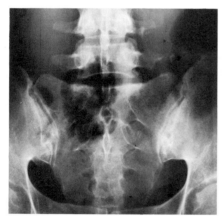

Anteroposterior projection.

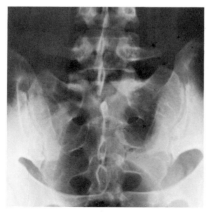

Posteroanterior projection.

LUMBOSACRAL JUNCTION AND SACROILIAC JOINTS
Frontal projections
Film: $8'' \times 10''$ or $10'' \times 12''$ lengthwise.

Position of patient

The semiaxial projection, which is required for the demonstration of the lumbosacral and sacroiliac joints, is made with the patient in the same position as for, and usually immediately following, the frontal projection of the lumbar vertebrae.

If the patient was in the prone position for the frontal projection, no change is required for the semiaxial projection. If he is in the supine position, the lower extremities may be extended to remove them from the path of the cranially angulated central ray, or the thighs may be abducted and adjusted in the vertical position or in a hyperflexed position in order to place the lumbosacral joint in a nearly vertical position.

In each of these positions, the central ray is directed through the lumbosacral junction. This joint is situated 1½ inches posterior to the midaxillary line at the intersection of the median sagittal plane and the transverse plane that passes midway between the iliac crests and the anterior superior iliac spines.

Supine extended position

With the patient supine and his lower extremities extended, direct the central ray through the lumbosacral joint at an average angle of 30 to 35 degrees toward the head.

An angulation of 30 degrees for the male patient and of 35 degrees for the female patient is satisfactory in a majority of subjects. By noting the contour of the lower back, unusual accentuation or diminution of the lumbosacral angle can be estimated and the central ray angulation varied accordingly.

Prone position

Lumbosacral joint. Direct the central ray through the joint to the midpoint of the film at an average angle of 35 degrees toward the feet; it will enter at, or just distal to, the spinous process of the fourth lumbar segment.

Sacroiliac joints. Direct the central ray vertically and center at the level of the anterior superior iliac spines; it will enter about 2 inches distal to the spinous process of the fifth lumbar segment.

Meese[1] recommends the prone position for examinations of the sacroiliac joints because, due to their obliquity, it places them in a position more nearly parallel with the divergence of the beam of radiation.

[1]Meese, T.: Die dorso-ventrale Aufnahme der Sacroiliacalgelenke, Fortschr. Roentgenstr. **85**:601-603, 1956.

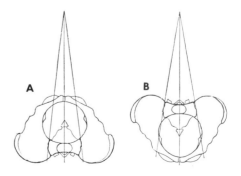

LUMBOSACRAL JUNCTION AND SACROILIAC JOINTS

Frontal projections—cont'd

Supine flexed positions

The anteroposterior flexed positions for the lumbosacral junction were described by Warner[1] and Samuel[2] in 1929. They found that flexion of the thighs, by tilting the pelvis forward and cranialward, straightens the lordotic curve and thus places the plane of the joint in a nearly vertical position. A less distorted view of the joint is obtained, when it is so placed, than is possible with central ray angulation alone.

Elevate the patient's head and shoulders on two firm pillows to relieve strain on the neck and chest muscles and to aid the patient in achieving full flexion in the Samuel position. Adjust the patient's gown or a draw sheet so that he will be well covered when his thighs are flexed and abducted.

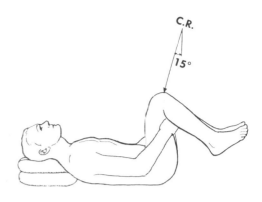

Have the patient flex his hips and knees and draw his feet up near his hips. Localize the lumbosacral junction, and center the central ray and film before adjusting the extremities in the final position.

Warner lithotomy position. Bring each thigh to the vertical position, abduct it enough to clear the path of the beam of radiation, and then support the foot on a stack of sandbags. Many patients are able to grasp the flexed knees and thus hold the thighs in the vertical position for the short time necessary for the exposure.

Direct the central ray through the lumbosacral joint at an angle of 15 degrees toward the head.

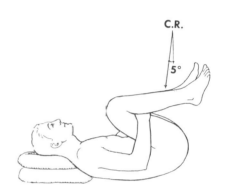

Samuel hyperflexed position. Have the patient grasp his flexed knees, abduct them widely so that the abdomen will not prevent full flexion, and then pull the thighs up as close as possible to his body. A majority of patients are able to maintain this position without difficulty.

Direct the central ray through the lumbosacral joint at an angle of 5 degrees toward the head.

[1]Warner, F.: Studien zur Pathologie des Lumbosakralgebietes, Verhandl. Deutsch. Ges. Unfallheilkunde, Sept., 1929.
[2]Samuel, M.: Ueber Ausbau und Bedeutung einer röntgenologischen Darstellung der Beckengelenk, Roentgenpraxis 1:944-947, 1929.

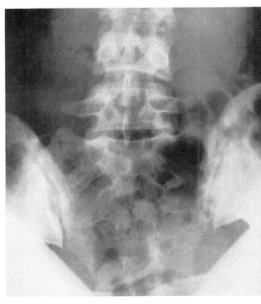

Lithotomy projection.

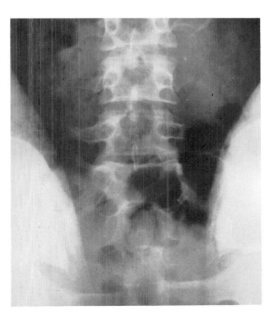

Hyperflexed projection.

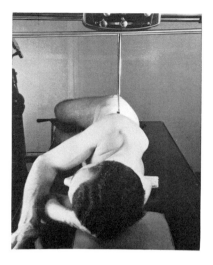

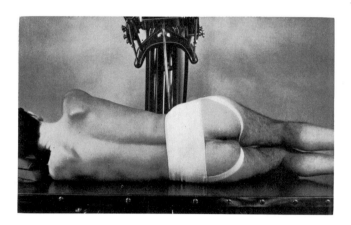

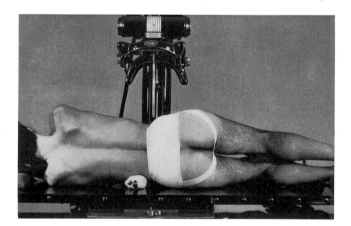

LUMBAR-LUMBOSACRAL VERTEBRAE
Lateral projections

Film: $14'' \times 17''$ for general survey examinations.

The high kilovoltage techniques that are permissible on most present-day radiographic equipment produce a more uniform overall film density, giving adequate exposure to the lumbosacral area without overexposure of the lumbar vertebrae. This permits the use of one film, and one exposure to the patient, for all patients except narrow-waisted, unusually wide-hipped persons, on whom it is necessary to take a localized projection of the lumbosacral junction.

Position of patient

The body position (recumbent or erect) used for the frontal projection is maintained for the lateral projection.

It is desirable to have the patient dressed in an open-back gown so that the spine can be exposed for final adjustment of the position.

Recumbent position
Position of part

Ask the patient to turn onto the indicated side and to flex his hips and knees to a comfortable position. When examining a thin patient, adjust a suitable pad under the dependent hip to relieve pressure.

Center the midaxillary line of the body to the midline of the table; the student must keep in mind that no matter how large or obese the patient, the long axis of the spine is situated in the midaxillary line.

Adjust the pillow so as to place the median sagittal plane of the head coextensive with that of the spine. With the patient's elbow flexed, adjust the dependent arm at right angles to his body. Ask the patient to grasp the side of the table with his opposite hand; then adjust its position to place the scapulae in the same vertical plane.

In order to prevent rotation, exactly superimpose the knees, elevate the dependent knee to hip level, and support it on a sandbag. A small sandbag may be placed between the knees, and others may be placed under and between the ankles for the patient's comfort.

Unless central ray angulation is to be used, place a suitable radioparent support under the lower thorax and adjust it so that the long axis of the spine is horizontal. Recheck the position for rotation. Rotation can be detected and easily corrected by standing so as to look down the back while adjusting the position.

When using a large film, center at the level of the iliac crest. When using two $10'' \times 12''$ films, the first is centered at the level of the third lumbar segment. For the lumbosacral area, move the film backward about 3 inches and center it at the level of the anterior superior iliac spines. The central ray is not moved from the midaxillary line of the body for the second exposure.

Central ray

After the spine has been adjusted in the horizontal position, direct the central ray vertically to the midpoint of the film.

LUMBAR-LUMBOSACRAL VERTEBRAE
Lateral projections
Central ray—cont'd

When the spine is not adjusted in the horizontal position, the central ray is directed at right angles to its long axis. The degree of central ray angulation depends upon the angulation of the lumbar column, which, in turn, depends upon the breadth of the pelvis. An average caudal angle of 5 degrees for male patients, and of 8 degrees for the wider-hipped, female patients, is satisfactory in a majority of cases.

Erect position
Position of part

With the film centered as for the posteroanterior projection, ask the patient to turn to the lateral position, and then center the midaxillary line of the body to the midline of the Potter-Bucky grid. Immobilize by placing a standard in front of the patient and having him grasp it with both hands at shoulder height.

Care must be taken to see that the patient stands normally erect. Subjects who have severe low back pain tend to relieve the discomfort by tilting the pelvis forward and upward. This movement reduces the lumbosacral angle and thus defeats the aim to demonstrate it in the orthostatic (erect) position. The weight of the body must be equally distributed on the feet.

Central ray

The central ray is directed horizontally to the midpoint of the film.

Structures shown

A lateral view of the lumbar bodies and their interspaces, the spinous processes, the lumbosacral junction, and the sacrum and coccyx. This projection gives a profile view of the upper four lumbar intervertebral foramina. The last lumbar intervertebral foramina (right and left) are not usually well visualized in this position because of their oblique direction. Oblique projections and the special Kovács position are used for these foramina.

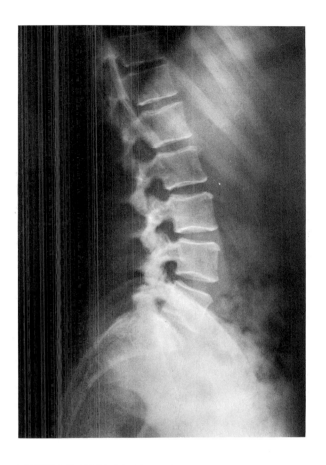

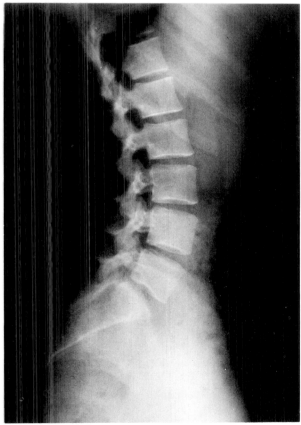

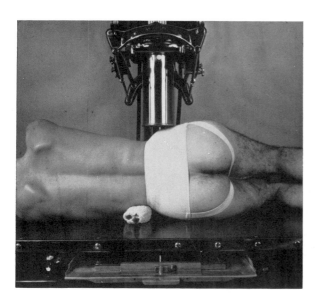

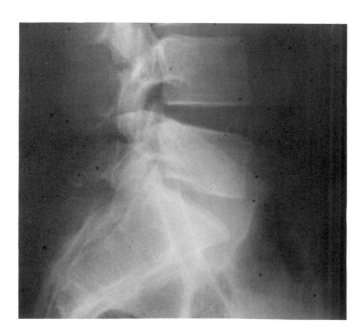

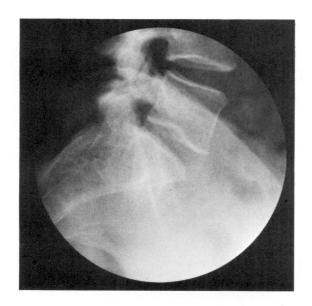

LUMBOSACRAL JUNCTION
Localized lateral projection

Film: $8'' \times 10''$ lengthwise.

Position of patient

Ferguson[1] recommended that the lumbosacral region be examined in the recumbent position because patients who have low back pain tend, when erect, to assume a protective position that reduces the lumbosacral angle. He further recommended that questionable cases be checked with a lateral projection made in the erect position as well as in the usual recumbent position.

Position of part

In order to center the laterally positioned lumbosacral joint to the film, align the patient's body so that the coronal plane passing 1½ inches posterior to the midaxillary line is centered to the midline of the table or of the vertical Potter-Bucky diaphragm.

With the patient in the recumbent position, adjust the pillow to place the median sagittal plane of the head coextensive with that of the spine. With the patient's elbow flexed, adjust the dependent arm in a position at right angles to the body. Have the patient grasp the side of the table with the opposite hand, and then adjust its position to place the scapulae in the same vertical plane.

It is desirable to have the hips fully extended for this study. When this cannot be done, extend them as much as possible and support the dependent knee at hip level on sandbags. Place sandbags under and between the ankles and knees.

Place a support under the lower thorax and adjust it so that the long axis of the spine is horizontal. Recheck the position and adjust the body so that there is no rotation.

With the cassette in the Potter-Bucky tray, center the film at the level of the transverse plane that passes midway between the iliac crests and the anterior superior iliac spines.

Central ray

Direct the central ray perpendicularly to the midpoint of the film.

When the spine is not adjusted in the horizontal position, the central ray is angled caudally, 5 degrees for males and 8 degrees for females; it enters midway between the level of the iliac crest and anterior superior iliac spine.

Structures shown

A lateral view of the lumbosacral joint, the lower one or two lumbar vertebrae, and the upper sacrum.

[1]Ferguson, A. B.: Roentgen diagnosis of the extremities and spine, enlarged ed. 1, New York, 1941, Harper & Row, Publishers.

LAST LUMBAR INTERVERTEBRAL FORAMINA
Oblique semiaxial projection
Kovács position[1]
Film: 8″ × 10″ lengthwise.

Position of patient

The patient is placed in the recumbent position and alternately turned onto the side being examined.

Position of part

Adjust the patient in the lateral position and align the body so that the coronal plane that passes 1½ inches posterior to the midaxillary line is centered to the midline of the table. Have the patient extend the uppermost arm and grasp the end of the table to aid in maintaining the thorax in the lateral position when the pelvis is rotated.

Keeping the patient's thorax exactly lateral, rotate the

[1]Kovács, Ákos: X-ray examination of the exit of the lowermost lumbar root, Radiol. Clin. **19:**6-13, 1950.

pelvis 30 degrees forward from the lateral position. Place a sandbag support under the flexed uppermost knee to prevent too much rotation of the hips. Check and adjust the degree of rotation with a protractor.

Adjust the position of the film so that its midpoint will coincide with the central ray.

Central ray

Tilt the tube to direct the central ray along a straight line extending from the superior edge of the uppermost iliac crest through the fifth lumbar segment to the inguinal region of the dependent side. According to the tilt of the spine, the central ray angulation will vary from 15 to 30 degrees toward the feet.

Structures shown

A profile view of the lowermost lumbar intervertebral foramen. Both sides are examined for comparison.

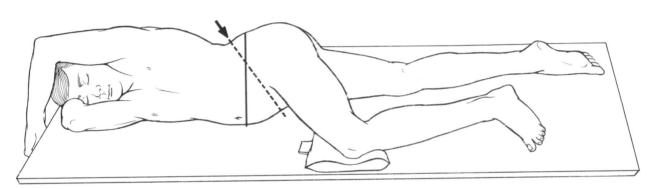

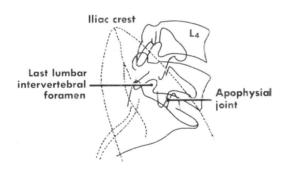

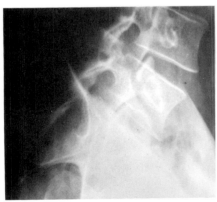

Kovács projection.

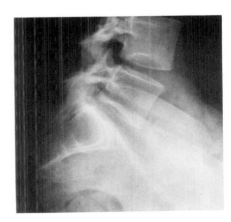

Direct lateral projection on opposite patient.

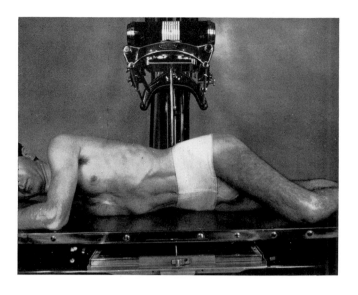

LUMBAR-LUMBOSACRAL APOPHYSIAL JOINTS
Posterior oblique projections
Anterior oblique views

The articular facets of the lumbar vertebrae form an angle of 45 degrees, and those between the last lumbar vertebra and the sacrum form an angle of 30 degrees, to the median sagittal plane in a majority of patients. The angulation does vary, however, not only from patient to patient but from side to side in the same patient. Exact adjustment of the part on the first examination makes it possible to determine any necessary change in rotation for further studies.

Film: 11″ × 14″ lengthwise; 8″ × 10″ for the last apophysial joints.

Position of patient

The patient may be examined in either the erect or the recumbent position. The latter is generally used because it facilitates immobilization.

Greater ease in positioning the patient, and a resultant higher percentage of success in duplicating results, make the semiprone position preferable to the semisupine position.

Position of part

Unless the patient is dressed in an open-back gown, cover the lower part of the body with a draw sheet and expose the back. With the patient prone, make a wax pencil mark over the spinous process of the third lumbar segment to indicate the centering point for the film; make a mark just distal to the spinous process of the fifth lumbar segment to indicate the centering point for the last joint. Make a mark 2 inches to each side of the first mark to localize the center of the spine when the patient is rotated to the oblique position.

Posterior oblique projection.

LUMBAR-LUMBOSACRAL APOPHYSIAL JOINTS

Posterior oblique projections
Anterior oblique views
Position of part—cont'd

Have the patient turn to a semiprone position and support himself on the forearm and flexed knee of the elevated side. Align the body so as to center the previously marked plane of the elevated side to the midline of the table.

With the use of a protractor or a cardboard triangle, check and, if necessary, adjust the degree of body rotation. It is adjusted at an angle of 45 degrees for the lumbar region, and at an angle of 30 degrees from the horizontal for the lumbosacral apophysial joint.

Center the film at the level of the previously marked localization point for the area being examined.

Central ray

Direct the central ray perpendicularly to the midpoint of the film.

Structures shown

An oblique view of the lumbar and/or the lumbosacral vertebrae, demonstrating the articular facets of the side farther from the film. The articulation between the twelfth thoracic and first lumbar vertebrae, having the same direction as those in the lumbar region, is shown on the larger film.

The last intervertebral foramen is usually well shown in oblique projections.

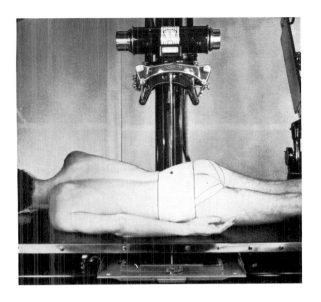

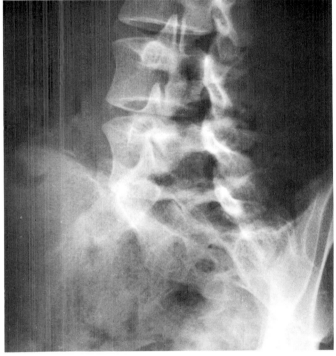

Posterior oblique projection.

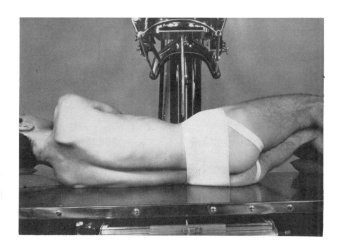

LUMBAR-LUMBOSACRAL APOPHYSIAL JOINTS
Anterior oblique projections
Posterior oblique views

Film: $11'' \times 14''$ lengthwise; $8'' \times 10''$ for last apophysial joint.

Position of patient

Oblique views are, when indicated, taken immediately following the frontal view and in the same body position—recumbent or erect. The recumbent position is described because it is more frequently used, but the directions can be easily adapted to the erect position.

Position of part

Have the patient turn from the supine position to the approximate degree of obliquity to be used. Center the spine to the midline of the table. In the oblique position, the lumbar spine overlies the longitudinal plane that passes along the dependent side 2 inches lateral to the spinous processes.

Ask the patient to place the dependent arm in a comfortable position and to grasp the side of the table with the opposite hand to aid in maintaining the position. Place suitable supports under the elevated shoulder, the hip, and the knee.

With the use of a protractor or a cardboard triangle, check and adjust the degree of body rotation. It is adjusted at an angle of 45 degrees for the demonstration of the articular facets in the lumbar region, and at an angle of 30 degrees from the horizontal plane for the demonstration of the lumbosacral facets.

Center the film at the level of the third lumbar segment for the lumbar region, and at the level of the transverse plane passing midway between the iliac crests and the anterior superior iliac spines for the last apophysial joint.

Central ray

Direct the central ray perpendicularly to the midpoint of the film.

Structures shown

An oblique view of the lumbar and/or the lumbosacral spine, demonstrating the articular facets of the side nearer the film. Both sides are examined for comparison.

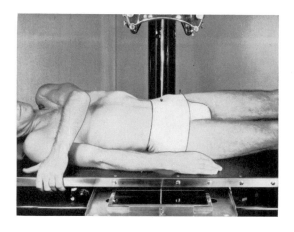

Anterior oblique projection.

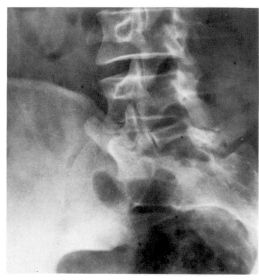

Anterior oblique projection.

LUMBAR INTERVERTEBRAL DISKS
Weight-bearing flexion and extension studies
Duncan-Hoen method of determining level of disk herniation

Film: 14″ × 17″ lengthwise.

Position of patient

This examination is made with the patient in the standing position. Duncan and Hoen[1] recommend that the posteroanterior position be used because, in this direction, the divergent rays are more nearly parallel with the interspaces.

With the patient standing before a vertical Potter-Bucky stand, adjust the height of the film so that its midpoint is at the level of the third lumbar vertebra. This centering will include several of the thoracic interspaces as well as all of the lumbar interspaces.

Position of part

Center the median sagittal plane of the patient's body to the midline of the Potter-Bucky stand and adjust the body in a true posteroanterior position. Let the arms hang unsupported by the sides.

One radiograph is made with right bending, and one with left bending. Have the patient lean directly laterally as far as is possible without rotation and without lifting his foot. The degree of leaning must not be forced, and the patient must not be supported in position.

Central ray

Direct the central ray to the midpoint of the film at an angle of 15 to 20 degrees toward the feet.

Structures shown

Two posteroanterior projections of the lower thoracic and the lumbar regions in lateral flexion for the demonstration of the mobility of the intervertebral joints. This method of examination is used in cases of disk protrusion to localize the involved joint as shown by limitation of motion at the site of the lesion.

Duncan and Hoen[1] also recommend that lateral views be made with the patient in extreme flexion and in extreme extension to demonstrate mechanical obstruction of the posterior portion of the intervertebral joints. The method of positioning for these studies is shown in the accompanying drawings. Again, the degree of leaning must not be forced, and the patient must not be supported in position.

[1]Duncan, William, and Hoen, Thomas: A new approach to the diagnosis of herniation of the intervertebral disc, Surg. Gynec. Obstet. **75**:257-267, 1942.

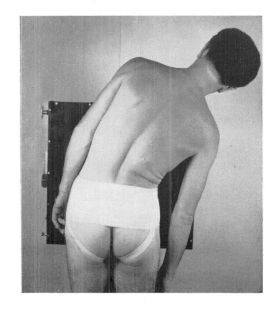

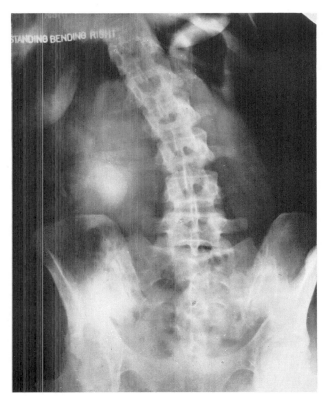

Courtesy Dr. Raymond W. Lewis.

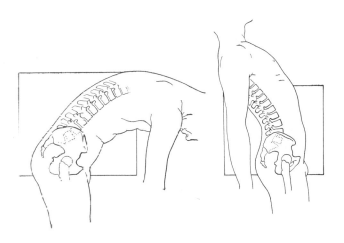

SACROILIAC JOINTS
Posterior oblique projection
Anterior oblique view

Film: 8″ × 10″ or 10″ × 12″ lengthwise.

Position of patient

Place the patient in a semiprone position, the side being examined adjacent to the table, and have him rest on the forearm and flexed knee of the elevated side. Place a small, firm pillow under the head.

Position of part

Adjust the rotation so that the upper side is elevated about 25 degrees, and then align the body so that a longitudinal plane passing 1 inch medial to the dependent anterior superior iliac spine is centered to the midline of the table. Adjust the shoulders to lie in the same transverse plane. Place sandbags under the ankles and under the flexed knee. Adjust the position of the elevated thigh so that the anterior superior iliac spines lie in the same transverse plane.

Using a 25- or 30-degree cardboard triangle to check the rotation, adjust the body so that the anterior superior iliac spines just touch the hypotenuse of the triangle. Check the degree of rotation at several points along the anterior surface of the body.

The forearm and flexed knee usually furnish sufficient support for this position. Respiration need not be suspended for the exposure unless the patient's breathing is labored.

Adjust the position of the film so that its midpoint will coincide with the central ray.

Central ray

1. With the central ray perpendicular to the plane of the film, center at the level of the anterior superior iliac spines.

2. With the central ray at an angle of 20 to 25 degrees toward the feet, center at the level of the transverse plane passing 1½ inches distal to the fifth lumbar spinous process; it will exit at the level of the anterior superior iliac spine.

Structures shown

A profile view of the sacroiliac joint nearer the film. Both sides are examined for comparison.

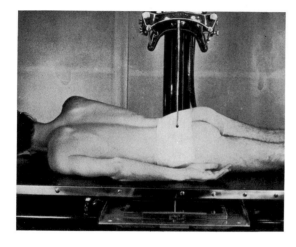

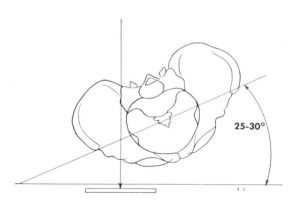

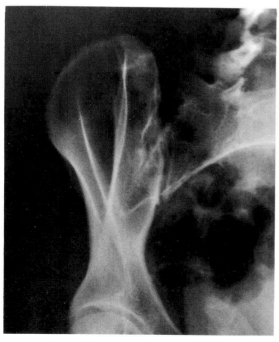

Central ray perpendicular.

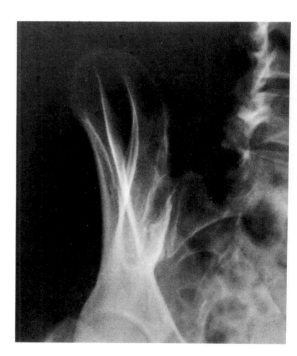

Central ray angled 25 degrees.

SACROILIAC JOINTS
Anterior oblique projection
Posterior oblique view

Film: 8″ × 10″ or 10″ × 12″ lengthwise.

Position of patient

Place the patient in the supine position and elevate the head on a firm pillow.

Position of part

Elevate the side being examined approximately 25 degrees and support the shoulder, the lower thorax, and the upper thigh on sandbags. Align the body so that the sagittal plane passing 1 inch medial to the anterior superior iliac spine of the elevated side is centered to the midline of the table. Place the dependent arm in a comfortable position, have the patient grasp the side of the table with the opposite hand to aid in maintaining the position, and then adjust his shoulders to lie in the same transverse plane.

Adjust the position of the elevated thigh—that is, pull it downward or push it upward—to place the anterior superior iliac spines in the same transverse plane. Place sandbag supports under the knee to elevate it to hip level.

Using a 25- or 30-degree cardboard triangle to check the position, adjust the degree of rotation so that the posterior surface of the body just touches the hypotenuse of the triangle. Check the rotation at several points along the back.

Respiration need not be suspended for the exposure unless the patient's breathing is labored.

Adjust the position of the film so that its midpoint will coincide with the central ray.

Central ray

1. With the central ray directed vertically, center at the level of the anterior superior iliac spines.

2. With the central ray at an angle of 20 to 25 degrees toward the head, center to a point 1½ inches distal to the level of the anterior superior iliac spines.

Structures shown

A profile view of the sacroiliac joint farther from the film, and an oblique view of the adjacent structures. Both sides are examined for comparison.

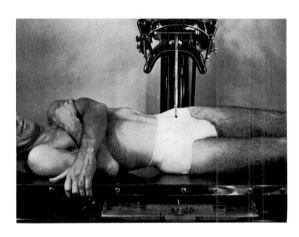

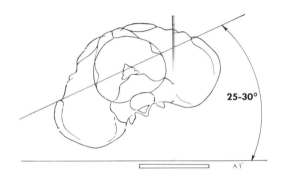

25-30°

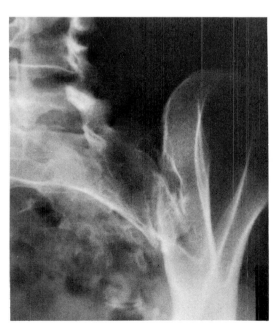

Central ray perpendicular.

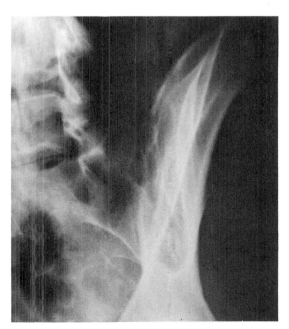

Central ray angled 25 degrees.

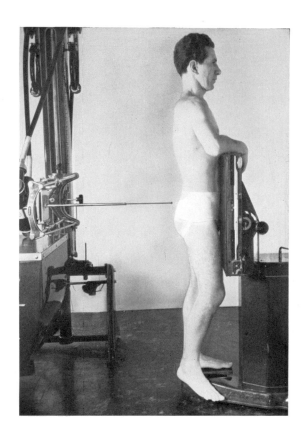

SACROILIAC JOINTS

Chamberlain method of demonstrating abnormal sacroiliac motion

Chamberlain[1] recommends the following procedure in cases of sacroiliac slip or relaxation:

1. A stereoscopic anteroposterior examination of the entire pelvis for the demonstration of any developmental asymmetry of the pelvis as a whole. This examination is made with the patient in the supine position.

2. A conventional lateral projection centered to the lumbosacral junction. Chamberlain[2] prefers to have this view made with the patient erect.

3. Two posteroanterior projections of the pubic bones, with the patient in the erect position and with weight-bearing on the alternate legs to demonstrate symphysis reaction by a change in the normal relation of the pubic bones in cases of sacroiliac slip or relaxation.

This examination requires two blocks or box stools approximately 6 inches high, the blocks being alternately removed to allow one leg to hang free.

Film: 8″ × 10″ lengthwise for each exposure.

Position of patient

Place the patient in the posteroanterior position, standing on the two blocks, before a vertical Potter-Bucky diaphragm. Adjust the height of the diaphragm so as to center the film to the symphysis pubis.

Position of part

Center the median sagittal plane of the body to the midline of the Potter-Bucky stand and adjust the body in a true posteroanterior position.

[1]Chamberlain, W. Edward: The symphysis pubis in the roentgen examination of the sacroiliac joint, Amer. J. Roentgen. **24:**621-625, 1930.
[2]Chamberlain, W. Edward: Personal communication.

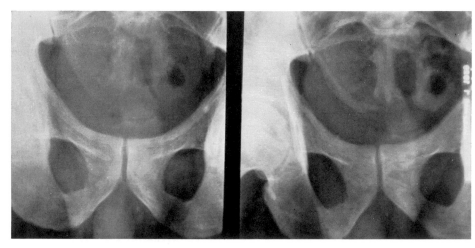

Anterior views in a normal male.

Courtesy Dr. W. Edward Chamberlain.

SACROILIAC JOINTS
Chamberlain method of demonstrating abnormal sacroiliac motion
Position of part—cont'd

The patient may be allowed to grasp the sides of the stand to steady himself, but he must not be allowed to aid in supporting his weight in this way; the full body weight must be alternately borne on one leg. Apply a compression band across the pelvis with enough pressure to immobilize the patient but not enough to aid in supporting the weight of the body. Respiration is suspended for the exposures.

For the first exposure, remove one of the blocks and let the leg hang free. The patient should be instructed to "let the leg hang like a dead weight" so that he will not overcome the desired effect through muscular resistance. For the second exposure, replace the first support and remove the opposite one. Chamberlain suggests that the identification marker be placed on the weight-bearing side.

Central ray

Direct the central ray horizontally to the midpoint of the film.

Structures shown

Two anterior views of the pubic bones, demonstrating any abnormal motion of the sacroiliac joints as shown by a change in the normal relation of the pubes to each other when the body weight is borne on one leg.

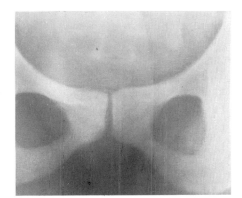 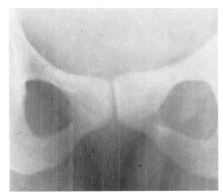

Anterior views in a normal female.

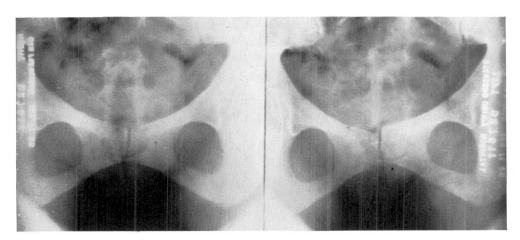

Anterior views in a patient with marked sacroiliac joint relaxation. The patient's weight was on the side bearing the marker.

Radiographs and diagnostic information courtesy Dr. W. Edward Chamberlain.

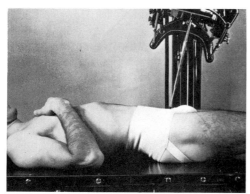

Central ray angulation for sacrum.

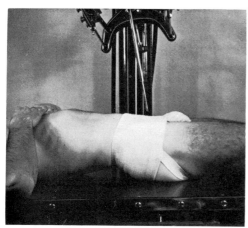

Central ray angulation for coccyx.

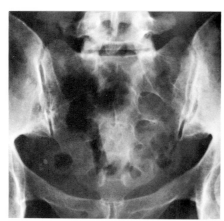

Supine projection of sacrum.

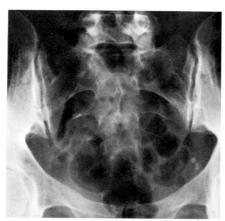

Prone projection of sacrum.

SACRUM AND COCCYX

Frontal projections

It is particularly desirable to have the colon free of gas and fecal material for examinations of the sacrum and coccyx. When bowel action is costive and preparation is possible, the patient should be instructed to take a nongas-forming cathartic or an enema, or both. The urinary bladder should be emptied immediately before the examination.

Film: $10'' \times 12''$ for sacrum; $8'' \times 10''$ for coccyx.

Position of patient

The patient is routinely adjusted in the supine position for the frontal view of the sacrum and coccyx in order to place the part as close as possible to the film. The prone position can be used without appreciable loss of detail, and should be used with patients who have a painful injury or a destructive disease.

Position of part

With the patient either supine or prone, center the median sagittal plane of the body to the midline of the table. Have the patient flex his elbows and place the arms in a comfortable, bilaterally symmetrical position. Adjust the shoulders to lie in the same transverse plane.

When the pelvis is rotated by a soft tissue abnormality (swelling or atrophy), adjust a radioparent support under the low side. Place a support under the ankles and, when the patient is supine, under the knees.

Position the film so that its midpoint will coincide with the central ray angulation.

Central ray

Sacrum. With the patient supine, direct the central ray 15 degrees toward the head and center it to the midpoint of the transverse plane that passes midway between the pubic symphysis and the anterior superior iliac spines. With the patient prone, angle the central ray 15 degrees toward the feet and center it to the clearly visible sacral curve.

Coccyx. With the patient supine, angle the central ray 10 degrees toward the feet and center to a point about 2 inches proximal to the pubic symphysis. With the patient prone, angle the central ray 10 degrees toward the head and center it to the easily palpable coccyx.

Structures shown

A frontal view of the sacrum or the coccyx projected free of self-superimposition.

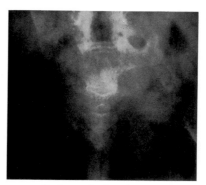

Supine projection of coccyx.

SACRUM AND COCCYX

Lateral projections

Film: $10'' \times 12''$ for sacrum and coccyx; $8'' \times 10''$ for the coccyx alone.

Position of patient

Ask the patient to turn onto the indicated side and flex his hips and knees to a comfortable position.

Position of part

For the sacrum, align the body so that the coronal plane passing 3 inches posterior to the midaxillary line is centered to the midline of the table.

The coccyx lies approximately 5 inches posterior to the midaxillary line; its exact position depends upon the pelvic curve. It can easily be palpated between the buttocks at the base of the spine, and the body can then be aligned to place the coccyx over the center line of the table.

Adjust the arms in a position at right angles to the body, and have the patient grasp the side of the table with the upper hand to aid in maintaining the position. Exactly superimpose the knees, and then elevate the lower knee to hip level and support it on sandbags. Place sandbags under and between the ankles, and between the knees.

Adjust a support under the body so as to place the long axis of the spine horizontal. Adjust the pelvis so that there is no rotation from the exact lateral position.

Position the film so that its midpoint is at the level of the anterior superior iliac spines for the sacrum, or at the level of the center of the coccyx.

Central ray

Direct the central ray vertically to the midpoint of the film.

Structures shown

A lateral view of the sacrum and/or the coccyx.

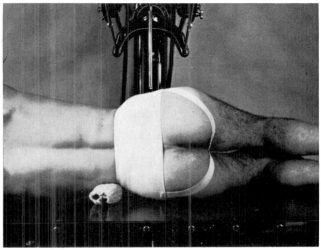

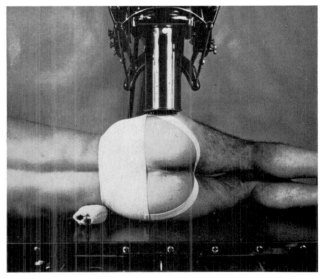

Centering for sacrum.

Centering for coccyx.

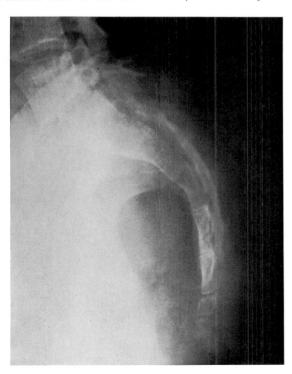

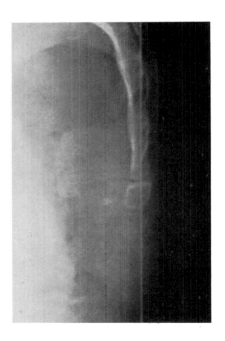

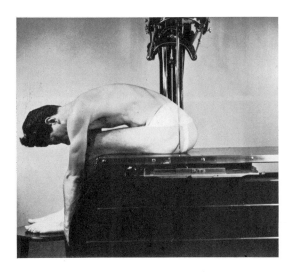

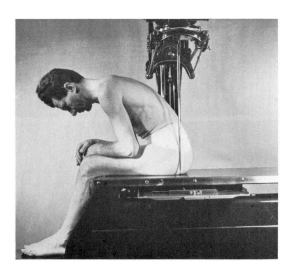

SACRAL CANAL—SACROILIAC JOINTS
Axial projection
Nölke position
Film: $8'' \times 10''$ or $10'' \times 12''$ crosswise.

Position of patient

In the examination of the sacral canal the patient is seated on the end of the table, and is then flexed in different degrees for the several regions of the canal. The exact degree of flexion depends upon the curvature of the sacrum.

Seat the patient far enough back on the table to center the midaxillary line of the body to the transverse axis of the Potter-Bucky tray. If the patient is too short to be comfortably seated so far back, the cassette can be shifted off center so that its midpoint will coincide with the region of the canal being projected. Support the feet on a chair or a stool.

Position of part

Adjust the position of the body so that its median sagittal plane is perpendicular to the midline of the table. Have the patient lean forward enough so that the upper, the middle, or the lower portion of the sacral canal is vertical, being careful not to let him lean laterally.

Have the patient grasp the sides of the table, or his legs or ankles, depending upon the degree of leaning, in order to maintain the position. Respiration need not be suspended for the exposure unless the patient's breathing is labored.

With the cassette in the Potter-Bucky tray, center to the vertically placed portion of the sacrum.

Central ray

Direct the central ray perpendicularly to the midpoint of the film.

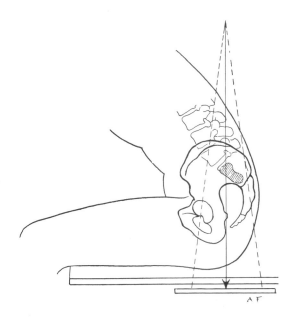

SACRAL CANAL—SACROILIAC JOINTS
Axial projection
Nölke position—cont'd
Structures shown

With the patient leaning forward in a position of acute flexion, as illustrated in the first photograph, the resultant radiograph shows the upper sacral canal projected into the angle formed by the ascending rami of the ischial bones just posterior to the pubic symphysis. The spinous process of the last lumbar segment is projected across the shadow of the canal.

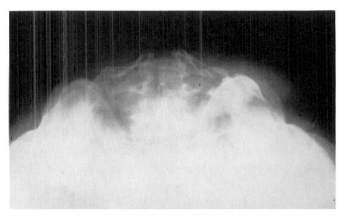

Acute flexion.

With the patient leaning forward in a position of slight flexion, as illustrated in the second photograph, the resultant radiograph shows the lower sacral canal, the junction of the sacrum and the coccyx, and the last lumbar vertebra.

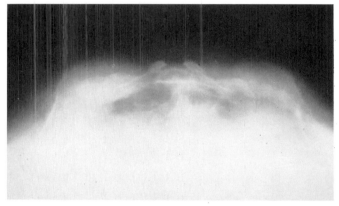

Slight flexion.

With the patient leaning forward in a position of moderate flexion, as illustrated in the third photograph, the resultant radiograph shows a cross section of the upper and lower sacral canal. The sacroiliac joints are also demonstrated in this position.

NOTE: In order to obtain a more uniform density throughout the radiograph, the posterior part of the region should be protected from overpenetration with a copper or an opaque plastic filter.

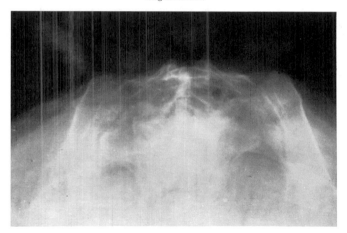

Moderate flexion.

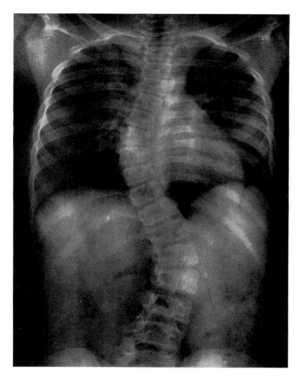

Supine position.

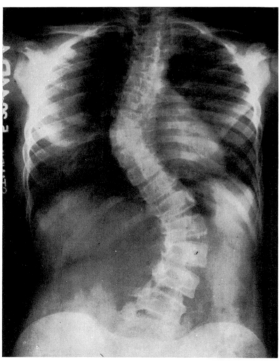

Standing position.
Radiographs courtesy Dr. Lawson E. Miller, Jr.

SCOLIOSIS SERIES
Ferguson method of distinguishing deforming curve from compensatory curve
Film: 14″ × 17″ placed lengthwise for each exposure.

Position of patient

Place the patient in the anteroposterior position, either seated or standing, before a vertical Potter-Bucky diaphragm. Have the patient sit or stand straight, and then adjust the height of the film so as to include about 1 inch of the iliac crests.

Position of part

For the first radiograph, the patient is adjusted in a normally seated or standing position in order to check the spinal curvature. Center the median sagittal plane of the body to the midline of the Potter-Bucky grid. Allow the arms to hang relaxed at the sides; if the patient is in the seated position, flex the elbows and rest the hands on the thighs.

For the second radiograph, elevate the hip or foot of the convex side of the curve approximately 3 or 4 inches by placing a block, a book, or sandbags under the buttock or the foot. Ferguson[1] specifies that the elevation must be sufficient to make the patient expend some effort in maintaining the position.

The patient must not be supported in these positions. A compression band is not employed. Respiration is suspended for the exposures.

The penetration should be increased approximately 5 kilovolts for the second position in order to compensate for the increase in thickness due to displacement of the abdominal viscera.

[1]Ferguson, Albert B.: Roentgen diagnosis of the extremities and spine, New York, 1939, Harper & Row, Publishers.

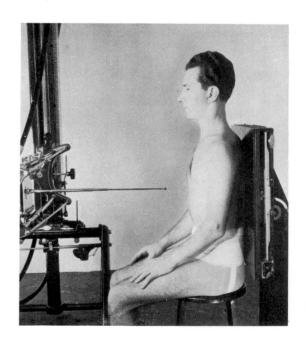

SCOLIOSIS SERIES
Ferguson method of distinguishing deforming curve from compensatory curve—cont'd

Central ray

Direct the central ray horizontally to the midpoint of the film.

Structures shown

Two posterior views (anteroposterior projections) of the thoracic and lumbar vertebrae, used for comparison to distinguish the deforming, or primary, curve from the compensatory curve in cases of scoliosis.

NOTE: Another widely used scoliosis series consists of four projections of the thoracic and lumbar spine: (1) a direct anteroposterior projection with the patient standing, (2) a direct anteroposterior projection with the patient supine, and (3) and (4) anteroposterior projections with alternate right and left flexion in the supine position. The right and left bending positions are described on the following page. For the scoliosis series, however, 14″ × 17″ films are used and are placed so as to include about 1 inch of the iliac crests.

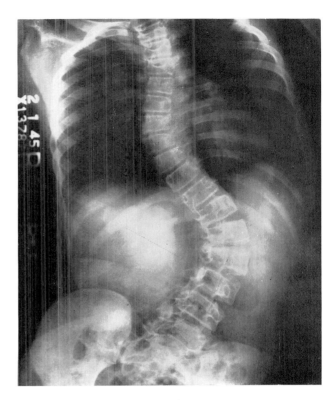

Right hip elevated.

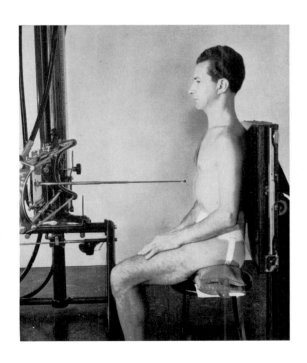

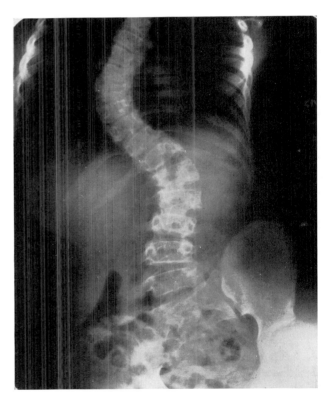

Left hip elevated.
Radiographs courtesy Dr. Lawson E. Miller, Jr.

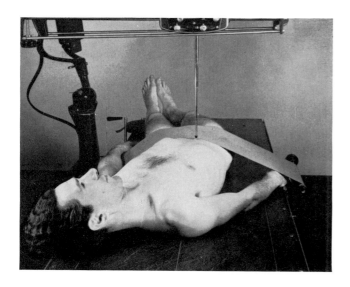

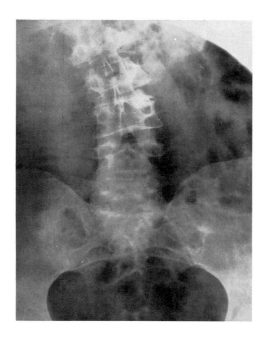

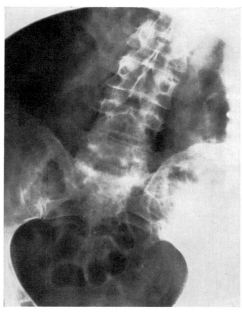

Radiographs courtesy Dr. Lawson E. Miller, Jr.

SPINAL FUSION SERIES
Supine right and left bending positions

Film: $10'' \times 12''$ or $14'' \times 17''$ placed lengthwise for each exposure.

Position of patient

Place the patient in the supine position and center the median sagittal plane of the body to the midline of the table.

Position of part

The first radiograph is made with maximum right bending, and the second with maximum left bending. In order to obtain equal bending force throughout the spine, cross the patient's leg on the side to be flexed over his opposite leg. Place one hand against the side of the lumbar region, draw the thighs lateralward enough to place the dependent heel near the edge of the table and immobilize with sandbags, and then draw the shoulders directly lateralward as far as is possible without rotating the pelvis.

After the patient is in position, a compression band may be applied to prevent movement. Respiration is suspended for the exposure.

Center the film to the mid-area of the region being examined.

Central ray

Direct the central ray vertically to the midpoint of the film.

Structures shown

Two posterior views (anteroposterior projections) of the lumbar vertebrae, made in maximum right and left flexion. These studies are employed (1) in cases of early scoliosis to determine the presence of structural change by unequal bend to right and left, (2) to localize a herniated disk as shown by limitation of motion at the site of the lesion, and (3) to demonstrate whether there is motion in the area of a spinal fusion. The latter examination is usually performed after a period of six months following the fusion operation.

The spinal fusion studies must be dark enough to demonstrate the degree of movement when they are superimposed. An increase of 5 kilovolts above the penetration customarily employed usually produces the desired density.

SPINAL FUSION SERIES
Lateral projection in flexion and extension

Film: $10'' \times 12''$ or $14'' \times 17''$ placed lengthwise for each exposure.

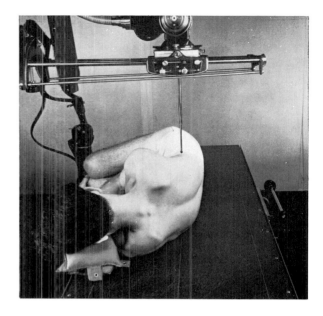

Position of patient

Adjust the patient in a lateral recumbent position. Center the coronal plane that lies approximately 2 inches posterior to the midaxillary line to the midline of the table.

Position of part

For the first radiograph, have the patient lean forward and draw his thighs upward so as to flex the spine as much as possible. This view requires 6 to 10 kilovolts more than the extension view because of the lateral displacement of the abdominal viscera in the flexed position.

For the second radiograph, have the patient lean backward, and then extend his hips and thighs as much as possible. After the patient is in position, a compression band may be applied across the pelvis to prevent movement.

Center the film at the level of the mid-area of the region being examined.

Respiration is suspended for the exposures.

Central ray

Direct the central ray vertically to the midpoint of the film.

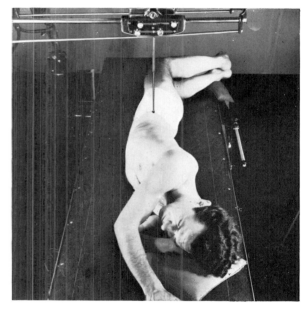

Structures shown

Two lateral views of the spine made in flexion and extension for the purpose of determining whether there is motion in the area of a spinal fusion, or to localize a herniated disk as shown by limitation of motion at the site of the lesion.

Spinal fusion studies must be dark enough to demonstrate the degree of movement when they are superimposed. An increase of 5 kilovolts above the penetration customarily employed usually produces the desired density.

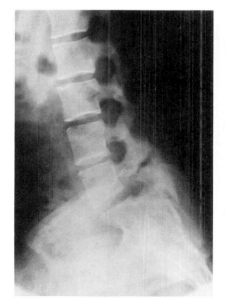

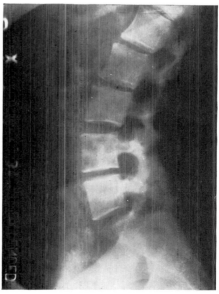

Radiographs courtesy Dr. Lawson E. Miller, Jr.

Glossary
Anatomic and medical terms

Plurals of some of the more common Greek and Latin nouns are formed as follows:

Singular	Plural	Example
— a	— ae	maxilla — maxillae
— ex	— ces	apex — apices
— ix	— ces	appendix — appendices
— is	— es	diagnosis — diagnoses
— ma	— mata	carcinoma — carcinomata
— on	— a	ganglion — ganglia
— um	— a	antrum — antra
— us	— i	ramus — rami

A

a-, an- (before a vowel). Prefixes signifying without, lack of; as, atypical, not characteristic of the type; anemia, lack of blood or of blood quality.

ab-. A prefix signifying away from, departure; as, abduct, movement away from the median plane or axis; abnormal, deviation from the usual structure or condition.

abdomen (ab-dō'men). The part of the body lying between the thorax and the pelvis; the cavity extending from the diaphragm to the pelvic floor.

abduct (ab-dukt'). To draw away from the median sagittal plane, as in moving an arm or leg laterally.

abnormal (ab-nor'mal). Irregular; deviation from the usual form or condition.

abrade (ab-rād'). To rub or scrape off the outer layer of a surface.

abrasion (ab-ra'zhun). The act of abrading; also, an area where the skin or mucous membrane has been abraded.

abscess (ab'ses). A localized pus collection in a cavity, resulting from tissue disintegration.

absorb (ab-sorb'). To suck in, as a sponge; to assimilate fluids or other substances from the skin, mucous surfaces, or absorbing vessels.

absorption (ab-sorp'shun). The sucking up or assimilation of fluids, gases, or other substances by the absorbing tissues and vessels of the body.

acanthiomeatal line (a-kan''the-o-me-ā'tal). An imaginary line extending from the external acoustic meatus to the acanthion.

acanthion (a-kan'the-on). A point at the center of the base of the anterior nasal spine.

accessory (ak-ses'or-e). Additional, supplementary; as, an accessory organ that contributes subordinately to the function of a similar but more important organ.

acinus (as'i-nus). Any one of the smallest lobules of a racemose gland; also, one of the saclike terminations of a passage, as the air sacs, or alveoli, of the lungs.

acoustic (a-koos'tik). Pertaining to sound or to the organs of hearing.

acromegaly (ak''ro-meg'al-e). A chronic disease characterized by permanent enlargement of the bones and soft tissues of the face as well as of the hands and feet.

acute (a-kūt'). Having a sudden onset and running a short but relatively severe course; as, an acute disease; opposed to chronic.

ad-. A prefix signifying toward; as, adduct, movement toward the central axis of the body.

Addison's planes (ad'i-sonz). The imaginary planes used to divide the abdomen into nine regions for descriptive purposes.

adduct (a-dukt'). To draw toward the median plane or axis, as drawing an extremity medialward.

adeno- (ad'en-o-), **aden-.** A gland; of or pertaining to a gland; as, adenitis, inflammation of a gland.

adenoma (ad''e-no'mah). A benign tumor of glandular origin.

adenopathy (ad''e-nop'ath-e). Any disease of the glands.

adherent (ad-hēr'ent). Clinging or sticking to or together; that which adheres, as a covering membrane.

adhesion (ad-he'zhun). The union or sticking together of two surfaces as the result of an inflammatory process; as, pleural adhesions.

adipose (ad'i-pōs). Fat; of a fatty nature; the fat in the cells of adipose tissue.

adnexa (ad-nek'sah). Appendages or conjoined parts; as, adnexa uteri, the ovaries and oviducts.

adrenal (ad-re'nal). Situated adjacent to the kidneys; pertaining to the adrenal glands or bodies, also called suprarenal glands.

aer- (ā'er-), **aer-i-, aer-o-.** Air; combining forms denoting relation to air or gas.

aerated (ā'er-at-ed). Filled with air, as the lungs; charged with air or gas.

afferent (af'er-ent). Conveying inward from the periphery to the center; applied to the nerves, and to blood and lymphatic vessels; opposed to efferent.

aggregate (ag're-gāt). Grouped or clustered together; as, an aggregate gland.

ala (ā'lah). A wing, or winglike process or part.

alar (ā'lar). Pertaining to an ala or alae; as, the alar processes of the sacrum.

-algia (-al'ji-ah). A suffix denoting pain; as, arthralgia, pain in a joint.

aliment (al'i-ment). That which nourishes; food or alima (a-li'mah), any nutritive substance.

alimentary (al''i-men'ta-re). Of or pertaining to nutrition or aliment; as, alimentary canal, the gastrointestinal tract.

alveolar (al-ve'o-lar). Pertaining to an alveolus, or alveoli, of the jaws or the lungs.

alveolus (al-ve'o-lus). A small cavity or pit; a socket for a tooth, an acinus or a compound gland, or the terminal air sac of a bronchiole.

ambi- (am'be-). A prefix meaning both; as, ambilateral, pertaining to or affecting both sides; bilateral.

amnion (am'ne-on). The thin, inner membrane of the closed sac, or bag of waters, surrounding the fetus in utero.

amphiarthrosis (am-fe-ar-thro'sis). An articulation admitting but little motion, as between the vertebral bodies.

ampulla (am-pul'ah). Any flasklike or saccular dilation of a canal; as, the rectal ampulla.

anal (ā'nal). Pertaining to the anus.

analgesia (an''al-je'ze-ah). Diminished sensibility to pain.

analogous (a-nal'o-gus). Having analogy; corresponding in function in certain particulars to an organ or part of different structures. See homologous.

anatomic (an''a-tom'ik). Of, pertaining to, or dealing with, body structure.

anatomy (a-nat'o-me). The science dealing with the structure of the body and the relation of the different parts.

anesthesia (an''es-the'ze-ah). Local or general loss of feeling or sensation; anesthesia may be produced by the administration of an anesthetic agent or by disease.

anesthetic (an''es-thet'ik). An agent capable of producing anesthesia.

aneurysm (an'u-rizm). An abnormal, saccular dilatation of the wall of a blood vessel, containing blood and usually forming a pulsating tumor.

angiography (an''je-og'ra-fe). The study of the blood and lymphatic vessels; the radiographic depiction of the blood vessels after the injection of a radiopaque contrast substance.

angioma (an''je-o'mah). A tumor composed largely of blood or lymph vessels.

ankylosis (ang''ki-lo'sis). Abnormal union of two or more normally separate bones; immobility of a joint.

anomaly (a-nom'al-e). A marked irregularity or deviation from the normal standard of structural formation.

ante- (an'te-). A prefix denoting before; as, anteversion, forward displacement of an organ; antenatal, occurring before birth.

anterior (an-ter'i-er). Pertaining to, designating, or situated in, the front part of the body or of an organ.

anteroposterior (an''ter-o-pos-ter'i-er). Directed or extending from front to back.

anthropologic base line. As established at the Munich Congress in 1877, the anthropologic base line of the skull passes from the lowest point of the inferior margin of the orbit to the center of the superior margin of the external auditory meatus. This line is also known as the Frankfurt horizontal plane, the German horizontal plane, Reid's base line, and the eye-ear plane. The infraorbitomeatal line, or Virchow's plane (*which see*), is more widely used in radiographic positioning because it is more easily localized, and it parallels the anthropologic base line closely enough for radiographic purposes.

anti- (an'ti-). A prefix signifying against, counter, opposite; as, antitoxin, against poison.

antiseptic (an''ti-sep'tik). Opposing decay or putrefaction; any substance that will prevent or arrest the growth of microorganisms without necessarily destroying them. Cf. disinfectant.

antrum (an'trum). A cavern or cavity within a bone, especially the maxillary air sinus.

anus (ā'nus). The terminal opening of the alimentary canal; the orifice through which fecal material is expressed.

aperture (ap'er-chūr). An opening, orifice, or mouth.

apex (a'peks). The tip, or the pointed extremity, of any conical structure.

apnea (ap-ne'ah). Suspended respiration; the transient cessation of breathing following a forced respiration; as deglutition apnea, temporary cessation of respiration activity during swallowing.

273

apophysial (ap-of-iz′e-al). Of or pertaining to an apophysis; apophyseal.

apophysis (a-pof′i-sis). Any outgrowth or offshoot; a process of bone, especially the articular processes of the vertebral arches.

appose (a-pōz′). To bring two surfaces in juxtaposition or proximity, as in the reduction of a fracture.

apposition (ap″o-zish′un). The contact of adjacent parts; the act of apposing, or the state of being apposed.

aqua (ak′wah). Latin for water; used in pharmacy in the sense of liquid or solution.

aqueduct (ak′wē-dukt). A canal for the transmission of a liquid; as, the aqueduct of Sylvius, the passage connecting the third and fourth ventricles of the brain.

aqueous (a′kwe-us). Of, or of the nature of, water; watery.

areola (a-re′-lah). A minute space or interstice in a tissue; the colored ring around the mammary nipple.

areolar (a-re′o-lar). Of or pertaining to an areola; containing interstitial areolae.

arteriography (ar-ter″e-og′ra-fe). The roentgenographic examination of the arteries during the injection of a contrast medium.

artery (ar′ter-e). Any one of the vessels conveying blood from the heart to various parts of the body.

arthritis (ar-thri′tis). Inflammation of the joints.

arthrosis (ar-thro′sis). Any joint or juncture uniting two bones.

articulation (ar-tik″u-la′shun). A joint between bones.

ascites (a-sī′tēz). A collection of serous fluid in the peritoneal cavity; abdominal dropsy.

asepsis (a-sep′sis). The methods of preventing, and of maintaining freedom from, infection; the state of being free from septic, or putrefactive, matter.

aseptic (a-sep′tik). Free from septic material; substances capable of destroying pathogenic germs. Cf. antiseptic.

-asis (-ă-sis). A combining form from -sis, used after nouns ending in *a* to denote action; as, metastasis, the transfer of a disease from a primary site of infection to another part or parts of the body.

aspirate (as′pi-rāt). To remove or draw off by suction; to tap; to treat by aspiration.

aspiration (as″pi-rā′shun). A drawing out by suction; the removal of fluids from a cavity by means of an aspirator; commonly called tapping.

assimilation (a-sim″i-lā′shun). The conversion or absorption of nutritive material into living tissue; anabolism or constructive metabolism.

asthenia (as-thē′ne-ah). Loss of strength; general debility.

asthenic (as-then′ik). Pertaining to asthenia, or weakness; a bodily habitus characterized by slender build and poor muscular development.

asthma (az′mah). A disease characterized by recurrent attacks of paroxysmal breathing, with a sense of suffocation.

ataxia (a-tak′si-ah). A condition characterized by inability to coordinate voluntary muscular movements.

atelectasis (at″e-lek′ta-sis). Defective aeration of the pulmonary alveoli at birth; collapse or partial collapse of one or more of the pulmonary lobes after birth.

atony (at′o-ne). Lack of normal tone or vitality; weakness; especially, deficient tonicity of contractile muscles.

atresia (ah-trē′zhe-ah). The absence or closure of a natural passage.

atrophic (a-trof′ik). Wasted; pertaining to, or characterized by, atrophy.

atrophy (at′ro-fe). A wasting away, or emaciation, of the body or of any part; a diminution in the size of an organ or part.

atypical (a-tip′i-kal). Unusual; not characteristic of the type.

auditory (aw′di-tō″re). Of or pertaining to the sense or organs of hearing.

auricle (aw′rik′l). The protruding portion of the external ear; the pinna, or flap of the ear; also, the small, pouched portion of each of the two atria of the heart.

auricular line (aw-rik′u-lar). One passing through the external auditory meatuses and perpendicular to the Frankfort horizontal plane.

auricular point. The center of the external acoustic meatus.

auto- (aw′tō). A prefix signifying self; as, autointoxicant, a virus generated within the body.

axial (ak′se-al). Pertaining to the axis of a body, a part, or a thing; directed along the axis, or center line.

axilla (ak-sil′ah). The armpit or the fossa beneath the junction of the arm and the shoulder.

axillary (ak′si-ler″e). Of or pertaining to the armpit, or axilla.

axis (ak′sis). A straight line, real or imaginary, passing through the center of a body or thing, and around which the body or part revolves or is supposed to revolve; also, the second cervical vertebra.

azygos (az′i-gos). An unpaired part, especially an azygous vein or an azygous lobe of the lung.

B

barium (bâr′e-um). A chemical element belonging to the alkaline earth metals; symbol, Ba; atomic weight 137.36. The soluble compounds or salts of barium are poisonous. Chemically pure (U.S.P.) barium sulfate is a heavy, white, insoluble compound of barium and sulfuric acid ($BaSO_4$), and is used as a contrast medium in roentgenography because of its high radiopacity.

basion (bā′se-on). The center of the anterior margin of the foramen magnum.

benign (be-nīn′). Of a mild character; as, benign tumor, not malignant.

bi- (bī-). [bis-, twice; di-, twice.]. A prefix signifying two or twice; as, bilateral, having, or pertaining to, two symmetric sides; biarcuate, twice curved.

bifurcate (bī′fur-kāt). To fork, or divide into two branches.

bifurcation (bī″fur-kā′shun). A division into two branches; also, the point of division.

bilateral (bī-lat′er-al). Two-sided; having, or pertaining to, two sides.

bio- (bī′o-). [*bios*, life.] A prefix signifying relation to life; as, biology, the science dealing with living organisms.

bismuth (biz′muth). A metallic element, the salts of which are used chiefly in medicine; by mouth in the treatment of certain gastrointestinal conditions, and by intramuscular injection in the treatment of syphilis. Bismuth salts are radiopaque.

BNA. Abbreviation for Basle Nomina Anatomica, or for the anatomic terminology adopted by the Anatomical Society at Basel, Switzerland, in 1895.

body section radiography. A technical procedure in which any selected plane of the body is depicted distinctly by moving the film and the x-ray tube in opposite directions to blur the superjacent and subjacent structures. Also called planigraphy, laminagraphy, stratigraphy, and tomography.

bolus (bō′lus). A round mass of anything, especially a soft mass of masticated food ready for swallowing.

bougie (bōō-zhē′). A tapering instrument used to dilate tubular passages.

brachial (brā′ke-al). Pertaining to the arm; as, brachialgia, pain in the arm.

brachiocubital (brā″ke-o-kū′bit-al). Pertaining to the arm and forearm.

brachy- (brak′e-). A prefix meaning short; as, brachyfacial, a short, broad face.

brachycephalic (brak″e-se-fal′ik). A head of the short, broad type.

brady- (brad′e-). A prefix meaning slow; as, bradycardia (also called brachycardia), abnormal slowness of heart action.

bregma (breg′mah). A point on the surface of the cranium at the junction of the coronal and sagittal suture.

bronchiectasis (brong″ke-ek′ta-sis). Dilatation of a bronchus or bronchi, which may be either saccular or cylindrical.

bronchiogenic (brong″ke-o-jen′ik). Of bronchial origin.

bronchitis (brong-kī′tis). Inflammation, acute or chronic, of the bronchial passages.

bronchography (brong-kog′ra-fe). The roentgenographic examination of the lungs and bronchial trees after the bronchi have been filled with a radiopaque contrast substance.

buccal (buk′al). Of or pertaining to a bucca, or cheek; as, buccal cavity, the space between the teeth and the cheeks.

bursa (bur′sah). A small, fluid-containing sac interposed between surfaces that glide upon each other and that would otherwise cause friction.

bursitis (bur-sī′tis). Inflammation of a bursa, sometimes attended with the formation of concretions or calculi.

C

c̄. Symbol for Latin *cum*, with.

calcareous (kal-kar′e-us). Consisting of, or containing, lime or calcium.

calcific (kal-sif′ik). Having or forming lime or calcium salts.

calcification (kal″si-fi-kā′shun). The deposition of lime salts in a tissue; the preliminary process in the formation of bone; a calcified part, or a calcific deposit.

calculus (kal'ku-lus). An abnormal concretion formed in any part of the body, usually in the various reservoirs of the body and in their passages; as, biliary calculi, or gallstones, located mainly in the gallbladder and the biliary ducts; urinary calculi, located in any part of the urinary tracts; renal calculi, occurring in the kidney.

callous (kal'us). Hard, horny; as, a thickened area of the skin, a callosity.

callus (kal'us). The plastic substance exuded around the fragments of a fractured bone, and ultimately converted into bone as it repairs the break.

Camper line. (Pieter Camper, Dutch physician, 1722-1789.) This line extends from the lower posterior border of the wing of the nose to the center of the tragus.

cancer (kan'ser). A malignant growth or tumor. See carcinoma.

cannula (kan'u-lah). A small, tubular instrument used for insertion, usually with a trocar, into a body cavity, as in a paracentesis.

canthus (kan'thus). The angle on each side of the eye where the upper and lower eyelids meet.

capillary (kap'i-ler-e). Any one of the minute, thin-walled vessels that connect the arterioles with the venules to form networks in practically all parts of the body.

carcinoma (kar"si-nō'mah). A malignant tumor originating in epithelial tissue and tending to spread, or metastasize, to other parts of the body; a cancer.

cardia (kar'de-ah). The upper, or esophageal, orifice of the stomach; pertaining to, or in relation to, the heart.

cardio- (kar'de-ō-), **cardi-** (kar'de-). A prefix indicating relation to the heart.

cardioangiography (kar"de-o-an"je-og'ra-fe). The roentgenographic demonstration of the heart and great vessels during the injection of an opaque contrast medium; angiocardiography.

cardiospasm (kar'de-o-spazm). Spasmodic contraction of the cardiac sphincter of the stomach.

caries (kā'ri-ēz). The molecular decay and subsequent suppuration of bone; a gradual disintegration, as distinguished from the mass destruction from necrosis; also, tooth decay.

cata- (kat'ah-). A prefix signifying down, lower, against, in accordance with; as, catabasis, the stage of decline of a disease; catastaltic, restraining, as an agent that tends to check a process.

cathartic (ka-thar'tik). A medicine producing evacuations by stool or catharsis; a mild purgative.

catheter (kath'e-ter). A tubular instrument for passage through a canal to withdraw fluid from a cavity or to distend the canal.

cauda (kaw'dah). A tail or tail-shaped appendage; as, cauda equina, the taillike termination of the spinal cord, which consists of the sacral nerves.

caudad (kaw'dad). In a caudal direction; toward the tail; opposed to cephalad.

-cele (-sēl). A suffix signifying a tumor or hernia; as, cystocele, a hernial protrusion of the urinary bladder.

celiac, coeliac (sē'le-ak). Pertaining to the abdomen; as, celiotomy, surgical incision into the abdominal cavity.

celiocentesis (sē"le-o-sen-tē'sis). The surgical puncture of the abdomen; tapping.

cellulitis (sel"u-lī'tis). Inflammation of cellular tissue, especially of the subcutaneous areas.

centesis (sen-tē'sis). Surgical puncture of a cavity; tapping.

centi- (sen'ti-). A prefix denoting a hundred or a hundredth part; used chiefly in the metric system, as in centimeter.

centigrade (sen'ti-grād). Graduated into one hundred equal divisions called degrees; centigrade thermometer (also called Celsius thermometer), a thermometer having 0° as the freezing point of water, and 100° as the boiling point of water. For conversion to degrees Fahrenheit, multiply degrees centigrade by nine-fifths and add 32.

cephalad (sef'al-ad). In a cranial direction, toward the head; opposed to caudad.

cephalic (se-fal'ik). Of or pertaining to the cranium; directed toward the head end of the body.

cephalo- (sef'al-o-), **cephal-**. A prefix indicating relation to the cranium; as, cephalotrypesis (sef"al-o-tri-pē'sis), trephination of the cranium.

cerebellum (ser-e-bel'um). The little brain; that part of the brain lying in the inferior occipital fossae below the cerebrum

and behind the fourth ventricle, the pons, and the upper part of the medulla.

cerebral (ser'e-bral). Of or pertaining to the brain; specifically, to the cerebrum.

cerebro- (ser'e-bro-). A prefix indicating relation to the brain; as, cerebrospinal, pertaining to or affecting the brain and the spinal cord.

cerebrum (ser'e-brum). The largest and main part of the brain, its two hemispheres filling the upper and greatest portion of the cranial cavity.

cervical (ser'vik-al). Of or pertaining to the neck or to any necklike part.

cervico- (ser'vi-ko-), **cervic-**. A prefix indicating relation to the neck or to the cervix of any organ; as, cervico-occipital, pertaining to the neck and the occiput; cervicitis, inflammation of the neck of the uterus.

cervix (ser'viks). The neck, or the necklike portion of any organ; as, cervix uteri, the narrow lower portion of the uterus.

cholangeitis, cholangitis (kol"an-jī'tis). Inflammation of the bile ducts.

cholangiography (ko-lan"je-og'ra-fe). The roentgenographic demonstration of the bile ducts after they have been filled with a radiopaque medium; cholangiography may be performed in the operation room while the biliary tract is exposed, or later in the radiology department.

chole- (kol'e-), **cholo-**. A prefix signifying relation to bile or to the biliary tract; as, cholecyst, the gallbladder; cholecystectomy, surgical removal of the gallbladder.

cholecystitis (kol"e-sis-tī'tis). Inflammation of the gallbladder.

cholecystography (kol"e-sis-tog'ra-fe). The roentgenographic demonstration of the gallbladder following the administration of a substance that will render the organ radiopaque.

choledochogram (ko-led-o'ko-gram). A radiograph of the common bile duct while it is filled with a contrast medium.

choledochography (ko-led-o-kog'ra-fe). The roentgenographic demonstration of the common bile duct while it is filled with an opaque medium administered by either ingestion or injection.

choledochus (ko-led'o-kus). The common bile duct.

cholegraphy (ko-leg'ra-fi). Radiologic examination of the biliary tract by means of a contrast medium.

cholelithiasis (kol"e-li-thī'a-sis). A condition favoring the formation of, or of being affected with, biliary concretions or calculi.

cholesteatoma (ko"les-te-a-tō'mah). A tumor containing cholesterol and fatty tissue, occurring in connection with the middle ear.

chondro- (kon'dro-), **chondr-**. A prefix signifying relation to cartilage; as, chondroma, a benign tumor composed of cartilage; chondrocostal, pertaining to the ribs and the rib cartilages.

chorea (ko-rē'ah). St. Vitus' dance, a nervous disease characterized by spasmotic twitching of the muscles; most common in children.

chorion (ko're-on). The outer membrane of the protective covering that envelops the fetus.

chronic (kron'ik). Continuing for a long time; as, a chronic disease, one which is characterized by a protracted course; opposed to acute.

cicatricial (sik"a-trish'al). Pertaining to, or having the character of, a scar or cicatrix.

cicatrix (sik'a-triks). A scar or scarlike mark; the contracted fibrous tissue that forms at the site of a wound during the process of healing.

cirrhosis (sir-ō'sis). A disease associated with an increase in fibrous tissue followed by contraction; specifically, a chronic disease of the liver in which the organ may diminish in size (atrophic cirrhosis), or may increase in size (hypertrophic cirrhosis).

cleido- (klī'do-), **cleid-**. A prefix indicating relation to the clavicle; as, cleidocostal, pertaining to the clavicle and the ribs; cleidarthritis, gouty pain in the clavicular region.

clysis (klī'sis). The washing out of a body cavity, as by lavage; an irrigation.

coagulation (ko-ag"u-lā'shun). The act or state of changing from a liquid to a gelatinous or solid mass; as, the clotting or coagulation of freshly drawn blood.

coalescence (ko"a-les'ens). A growing together or fusion of parts, as in a wound.

cohesion (ko-he'zhun). The molecular attraction or force that causes the particles of a substance to cohere, or cling together, as in a mass.

colitis (ko-lī′tis). Inflammation of the colon.

collateral (ko-lat′er-al). Having indirect relation to; secondary or accessory in function.

colo- (ko′lo-; kol′o-). A prefix denoting relation to the colon; as, colocentesis, surgical puncture of the colon.

columella (kol′′u-mel′ah). A little column; any part likened to a column; as, columella nasi, the nasal septum.

coma (ko′mah). A state of profound unconsciousness caused by disease or injury, and from which the patient cannot be aroused.

comatose (kōm′a-tōs). Resembling or affected with coma; lethargic.

comminuted (kom′′i-nūt′ed). Broken into small pieces; splintered, as in a comminuted fracture.

compound (kom′pound). A distinct, homogeneous substance composed of two or more chemically combined elements that have lost their original identity and cannot be separated by other than chemical means. Cf. mixture; solution.

compound fracture. One having an open wound extending into the site of the fracture.

concentric (kon-sen′trik). Having a common center, as graduated circles, one within the other; also, directed toward, or converging at, a common center; opposed to eccentric.

condyle (kon′dīl). A rounded, knucklelike articular process on a bone; applied mainly to rounded articular eminences that occur in pairs, as those of the occipital bone, the mandible, and the femur.

confluent (kon′flu-ent). Coming together; meeting or merging.

congenital (kon-jen′i-tal). Existing at birth; acquired or developed in the uterus.

congestion (kon-jes′chun). An abnormal accumulation of blood in any part or organ; hyperemia.

coniosis (ko′′ne-ō′sis). A pulmonary disease caused by the inhalation of dust.

consolidation (kon-sol′′i-dā′shun). A process of solidification in porous tissue as a result of disease, as of the lung in pneumonia and tuberculosis.

constriction (kon-strik′shun). A narrowing of the lumen or orifice of a passage; a stricture.

contagion (kon-tā′jun). The communication of disease by direct or indirect contact; a contagious disease, one that is readily transmissible from one to another without immediate contact.

contagious (kon-tā′jus). Transmissible by mediate or immediate contact; generating disease; conveying contagion.

contra- (kon′trah-). A prefix signifying against, in opposition; as, contraindication, a symptom that opposes a treatment otherwise advisable.

contralateral (kon′′tra-lat′er-al). Occurring on, or associated in function with a similar part on, the opposite side.

contusion (kon-tū′zhun). A bruise; injury to subcutaneous tissue, with effusion of blood throughout the area, but without breaking the skin.

coracoid (kor′a-koid). The process of bone projecting upward and forward from the upper part of the neck of the scapula, called the coracoid process because of its resemblance to a crow's beak.

coronal (ko-rō′nal; kor′o-nal). Of or pertaining to the crown of the head; passing in the direction of the coronal suture, as a frontal or coronal plane.

coronoid (kor′o-noid). Shaped like the beak of a crow; the process on the anterior surface of the upper extremity of the ulna.

corpus (kor′pus). Latin for body; the main part of any organ; a mass of specialized tissue.

costal (kos′tal). Of or pertaining to a rib or ribs.

costo- (kos′to-). A prefix signifying relation to the ribs; as, costogenic, originating in a rib.

costophrenic (kos′′to-fren′ik). Pertaining to the ribs and the diaphragm; as, costophrenic angle, the angle formed by the ribs and the diaphragm, and occupied by the phrenicostal sinus of the pleural cavity.

cox- (koks), **coxo-.** Prefixes denoting relation to the hip or hip joint; as, coxalgia, pain in the hip; coxofemoral, pertaining to the hip and the thigh.

coxa (kok′sah). The hip or hip joint.

cranial (kra′ne-al). Of or pertaining to the cranium.

cranio- (kra′ne-o-). A prefix denoting relation to the cranium; as, craniofacial, pertaining to the cranium and face.

craniotrypesis (kra′′ne-o-tri-pē′sis). Trephination of the cranium, as in preparation for pneumoventriculography.

crater (kra′ter). A pit; a bowl-shaped depression.

crepitation (krep′′i-tā′shun). A crackling or grating sound, such as that produced by rubbing together the two ends of a fractured bone; also, crepitant râles, the crackling sound heard on auscultation in certain lung diseases.

crepitus (krep′i-tus). A crackling noise; crepitation; the noise produced by rubbing fragments of fractured bones.

crisis (kri′sis). The turning point in a disease; the change that indicates whether the symptoms will begin to subside or to increase in severity.

cum (kum). Latin for with. Its symbol is c̄.

cumulative (kū′mu-lā′′tiv). Composed of added parts; increasing in intensity of action after successive additions; cumulative force or action.

cutaneous (kū-tā′ne-us). Of or pertaining to the skin or cutis.

cutis (kū′tis). The corium or dermis, the true skin as distinguished from the epidermis.

cyanosis (sī′′a-nō′sis). A bluish or purplish coloration of the skin and mucous membrane due to deficient oxygenation of the blood.

cyst (sist). Any normal fluid-containing sac or pouch, such as the gallbladder and the urinary bladder; also, any encapsulated or encysted collection of fluid or semifluid material formed as a result of disease.

cystitis (sis-tī′tis). Inflammation of the urinary bladder.

cystography (sis-tog′ra-fe). The roentgenographic examination of the urinary bladder after it has been filled with a contrast medium.

cystoscopy (sis-tos′ko-pe). The visual inspection of the interior of the urinary bladder by means of a cystoscope.

D

dacryo- (dak′ri-o-), **dacry-** (dak′ri-). A combining form denoting relation to tears, or to the lacrimal apparatus; as, dacryocyst, the lacrimal sac; dacryocystography, radiography of the lacrimal drainage system.

debility (de-bil′i-te). Weakness; lack or loss of strength.

deciduous (de-sid′u-us). Temporary; that which falls off or is shed; as, deciduous teeth.

decubitus (de-kū′bi-tus). Lying down; as, dorsal decubitus, lying on the back.

defecation (def′′e-kā′shun). The act or process of expressing fecal material from the bowel.

deglutition (de′′glū-tish′un; deg′′lu-tish′un) Swallowing; the act or process of swallowing.

demarcation (dē′′mar-kā′shun). The act or process of marking off boundaries; a line of separation, as between healthy and diseased tissue.

dens (denz). The odontoid process of the second cervical vertebra; also, a tooth.

dentition (den-tish′un). The eruption, or cutting, of teeth; the form and general arrangement of the teeth.

denture (den′tūr). A full set of teeth; specifically, of artificial teeth.

depression (de-presh′un). A hollow area; a concavity; also, a decrease of functional activity or mental vitality.

dermato- (der′ma-to-). A prefix denoting relation to the skin; as, dermatoma, a skin tumor.

dermis (der′mis). The skin; specifically, the corium, or true skin.

detergent (de-ter′jent). Any cleansing agent; a medicine used to cleanse wounds.

dextral (deks′tral). Of or pertaining to the right side; opposed to sinistral.

dextro- (deks′tro-). A prefix denoting relation to the right side; as, dextrocardia, transposition of the heart to the right side of the chest.

dextrosinistral (deks′′tro-sin′is-tral). Extending from right to left; as, a dextrosinistral plane.

diagnosis (dī′′ag-nō′sis). The art or act of determining the character of a disease from the existing symptoms; also, the conclusion reached.

diaphysis (dī-af′i-sis). The shaft, or main part, of a long bone.

diarrhea (dī′′a-rē′ah). Frequent discharge of loose or fluid fecal material from the bowels.

diarthrosis (dī′′ar-thrō′sis). A joint that permits free movement, such as the hip or shoulder joint.

diastole (di-as'to-le). The phase of rhythmic dilatation or relaxation of the heart and arteries; correlative to systole.

digestion (di-jes'chun). The process of converting food into chyme and chyle so that it can be absorbed and assimilated.

diploe (dip'lo-e). The cancellous osseous tissue occupying the space between the two tables of the cranial bones.

dis- (dis-). A prefix denoting absence, reversal, or separation.

disarticulation (dis″ar-tik″u-la'shun). Amputation at a joint, with separation of the joint.

disinfectant (dis″in-fek'tant). Any agent (heat or chemical) that destroys disease germs but does not, ordinarily, injure spores. Cf. germicide.

dispersion (dis-per'shun). The act of separating, or the state of being separated, as the finely divided particles of a substance dispersed through a suspension medium.

distal (dis'tal). Remote from the origin or head of a part; as, the distal end of a long bone; opposed to proximal.

diverticulitis (di″ver-tik″u-li'tis). Inflammation of a diverticulum or diverticula.

diverticulosis (di″ver-tik″u-lo'sis). Multiple diverticula of any cavity or passage, most commonly of the colon.

diverticulum (di″ver-tic'u-lum). A blind sac or pocket branching off from a main cavity or canal.

dolicho- (dol'i-ko-). A prefix meaning long and narrow; as, dolichofacial, a long, narrow face.

dolichocephalic (dol″i-ko-se-fal'ik). Having a long, narrow head.

dorsal (dor'sal). Pertaining to, or situated near, the back of the body or an organ; opposed to ventral.

dose (dos). The proper quantity of a medicine to be taken at one time or within a specified time; the quantity of x-radiation administered therapeutically at one time or over a period of time.

dropsy (drop'se). An abnormal accumulation of fluid in cellular tissue or in a cavity of the body.

drug (drug). Any chemical substance used, either internally or externally, in the treatment of disease.

dys- (dis-). A prefix denoting (1) difficulty or pain; as, dyspnea, labored or painful breathing; (2) abnormal or impaired; as, dysarthrosis, malformation of a joint; dystrophia, defective nutrition.

dyspnea (disp-ne'ah). Labored or painful breathing.

dysuria (dis-u'ri-ah). Difficult or painful urination.

E

ec- (ek-). A prefix meaning out or out of; as, eccyesis, extrauterine pregnancy; ecchymosis, extravasation of blood, also the resulting discoloration of the skin.

eccentric (ek-sen'trik). Situated off center; not having the same center; opposed to concentric.

ecto- (ek'to-), **ect-**. A prefix denoting without, on the outer side, external; as, ectopic, out of the normal position; ectocondyle, the external condyle of a bone.

-ectomy (-ek'to-me). A suffix denoting the surgical removal of; as, cholecystectomy, the removal of the gallbladder.

edema (e-de'mah). An abnormal accumulation of fluid in the tissues or cavities of the body, resulting in a puffy swelling when present in subcutaneous tissues, in distention when in the abdominal cavity; dropsy.

edentulous (e-den'tu-lus). Without teeth; edentate.

efferent (ef'er-ent). Conveying outward from the center toward the periphery; applied to the nerves, and to blood and lymphatic vessels; opposed to afferent.

effusion (ef-u'zhun). The escape of fluid from the vessels into the tissues or cavities of the body.

egest (e-jest'). To expel or excrete waste material from the body; opposed to ingest.

elephantiasis (el″e-fan-ti'a-sis). A chronic disease in which the affected part undergoes extensive enlargement and the skin becomes thick, rough, and fissured, so that it resembles an elephant's hide.

em-, en-. Prefixes meaning in; as, empyema, pus in a cavity; encysted, enclosed in a sac.

emaciation (e-ma″si-a'shun). Wasted; the condition of becoming lean or emaciated.

embolism (em'bo-lizm). The obstruction of a blood vessel by an embolus or plug carried in from a larger vessel, most usually a blood clot.

embolus (em'bo-lus). A clot of blood, an air bubble, or other obstructive plug conveyed by the bloodstream and lodging in a smaller vessel. Cf. thrombus.

emesis (em'e-sis). The act of vomiting.

emetic (e-met'ik). Any means employed to produce vomiting; a medicine that causes vomiting.

emphysema (em″fi-se'mah). Swelling produced by an accumulation of gas or air in the interstices of connective tissues; also, dilatation of the pulmonary alveoli.

empyema (em″pi-e'mah). An accumulation of pus in a body cavity; most frequently, in the pleural cavity.

emulsion (e-mul'shun). An oily or resinous substance suspended in an aqueous liquid by a mucilaginous or other emulsifying agent.

en-, em-. Prefixes meaning in.

encephalo- (en-sef'a-lo-). A prefix signifying relation to the brain.

encephalography (en-sef″a-log'ra-fe). The roentgenographic examination of the brain after the ventricles have been filled with a contrast medium; pneumoencephalography.

encysted (en-sist'ed). Enclosed in a sac or cyst.

endo- (en'do-). A prefix meaning within; occupying an inward position; as, endocarditis, inflammation of the lining membrane of the heart; endoscope, an instrument that permits visual examination of the interior of a hollow viscus, such as the urinary bladder.

endocrine (en'do-krin). Secreting internally, as the ductless glands; pertaining to the endocrine glands, such as the pituitary, the thyroid, the thymus, the pineal body, and the spleen.

endosteal (en-dos'te-al). Of or pertaining to the endosteum, the vascular tissue lining the medullary cavity of bones.

enema (en'e-mah). A fluid injected into the rectum for the purpose of cleansing the bowel or of administering food or a drug.

enteric (en-ter'ik). Of or pertaining to the intestines.

enteritis (en-ter-i'tis). Inflammation of the intestine; specifically, of the small intestine.

entero- (en'ter-o-), **enter-**. A prefix denoting relation to the intestine; as, enteroptosis, a dropping, or downward displacement, of the intestines.

enterostomy (en″ter-os'to-me). The surgical formation of an opening into the intestine through the abdominal wall; as, gun-barrel enterostomy, the operation in which each segment of the divided intestine is brought to a separate opening on the surface of the abdominal wall.

enuresis (en'u-re'sis). The involuntary discharge of urine; incontinence of urine.

epi- (ep'i-) **ep-**. A prefix meaning upon, above, on the outside, over; as, epicostal, situated upon a rib; epigastric, situated above the stomach; epidermis, the outermost layer of skin.

epiphysis (e-pif'i-sis). A center of ossification separated during growth from the main body of a bone by cartilage that subsequently ossifies to unite the two parts of the bone, the epiphysis and the diaphysis.

epiphysitis (e-pif″i-si'tis). Inflammation of an epiphysis or of the cartilage separating it from the diaphysis.

erosion (e-ro'zhun). An irregular or uneven wearing or eating away, beginning at the surface of a part, as an ulcerative or necrotic process.

eructation (e″ruk-ta'shun). The act of discharging or belching gas from the stomach; a belch.

erythema (er″i-the'mah). A morbid redness of the skin due to capillary congestion resulting from irritation or any form of inflammatory process.

etiology (e″ti-ol'o-je). The science or doctrine of causation; the investigation or assignment of the cause of a disease.

eu- (u-). A prefix signifying well; as, eupnea, normal breathing; opposed to dys-.

evagination (e-vaj″i-na'shun). Turned inside out; the protrusion of a part or organ.

eventration (e″ven-tra'shun). The protrusion of the intestines from the abdomen.

eversion (e-ver'shun). The act of turning, or the state of being turned, outward or inside out.

evert (e-vert'). To turn outward or inside out.

ex- (eks-). A prefix denoting out, out of, or away from; as, excavation, a hollowing out; excrete, the throwing off of waste material.

excreta (eks-kre'tah). Waste materials excreted or separated out by an organ; waste products cast out from the body.

excretion (eks-krē'shun). The throwing off of waste matter.

excretory (eks'kre-tō''re). Of or pertaining to excretion.

exo- (ek'so-), **ex-**. A prefix meaning outward or outside; as, exogenous, growing from or on the outside of a part of the body; originating outside the body.

exostosis (eks''os-tō'sis). A spur, or osseous outgrowth, from a bone or tooth.

extension (eks-ten'shun). The movement of a joint or joints that brings the parts of an extremity or of the body into or toward a straight line.

extra- (eks'tra-). A prefix meaning on the outside, beyond, in addition; as, extragastric, situated or occurring outside the stomach.

extravasation (eks-trav''a-sā'shun). The escape of fluid from a vessel into the surrounding tissues; said of blood, lymph, and serum.

extrinsic (eks-trin'sik). Originating outside of the part involved.

exudate (eks'u-dāt). An adventitious material exuded or thrown out upon injured or diseased tissues.

F

facet (fas'et). Any plane, circumscribed surface; as, an articular facet on a bone.

Fahrenheit (fah'ren-hīt). Pertaining to the thermometric scale invented by Gabriel Daniel Fahrenheit. On the Fahrenheit thermometer, the freezing point of water is 32 degrees above the zero point, and the boiling point of water at 212 degrees. Cf. centigrade.

febrile (fē'bril). Pertaining to fever; feverish.

fecal (fē'kal). Relating to, or of the nature of, feces.

feces (fē'sēz). The excrement, or waste products, of food digestion discharged from the bowels.

fenestra (fe-nes'trah). A small aperture, or opening, as in certain bones.

fetid (fet'id). Having an offensive smell.

fetography (fē-tog'ra-fe). The roentgenographic examination of the fetus in utero.

fibroma (fī-brō'mah). A benign tumor composed mainly of fibrous tissue.

fibrosis (fī-brō'sis). The formation of fibrous tissue in any organ or region; the replacement of normal tissue with fibrous tissue.

fissure (fish'ūr). Any narrow furrow, cleft, or slit, normal or otherwise.

fistula (fis'tu-lah). An abnormal passage leading from an abscess cavity or from a hollow organ to the surface of the body, or from one hollow organ to another.

flaccid (flak'sid). Without firmness or tone; flabby, as a flaccid muscle.

flatulence (flat'u-lens). The gaseous distention of the stomach or intestines.

flatus (flā'tus). Gas generated in the stomach or intestines.

flexion (flek'shun). The bending of a joint in which the angle between the parts is decreased; forward bending; opposite of extension.

flocculent (flok'u-lent). Containing soft flakes or shreds, as in a flocculent precipitate.

flux (fluks). The flow of a liquid; an excessive discharge, as from the bowels.

fontanel (fon'ta-nel). Any one of the intervals or soft spots between the angles of the parietal bones and the adjacent bones of the cranium in an infant.

formula (for'mu-lah). The prescribed ingredients, with proportions, for the preparation of a medicine; a prescription; also, a combination of symbols to express the chemical constituents of a body.

fossa (fos'ah). A pit, cavity, or depression; as, the acetabular fossa, the supraclavicular fossa, and the nasal fossae.

fovea (fo've-ah). A pit or cup-shaped depression.

Fowler's position (fow'lerz). A position in which the head end of the body is elevated, usually about 30 degrees.

Frankfurt plane or line. *See* anthropologic base line.

fremitus (frem'i-tus). A palpable vibration or thrill; as, tussive fremitus, the vibration felt through the head on humming with the mouth closed.

frenulum (fren'u-lum). A small fold of mucous membrane serving to support or restrain the movements of a part.

frontal plane. A plane or section passing from side to side, parallel with the coronal suture, at right angles to the median sagittal plane of the body; a coronal plane.

fundus (fun'dus). The base of a hollow organ; the part farthest from the opening, as the cardiac end of the stomach.

furuncle (fū'rung-k'l). A boil.

G

gall (gawl). The bitter, brownish or greenish yellow fluid secreted by the liver; the bile.

ganglion (gang'gle-un). Any aggregation of nerve cells forming a nerve center; also, a small cystic tumor occurring on a tendon, usually about the wrist or ankle.

gangrene (gang'grēn). Necrosis of tissue due to interference with the blood supply to the part, usually accompanied with putrefaction.

gas gangrene. Gangrene occurring chiefly in lacerated wounds, and in which the tissues become impregnated with gas produced by a mixed infection of bacteria, including the gas bacillus.

gastr- (gas'tr-), **gastro-**. A prefix signifying relation to the stomach; as, gastritis, gastroenterostomy.

gastric (gas'trik). Of or pertaining to the stomach.

gastroentero- (gas''tro-en'ter-o-), **gastroenter-**. A prefix denoting relation to the stomach and intestine; as, gastroenteroptosis, the prolapse or downward displacement of the stomach and intestines.

gavage (gah''vahzh'). Feeding by stomach tube.

-genic (-jen'ik). A combining form meaning causing, giving origin to, or arising from; as, osteogenic, originating in bone.

German horizontal. The base line of the cranium; the anthropologic base line.

germicide (jer'mi-sīd). Any agent that destroys germs. Cf. antiseptic; disinfectant.

gingivae (jin-ji've); sing. gingiva (jin-ji'vah). The gums.

gingival (jin'ji-val). Of or pertaining to the gums.

glabella (glah-bel'ah). The smooth space on the forehead between the superciliary arches, which correspond in position with the eyebrows.

glabelloalveolar line (glah-bel''o-al-vē'o-lar). An imaginary line extending from the glabella to the upper alveolus; the localization plane of the face.

glabellomeatal line (glah-bel''o-me-a'tal). An imaginary line extending from the glabella to the external acoustic meatus; the localization line used in the Caldwell sinus position.

glenoid (gle'noid). A smooth, shallow depression; specifically, the glenoid fossa of the scapula.

glioma (glī-o'mah). A malignant tumor originating in nerve tissue.

glossa (glos'ah). Greek for tongue.

glossal (glos'al). Of or pertaining to the tongue; lingual.

gonion (go'ne-on). The tip of the angle of the mandible.

Graham test. The roentgenographic examination of the gallbladder following the administration of a contrast medium.

granulation (gran-u-lā'shun). The formation of small grains or particles; any small, granulelike mass of abnormal tissue projecting from the surface of an organ; also, the formation in a wound of small, rounded granules of new tissue during the healing process.

gravel (grav'el). A deposit of small, stonelike concretions in the kidneys and urinary bladder; calculi.

groin (groin). The depression between the lower part of the abdomen and the thigh, or the region around the depression; the inguen, or the inguinal region.

groove (groov). A shallow, linear depression, or furrow, in a part, especially in bone.

gumma (gum'ah). A soft, gummy, granulomatous tumor of syphilitic origin, occurring in the third stage of the disease.

gynecology (jin''e-kol'o-je). The branch of medicine that treats of women's diseases, those occurring in the genital, urinary, and rectal regions.

H

habitus (hab'it-us). [Latin for habit.] A fixed practice established by frequent usage; also, bodily appearance; the general form or architecture of the body.

haustrum (haws'trum); pl. **haustra** (-trah). Any one of the recesses formed by the sacculations of the colon.

hem-, haem-, hemo-. A prefix denoting blood, or relation to blood; as, hematuria, the presence of blood in the urine.

hemangioma (he-man''je-o'mah). A tumor consisting of newly formed blood vessels.

hematoma (he''mah-tō'mah). A tumor or swelling containing effused blood.

hemi- (hem'i-). A prefix signifying one-half; pertaining to or affecting one side of the body; as, hemiplegia, paralysis of one side of the body.

hemoptysis (he-mop'ti-sis). The presence of blood in the sputum; the expectoration of blood.

hemorrhage (hem'o-rij). A discharge of blood from the vessels in any region; bleeding.

hemorrhoid (hem'o-roid). A vascular tumor situated at the orifice of, or within, the anal canal.

hepatic (he-pat'ik). Of or pertaining to the liver.

hepato- (hep'a-to-), **hepat-**. A prefix signifying relation to the liver; as, hepatomegalia, enlargement of the liver.

hernia (her'ne-ah). The protrusion of a part of an organ through either a normal or an abnormal opening in the wall of its natural cavity; a rupture.

herniation (her-ne-ā'shun). A hernial protrusion; the formation of a hernia.

herpes (her'pēz). Acute inflammation of the skin or mucous membrane, in which clusters of small vesicles form and tend to spread.

hetero- (het'er-o-). A prefix signifying other, other than usual; difference or dissimilarity between constituents; to or from a different source; opposite of homo-.

heterogeneous (het″er-o-jē'ne-us). Differing in kind or nature; composed of unlike elements or ingredients, or having dissimilar characteristics; opposed to homogeneous.

heterogenous (het″er-oj'e-nus). Arising or originating outside the body; opposed to autogenous.

hiatus (hi-ā'tus). An opening; a space, gap, or fissure for the transmission of a nerve, a vessel, or a tubular passage.

hilum (hi'lum). The depression on a gland or organ that marks the site of entrance and exit of the nerves, vessels, and ducts; as, the hilum of the kidney or of the lung.

hilus (hi'lus). Same as hilum.

homeo-, homoeo- (ho'me-o-). A prefix meaning like, similar; as, homeomorphous, of similar structure and form.

homo- (ho'mo-). A prefix meaning one and the same, common, similar; as, homodox, homocentric, homologue; opposed to hetero-.

homogeneous (ho″mo-jē'ne-us). Of the same kind or nature; composed of similar elements or ingredients, or having similar uniform characteristics; opposed to heterogeneous.

homologous (ho-mol'o-gus). Corresponding in position or structure, but not necessarily resembling in function. Cf. analogous.

hydro- (hi'dro-). A prefix meaning water, or denoting some relation to water or to hydrogen.

hydrocele (hi'dro-sēl). An accumulation of fluid, usually in a sacculated cavity such as the scrotum.

hydrocephalus (hi″dro-sef'a-lus). A condition characterized by an excessive amount of cerebrospinal fluid in the cerebral ventricles, accompanied by dilatation of the ventricles, and causing atrophy of the brain substance and enlargement of the head.

hydronephrosis (hi″dro-nef-rō'sis). An accumulation of urine in the pelvis of the kidney, due to obstruction of the ureter, with resultant dilatation of the pelvis and atrophy of the organ itself.

hydrops (hi'drops). An excessive accumulation of fluid in a cavity of the body; dropsy.

hyper- (hi'per-). A prefix meaning over; above in position; beyond the usual or normal extent or degree; excessive; opposite of hypo-.

hypermotility (hi″per-mo-til'i-te). Excessive movement, or motility, of involuntary muscles, especially those of the gastrointestinal tract.

hyperpnea (hi″perp-nē'ah). Abnormally rapid respiratory movements.

hypersthenic (hi″per-sthen'ik). Excessive strength or tonicity of the body, or of any part; the type of bodily habitus characterized by massive proportions.

hyperthyroid (hi″per-thī'roid). Pertaining to hyperthyroidism; excessive functional activity of the thyroid gland.

hypertrophic (hi″per-trof'ik). Pertaining to, or affected with, hypertrophy.

hypertrophy (hi-per'tro-fe). A morbid increase in the size of an organ or part.

hypo- (hi'po-). A prefix meaning under; below or beneath in position; less than the usual or normal extent or degree; deficient; opposite of hyper-.

hyposthenic (hi″pos-then'ik). Lack of strength or tonicity;

the type of bodily habitus characterized by slender build, a modification of the more extreme asthenic type.

hypothyroid (hi″po-thī'roid). Pertaining to hypothyroidism; deficient functional activity of the thyroid gland.

hysteresis (his'ter-ē'sis). A lagging or retardation of one of two associated phenomena; failure to act in unison.

hystero- (his'ter-o-), **hyster-**. A prefix denoting relation to the uterus; as, hysterectomy, the surgical removal of the uterus.

hysterography (his″ter-og'ra-fe). The roentgenographic examination of the uterus after the injection of a contrast medium; uterography.

hysterosalpingography (his″ter-o-sal-ping-gog'ra-fe). The roentgenographic examination of the uterus and the oviducts after the injection of a contrast medium; uterosalpingography.

I

-iasis (-ī'a-sis). A suffix denoting a morbid or diseased condition; as, elephantiasis, nephrolithiasis, dracontiasis.

idio- (id'i-o-). A combining form denoting self-produced; as, idiopathic self-originated, of unknown cause.

ileac (il-e-ak). Pertaining to the ileum, or to ileus. Cf. iliac.

ileo- (il'e-o-). A prefix denoting some relation to the ileum; as, ileocolic, ileocecal, ileotomy.

ileum (il'e-um). The terminal three-fifths of the small intestine, the part extending from the jejunum to the cecum. Cf. ilium.

ileus (il'e-us). A condition due to intestinal obstruction, marked by severe pain in, and distention of, the abdomen; volvulus.

iliac (il'e-ak). Of or pertaining to the ilium. Cf. ileac.

ilium (il'e-um). The wide upper one of the three bones composing each half of the pelvic girdle. Cf. ileum.

im-, in-. Prefixes meaning in, within, or into, as in immersion, injection; also, not, non-, un-, as in imbalance, inactive, incurable.

impacted (im-pak'ted). Firmly wedged or lodged in position; forcibly driven together, as the two ends of a bone in an impacted fracture.

incipient (in-sip'e-ent). Beginning to exist; commencing; as, the incipient or initial stage of a disease.

incisura (in″si-sū'rah). A notch or cleft; a deep indentation.

incisure (in-sizh'ūr). A notch; a cut or gash.

incontinence (in-kon'ti-nens). The inability of any of the organs to restrain a natural evacuation; involuntary discharges; as, incontinence of urine or feces.

induration (in″du-rā'shun). Hardening or hardened tissue due to inflammation or congestion.

infarct (in'farkt). A circumscribed area of necrosis of tissue, resulting from obstruction of the local blood supply by an embolus or a thrombus.

infection (in-fek'shun). The communication of disease germs to the body tissues by any means.

infectious (in-fek'shus). Contaminated, or charged with disease germs; readily communicable by infection but not necessarily contagious. Cf. contagious.

inferior (in-fer'i-er). Situated lower or nearer to the bottom or base; below.

inferosuperior (in″fer-o-su-per'i-er). Directed or extending from below upward; caudocranial.

infiltration (in″fil-trā'shun). The filtering into, or penetration of, the tissues by a substance not normal to them.

inflammation (in″fla-mā'shun). A morbid condition produced in the tissues by an irritant; a natural reaction to irritation wherein plasma and blood cells are exuded at the site of infection or injury in an attempt to heal the damage; it is manifested by redness, swelling, and pain.

infra- (in'frah-). A prefix meaning below; as, infraorbital, situated below the orbit.

infraorbitomeatal line (in″frah-or'bit-o-me-a'tal). Also known as Virchow's plane (fēr'kōz). A line that extends from the center of the inferior orbital margin to the center of the tragus, and that is used in radiography for the adjustment of the base of the cranium. Because this line closely parallels the anthropologic base line, it is frequently denoted by this and the other terms applied to the anthropologic base line.

infundibulum (in″fun-dib'u-lum). Any conical or funnel-shaped structure or passage.

infusion (in-fū'zhun). The process of introducing a solution into a vessel or a hollow viscus by gravity pressure. Cf. injection; instillation; insufflation.

ingest (in-jest'). To take in for digestion; to eat; to take anything by mouth.

inguinal (ing'gui-nal). Of or pertaining to the region of the inguen or groin, the region between the abdomen and thigh.

inion (in'i-on). The external occipital protuberance.

injection (in-jek'shun). The forcible introduction, usually by syringe, of a liquid, a gas, or other material into a part of the body, a vessel, a cavity, an organ, or subcutaneous tissue. Cf. infusion; instillation; insufflation.

inorganic (in''or-gan'ik). Not organic in origin; pertaining to, or composed of, substances other than animal or vegetable; inanimate matter; as, inorganic elements.

inspissated (in-spis'a-ted). Thickened by evaporation or by the absorption of the fluid content; as, inspissated pus.

instillation (in''stil-lā'shun). To drop in; the process of introducing a liquid into a cavity drop by drop. Cf. infusion; injection; insufflation.

insufflation (in''su-flā'shun). The act of blowing air or gas (or a powder or vapor) into a cavity of the body, as into the colon for a double-contrast enema. Cf. infusion; injection; instillation.

inter- (in'ter-). A prefix signifying between; as, interlobar, situated between two lobes. Cf. intra-.

intercostal (in''ter-kos'tal). Pertaining to, or situated in, the spaces between the ribs.

interpediculate (in''ter-pe-dik'u-lāt). Of or pertaining to the space between the pedicles of the neural arch.

interpupillary line (in''ter-pu'pi-ler''e). An imaginary line passing through the pupils of the eyes; used in radiography in the adjustment of the head in an exact lateral position.

interstice (in-ter'stis). A small gap, or space, in a tissue; an interval.

interstitial (in''ter-stish'al). Of or pertaining to the spaces, or interstices, of a tissue.

intra- (in'trah-). A prefix meaning within or into; as, intralobar, within a lobe; intravenous, injected into a vein. Cf. inter-.

intrinsic (in-trin'sik). Situated or originating entirely within an organ or part. Opposite of extrinsic.

invaginated (in-vaj'i-nāt''ed). The condition of being drawn inward so as to become ensheathed, as a covering membrane turning backward to form a double-walled cavity.

invert (in'vert). To turn inward; as, to invert the foot.

involuntary (in-vol'un-ter''e). Movement not under the control of the will, as that of the cardiac, gastrointestinal, and other involuntary muscles.

ipsilateral (ip''si-lat'er-al). [L. *ipse*, self.] Located on, or pertaining to, the same side.

-itis (-ī'tis). A suffix signifying inflammation of the specified part; as, arthritis, appendicitis, bronchitis.

J

jaundice (jawn'dis). A morbid condition caused by obstruction of the biliary passages; it is characterized by a yellowish discoloration of the skin, the eyes, and the secretions of the body due to absorption of the accumulation of bile pigments from the blood.

jejuno- (je-ju'no-), **jejun-.** A prefix signifying some relation to the jejunum; as, jejunoduodenal, jejunitis, jejunectomy, jejunostomy.

jejunum (je-ju'num). The middle division of the small intestine, extending from the duodenum to the ileum.

joint mouse (joint mous). A small, movable calcific body in or near a joint, most commonly the knee joint.

jugular (jug'u-lar). Of or pertaining to the region of the throat or neck, specifically, to the jugular vein.

juxta- (juks'tah-). A prefix meaning by the side of, near; as, juxtaspinal, juxtapyloric, juxta-articular, situated or occurring near the part specified.

juxtaposition (juks''tah-po-zish'un). A placing or being placed end to end or side by side; apposition.

K

keloid (kē'loid). A new growth or tumor of the skin consisting of dense, fibrous tissue, usually due to hypertrophy of a cicatrix, or scar.

KUB, K.U.B. Abbreviation for kidney, ureter, and bladder.

kymograph, roentgen (kī'mo-graf). An apparatus for use in the radiographic recording of the involuntary movements of such viscera as the heart, the stomach, and the diaphragm.

kyphoscoliosis (kī''fo-sko''li-ō'sis). Backward and lateral curvature of the spine.

kyphosis (kī-fō'sis). Acute curvature of the spine, usually of the thoracic region, with the convexity backward; humpback.

kyphotic (kī-fot'ik). Relating to, or affected with, kyphosis.

L

labial (lā'be-al). Of or pertaining to the lips, or labia.

labium (lā'bi-um). A lip; any lip-shaped part.

lacerated (las'er-āt''ed). Torn or mangled; not clean-cut; a wound inflicted by tearing.

lacrimal (lak'ri-mal). Pertaining to, or situated near, the lacrimal, or tear, gland; as, lacrimal duct, lacrimal bone.

lacuna (la-kū'nah). A small pit or depression; a minute cavity.

lambda (lam'dah). The eleventh Greek letter (Λ, λ); the point of junction of the lambdoidal and sagittal sutures of the cranium, the site of the posterior fontanel.

lamina (lam'i-nah). A thin, flat plate or layer; the flattened posterior portion of the neural arch, which extends from the pedicle to the median sagittal plane, where it unites with the contralateral lamina or neurapophysis.

laminagraphy (lam''i-nag'ra-fe). Same as body section radiography (*which see*).

laminated (lam'i-nāt''ed). Separated into or made up of thin, flat plates or layers; arranged in layers.

laminectomy (lam''i-nek'to-me). The excision of the posterior part of the neural arch.

laparo- (lap'a-ro-), **lapar-.** A prefix signifying relation to the flank, the side of the body extending between the ribs and the ilium; or, more loosely, to the abdominal wall; as, laparotomy, the surgical incision into the abdominal wall.

laryngo- (lăr-in'go-), **laryng-.** A prefix denoting relation to the larynx; as, laryngotracheal, laryngitis.

laryngogram (la-rin'go-gram). A radiograph of the larynx.

laryngography (lăr''in-gog'ra-fe). The roentgenographic examination of the larynx with the aid of a contrast medium.

larynx (lăr'ingks). The modified upper extremity of the trachea; the organ of voice.

latent (lā'tent). Not apparent or manifest; dormant.

laterad (lat'er-ad). Directed toward the side.

lateral (lat'er-al). Pertaining to the side.

lavage (lah''vahzh'). The washing out of an organ, especially, the irrigation of the stomach.

laxative (laks'a-tiv). A mild cathartic.

lesion (lē'zhun). Any injury or local pathologic change in the structure of an organ or part.

lien (lī'en). Latin for spleen.

lienal (lī-ē'nal). Of or pertaining to the spleen.

lienitis (lī''e-ni'tis). Inflammation of the spleen.

lieno- (lī-ē'no-), **lien-.** A prefix signifying relation to the spleen; as, lienorenal, pertaining to the spleen and the kidney.

lienography (lī''en-og'ra-fe). The roentgenographic examination of the spleen after the injection of a contrast medium.

linea (lin'e-ah). Latin for line; any normal strip, mark, or narrow ridge.

lingua (ling'gwah). Latin for tongue.

lingual (ling'gwal). Of or pertaining to the tongue; glossal.

lipo- (lip'o-), **lip-.** A prefix meaning fat, fatty; as, lipomyoma, a tumor composed of muscular and fatty elements.

lipoma (li-pō'mah). A tumor composed of fatty tissue.

-lith (-lith). A suffix meaning a concretion or calculus; as, phlebolith, a concretion or calculus in a vein.

lithiasis (li-thī'a-sis). The formation of concretions or calculi in the body, especially in the urinary passages and the gall bladder.

litho- (lith'o-), **lith-.** A prefix meaning calculus or concretion; as, lithonephritis, inflammation of the kidney caused by the presence of calculi.

lithotomy position (lith-ot'o-me). A position in which the body is supine, the legs flexed on the thighs, and the thighs flexed on the abdomen and abducted; also called the dorsosacral position.

localize (lō'kal-īz). To restrict or limit to one area or part.

localized (lō'kal-īzd). Restricted to a limited area; not general.

locular (lok'u-lar). Divided into small compartments or loculi; pertaining to a loculus or loculi.

loculus (lok'u-lus). A small cavity, compartment, or chamber; a recess or cell, as the cells of the ethmoidal sinuses.

longitudinal (lon''ji-tū'di-nal). Extending lengthwise, as distinguished from transverse; axial, as the longitudinal plane of the posterior teeth extends anteroposteriorly with the long axis of the mandible.

lordosis (lor-dō′sis). Curvature of the spine with a forward convexity.

lumbar (lum′ber). Of or pertaining to the loin; the vertebrae situated in the region of the loin.

lumen (lū′men). The cavity or clear space of a tubular passage such as an artery, a bronchus, or the intestine.

luxation (luks-ā′shun). The act or condition of being dislocated or luxated; dislocation.

lymph (limf). A transparent, nearly colorless fluid contained in the lymphatics.

lymphatics (lim-fat′iks). The lymphatic system; the lymphatic glands, and the lymphatic vessels, which pervade the body and which collect and convey the lymph.

M

macerate (mas′er-āt). To soften and separate the parts of, by soaking or steeping, with or without heat.

maceration (mas″er-ā′shun). The process of becoming macerated.

macro- (mak′ro-), **macr-**. A prefix signifying excessive development, especially elongation; as, macrocephalic, an unusually large head; also, morbid enlargement; as, macrencephaly, hypertrophy or enlargement of the brain; opposed to micro-.

magenblase (mah″gen-blah′zä). A German term applied to the radiographic shadow of the gas-filled fundic portion of the stomach.

mal- (mahl-). A prefix meaning ill, bad, badly; as, malalignment, malfunction, maldevelopment.

mal (mahl). Disease; usually qualified, as, mal de mer, petit mal.

malacia (mă-lā′shi-ah). Morbid softening of any tissue; as, osteomalacia, softening of bone.

malignant (ma-lig′nant). Virulent; having a tendency to cause death; as, a malignant tumor.

mammary (măm′ah-re). [L. mamma, breast.] Of or pertaining to the breast, or mamma (măm′ah).

mammilla (mă-mil′ah). The mammary nipple; any nipple-shaped part.

mammillary line (măm′i-ler″e). An imaginary line passing vertically through the mammilla, or one passing transversely through the mammillae.

mammography (măm-og′ra-fe). The radiologic examination of the breasts; also called mastography.

masto- (mas′to-), **mast-**. [G. mastos, breast.] A prefix denoting relation to the breast, as in mastocarcinoma, mastitis.

mastography (mas-tog′ra-fe). Same as mammography.

maximal (mak′si-mal). The greatest appreciable or allowable; opposite of minimal.

meatus (me-ā′tus); pl. **meatuses** (-iz). A natural passage or canal, especially the external orifice of such a passage.

mediad (mē′di-ad). Directed toward the median sagittal plane.

medial (mē′di-al). Situated in or occurring near the middle in relation to another part; nearer the center, or the median sagittal plane.

median (mē′di-an). Having a central position; in the middle; mesial.

mediastinum (mē″di-as-tī′num). The space between the pleural sacs of the lungs, the sternum, and the thoracic spine; it contains the heart and all the thoracic viscera except the lungs.

mediate (mē′di-it). Indirect; effected by a secondary or intervening cause or medium; not immediate.

mediate (mē′di-āt). To effect by mediation; to intervene.

medulla (me-dul′ah). The marrow of bones; the inner substance of an organ, such as that of the kidney; also, the tapering terminal portion of the brain, the medulla oblongata.

medullary (med′ŭ-ler″e). Pertaining to any medulla; consisting of or resembling marrow.

mega- (meg′ah-), **meg-**. A prefix meaning large, as in megacephalic; also, a million times, as in megohm.

megacolon (meg″ah-kō′lon). Abnormally large colon.

megalo- (meg′a-lo-), **megal-**. A prefix meaning large, great, abnormal enlargement; as, megalo-esophagus, megalakria, acromegaly.

meninges (me-nin′jēz). The three membranes (dura mater, arachnoid, and pia mater) that form the protective covering of the brain and spinal cord.

meniscus (me-nis′cus). An interarticular, crescent-shaped fibrocartilage, especially of the knee.

mental (men′tal). [L. mentum, chin; mens, mind.] Of or pertaining to the chin or to the mind.

mesati- (mes′ah-ti-). A prefix meaning medium, or mid-most; as, mesatipelvic, having a medium-sized pelvis.

mesaticephalic (mes″ah-ti-se-fal′ik). Having a head of medium or average proportions; midway between brachycephalic and dolichocephalic; same as mesocephalic.

mesentery (mes′en-ter″e). The fold of peritoneum that invests the intestines and attaches them to the posterior wall of the abdominal cavity.

mesiad (mē′zi-ad). Toward, or directed toward, the middle or the mesial plane; opposed to laterad.

mesial (mē′zi-al). Situated near or toward the median sagittal plane; medial.

mesiodistal (mē″zi-o-dis′tal). Directed lateralward or backward from the center or median line of the dental arch.

mesion (mē′zi-on). The plane that divides the body into right and left halves; the median sagittal plane.

meso- (mes′o-). A prefix meaning medium, moderate, or middle; as, mesosoma, having medium stature; mesosyphilis, the secondary stage of syphilis; mesotropic, located in the center of a cavity.

mesocephalic (mes″o-se-fal′ik.) A head of medium or average size; same as mesaticephalic.

meta- (met′ah-), **met-**. A prefix signifying change or transfer, as in metabolism, metabasis; along with, after, or next, as in metatarsus.

metaphysis (me-taf′ĭ-sis). The zone of spongy bone between the cartilaginous epiphyseal plate and the diaphysis of a long bone.

metastasis (me-tas′tah-sis). The transfer of a disease from one organ or region to another, as a malignant tumor spreading from the initial location to secondary locations in the body; also, the secondary growth so produced.

metastasize (me-tas′tah-size). To form new or secondary sites of infection in other parts of the body by metastasis, as a tumor.

metra (mē′trah) The uterus.

metro- (mē′tro-), **metr-**. A prefix denoting relation to the uterus, as in metrocarcinoma, metritis.

micro- (mī′kro-), **micr-**. A prefix meaning small, minute, as in microbe, microcephaly; also, one-millionth part of, as in microfarad.

microcephalic (mī″kro-se-fal′ik). Having an unusually small head.

micturition (mik″tū-rish′un). The act of urinating.

miscible (mis′i-b′l). Susceptible of being readily mixed; mixable.

mixture (miks′chur). A heterogeneous substance made up of two or more ingredients that retain their own properties and can be separated by mechanical means. Cf. compound; solution.

mobility (mo-bil′i-te). The capacity or facility of movement of an organ, such as the stomach, gallbladder, or kidney. Cf. motility.

mono- (mon′o-) **mon-**. A prefix meaning one, single, alone; as, monoplegia, paralysis affecting but one part of the body.

morbid (mor′bid). Disease; of or pertaining to an abnormal or diseased condition.

moribund (mor′i-bund). Near death; a dying state.

mortification (mor″ti-fi-kā′shun). Death of a part or localized area of tissue; gangrene.

motility (mo-til′i-te). The capacity to move or contract spontaneously; contractility. Cf. mobility.

mucoid (mū′koid). Resembling mucus.

mucosa (mū-kō′sah). Mucous membrane.

mucosal (mū-kō′sal). Of or pertaining to mucous membrane.

mucous (mū′kus). Of or pertaining to mucus.

mucus (mū′kus). The viscid, watery fluid secreted by the mucous glands.

Müller maneuver. (Johannes Peter Müller, German physiologist, 1801-1858.) Forced inspiration against a closed glottis. The maneuver is performed by closing the mouth, holding the nose, and attempting to breathe in.

multi- (mul′ti-). A prefix meaning many, much; as, multilobular, composed of many lobes.

multipara (mul-tip′a-rah). A woman who has borne two or more children.

mummify (mum'mi-fī). A term which, as used in nursing and roentgenographic procedures, means to wrap the body mummy fashion with a sheet, binding the arms to the sides, in order to restrain movement during an examination or treatment.

myel (mī'el). The spinal cord; myelon.

myelitis (mī''e-lī'tis). Inflammation of the spinal cord or of the bone marrow.

myelo- (mī'e-lo-), **myel-**. A prefix denoting relation to the bone marrow or to the spinal cord; as, myeloma, myelomeningitis.

myelography (mī''e-log'ra-fe). The roentgenographic examination of the spinal cord following the injection of a contrast medium into the spinal canal.

myo- (mī'o-), **my-**. A prefix signifying relation to a muscle or muscles; as, myocarditis, myositis.

myoma (mī-ō'mah). A tumor consisting of muscular elements.

N

nares (na'rēz); sing. naris (na'ris). The openings of the nasal passages; the anterior nares are commonly called the nostrils.

nasion (na'zi-on). The midpoint of the frontonasal suture.

naso- (na'zo-). A prefix denoting relation to the nose; as, nasofrontal, nasopharyngeal.

nates (na'tēz). The buttocks.

nausea (naw'she-ah). A feeling of sickness at the stomach, associated with a desire to vomit.

navel (na'vel). The cicatrix, or scar, in the center of the abdomen, marking the point of attachment of the umbilical cord; the umbilicus.

necrosis (ne-kro'sis). Death or mortification of a part or of a circumscribed area of tissue.

necrotic (ne-krot'ik). Affected with, or pertaining to, necrosis, or death of tissue.

neo- (ne'o-). A prefix meaning new or recent; as, neonatus, a newborn infant.

neoplasm (ne'o-plasm). Any new or morbid growth, such as a tumor.

nephro- (nef'ro-), **nephr-**. A prefix denoting relation to the kidney; as, nephrolith, nephritis, nephrectomy.

nephrolithiasis (nef''ro-li-thi'a-sis). A condition caused by an accumulation of calculi in the kidney.

nephroptosis (nef''rop-to'sis). Abnormal dropping or downward movement of the kidney.

neural (nū'ral). Pertaining to a nerve of the nervous system.

neuro- (nū'ro-), **neur-**. A prefix denoting relation to the nerves, as in neurofibroma, neuralgia, neuritis.

niche (nich). A small recess or hollow space in a wall; an abnormal saccular prominence on the wall of the stomach due to an ulcer crater.

nodular (nod'u-lar). Pertaining to, or having the form of, a node or nodule.

nodule (nod'ūl). A small, rounded prominence; a little bump.

norm (norm). A fixed or authoritative standard; a rule; a pattern or model; a type.

normal (nor'mal). Conforming to an established norm or principle; regular; natural; functioning properly.

normal salt solution. A normal or, more correctly, a physiologic salt solution is approximately isotonic with the body fluids; it is a 0.9% solution of sodium chloride, which is common table salt.

nullipara (nu-lip'ar-ah). A woman who has never borne a child.

O

obstetrics (ob-stet'riks). The science dealing with pregnancy and parturition; the management of childbirth.

occiput (ok'si-put). The back part of the cranium.

occlusal (o-klu'sal). Of or pertaining to the biting surface of a tooth or the teeth.

occlusal line. An imaginary line passing through the head at, and parallel with, the biting surface of the teeth.

occlusion (o-klu'zhun). The act of closing or occluding, or the state of being closed or occluded, as in a stricture of a normal passage; also, the bringing into contact of the opposing surfaces of the upper and lower teeth.

oedema (e-dē'mah). See edema.

-ology (-ol'o-je). A suffix meaning a science or branch of knowledge; as, radiology, the science dealing with the diagnostic and therapeutic application of roentgen and radium radiation.

-oma (-o'mah); pl. **-omata** (o'mah-tah), or **-omas** (-o'maz). A suffix denoting a morbid condition of some type, usually a tumor, such as carcinoma, fibroma, myoma, sarcoma.

omentum (o-men'tum). The free folds of peritoneum that connect the stomach with the adjacent organs, the apronlike great omentum hanging downward in front of the small intestines.

optimal (op'ti-mal). The best; the most conducive to success.

optimum (op'ti-mum). The condition that is best or most favorable; the most suitable degree, quantity, or factor for the attainment of a given end.

oral (o'ral). Of or pertaining to the mouth, or to speech sound.

orbitomeatal line (or''bi-to-me-ā'tal). An imaginary line extending from the outer canthus to the center of the tragus; it is used in radiography for localization purposes.

organic (or-gan'ik). Of or pertaining to an organ or organs; consisting of, or affecting, organic structure; also (chemistry) pertaining to carbon compounds, those of artificial origin as well as those derived from living organisms.

orifice (or'i-fis). The opening, or aperture, of any body cavity.

ortho- (or'tho-), **orth-**. A prefix meaning straight or normal; correct or true; as, orthodontic, orthographic, orthuria, orthostatic, standing upright, caused by or pertaining to standing erect.

orthodiagraph (or''tho-di'a-graf). A radioscopic apparatus for tracing the exact size of an organ, especially the heart, by restricting the radiation to the margin of the organ with a small movable aperture; the shadow thus cast, and the tracing obtained, represent the true size of the organ due to the utilization of only the parallel rays.

orthopedics (or''tho-pe'diks). The branch of surgery dealing with the correction or prevention of deformities, and with the treatment of diseases of the bones.

os (os); pl. **ora** (o'rah). [L. *oris*, mouth.] A mouth; any mouthlike orifice; as, os uteri.

os (os); pl. **ossa** (os'ah). [L. *ossis*, bone.] A bone; as, os calcis, os coxae, os magnum.

os innominatum (os in-nom''i-nā'tum). The innominate bone; os coxa.

-osis (-o'sis); pl. **-oses** (-o'sēz). A suffix denoting state or condition; as, psychosis, stenosis, sclerosis.

ossification (os'i-fi-kā'shun). The formation of bone; the process of changing into bone.

osteo- (os'te-o-), **oste-**. A prefix denoting relation to bone; as, osteoma, a benign bony tumor.

osteomalacia (os''te-o-mal-a'shi-ah). A chronic disease characterized by gradual softening of the bones, with resultant deformities.

osteomyelitis (os''te-o-mi-el-i'tis). Inflammation of the marrow and medullary portion of a bone.

osteoporosis (os''te-o-po-ro'sis). A condition characterized by the absorption or rarefaction of bone so that the tissue becomes thin and porous.

ostium (os'ti-um). A small mouthlike orifice, especially the opening into a tubular passage such as an oviduct.

(o)-stomy. [G. *stomos*, mouth.] A suffix signifying the surgical formation of an artificial mouth or opening into some part, or between two parts; as, enterostomy, the formation of an opening into the intestines through the abdominal wall; gastroenterostomy, the formation of an artificial opening between the stomach and the small intestine.

otic (o'tik). Of or pertaining to the ear; auditory.

otitis (o-ti'tis). Inflammation of the ear; as, otitis media, inflammation of the middle ear.

(o)-tomy. [G. *-tomia*, cutting.] A suffix signifying the surgical incision of, usually for the purpose of draining; as, cholecystotomy, nephrotomy, osteotomy.

oviduct (o'vi-dukt). The duct, or passage, extending, one on each side, from the uterus to the ovary; the fallopian tubes.

oxycephalic (ok''si-se-fal'ik). Having an unusually high vertex; a steeple-shaped head.

P

pachy- (pak'e-). A prefix meaning thick, dense; as, pachypleuritis, inflammation of the pleura attended with thickening of the membranes.

pachycephalic (pak''e-se-fal'ik). Having unusually thick, dense cranial walls.

Paget's disease (paj'ets). Osteitis deformans; a chronic disease of the bones, characterized by irregular rarefaction and thickening, enlargement, and deformity.

palsy (pawl'ze). A loss of power of voluntary movement or sensation, partial or complete, of any part of the body; paralysis.

para- (par'ah-), **par-**. A prefix denoting: irregular or abnormal, as in paranoia, parachroia, parachroma, resembling in form (said of diseases), as in paraparesis, parapneumonia, paratyphoid; near, beside, alongside of, as in paracystic, parathyroid; accessory to, as in paranasal sinuses. Cf. peri-.

paracentesis (par''ah-sen-te'sis). The surgical puncture of a cavity of the body for the withdrawal of fluid; tapping.

paralysis (pah-ral'i-sis). A loss of function or sensation, partial or complete, in any part of the body through injury or disease of the nerve supply; palsy.

paralysis agitans (aj'i-tanz). A chronic, progressive disease of old age, characterized by muscular tremor, weakness, and a peculiar gait; shaking palsy or Parkinson's disease.

parenchyma (pah-reng'ki-mah). The essential, functional tissue of an organ as distinguished from its stoma or framework.

paries (pā'ri-ēz); pl. **parietes** (pah-rī'e-tēz). A wall, especially the wall of a hollow organ or a cavity.

parietal (pah-rī'e-tal). Of or pertaining to the parietes, or walls of a cavity.

parotid (pah-rot'id). Situated near the ear; specifically, the parotid gland, the largest of the salivary group, which is located on the side of the face in front of and below the ear.

parotitis (par''ot-i'tis). Inflammation of the parotid glands; mumps.

parturition (par''tū-rish'un). The process of bringing forth young; labor; childbirth.

patent (pā'tent). Open, patulous, unoccluded, as the lumen of a vessel.

p.c. Abbreviation for Latin *post cibum*, after food.

patho- (path'o-), **path-**. A prefix denoting disease; as, pathogenic, causing or giving origin to disease.

pathology (pah-thol'o-je). The science treating of the essential nature of diseases, the structural and functional alterations caused by them; also, the condition or changes produced by disease.

pediatrics (pe''de-at'riks). The science that treats of the diseases of children.

pedicle (ped'i-k'l). [L. *pediculus*, little foot.] A short stem or stalklike part; a pedicle or peduncle; specifically, the anterolateral part of each side of the neural arch, connecting the laminae with the body of the vertebra.

pedicular (pe-dik'u-lar). [L. *pedicularis*, louse.] Pertaining to lice; lousy.

pediculate (pe-dik'u-lāt). (L. *pediculatus*.) Of or pertaining to a pedicle or pedicles.

pedunucular (pe-dung'ku-lar). Of or pertaining to a peduncle or pedicle.

pelvimetry (pel-vim'e-tre). The measurement of the size and capacity of the pelvis.

peri- (per'i-). A prefix meaning around, about, all around, near; as, periapical, around the apex of a tooth.

periosteum (per''i-os'te-um). The fibrous membrane that closely invests all parts of the surface of a bone, except the articular surfaces.

periphery (pe-rif'er-e). The external part of an organ; the circumference.

peristalsis (per''i-stal'sis). The rhythmic contractions by which tubular passages such as the alimentary canal force their contents onward.

petrous (pet'rus; pē'trus). Resembling a stone or rock; specifically, pertaining to the petrosa or petrous portion of the temporal bone.

pH. A symbol used to denote the negative logarithm of the hydrogen ion concentration in gram atoms per liter.

phleb- (fleb-), **phlebo-**. A suffix denoting relation to a vein; as, phlebitis, phlebolith.

phlebogram (fleb'o-gram). A radiograph of the veins following the injection of a radiopaque substance; also called a venogram.

phonate (fō'nāt). To utter throaty or laryngeal, usually prolonged, vowel sounds with minimum aid from the lips.

phrenic (fren'ik). [G. *phren, phrenos*, the diaphragm, the mind.] Of or pertaining to the diaphragm, or to the mind.

phrenico- (fren'-ko). A prefix signifying some relation to the phrenic nerve; as, phrenicotomy.

phreno- (fren'o-), **phren-**. A prefix denoting relation to the diaphragm; as, phrenogastric, phrenohepatic; or to the mind; as, phrenopathy, phrenoplegia.

physiology (fiz''i-ol'o-je). The science that treats of the functions of tissues and organs, as distinguished from anatomy, which deals with their structure.

placenta (plah-sen'tah). A flat, cakelike mass; specifically, the vascular organ through which the fetus communicates with the mother by means of the umbilical cord.

placentography (plas''en-tog'ra-fe). The roentgenographic examination of the gravid uterus for localization of the placenta.

plane (plān). Any flat surface, real or imaginary.

planigraphy (plah-nig'ra-fe). Same as body section radiography.

platy- (plat'i-), **plat-**. A prefix meaning broad, flat; as, platycephalic, having a broad, flat head.

pleural (ploor'a-). Of or pertaining to the pleura or pleurae.

pleurisy (ploor'-se). Inflammation of the pleura, usually attended with exudation into the pleural cavity.

plica (pli'kah). A fold; as, plica sublingualis, the fold of mucous membrane on each side of the floor of the mouth overlying the sublingual gland.

-pnea (-p'ne'ah). A suffix meaning breath; as, eupnea, dyspnea.

pneumo- (nū'mo-). [G. *pneumon*, lung; *pneuma*, air.] A prefix denoting relation to the lungs, or to air or other gas; as, pneumonia, pneumonic, pneumothorax, pneumocystography, pneumoperitoneum.

pneumothorax (nū''mo-tho'raks). An accumulation of air or other gas in the pleural cavity, usually induced for therapeutic purposes, but occasionally, spontaneously as a result of injury or disease.

poly- (pol'e-). A prefix meaning many, much, often; as, polycystic, polygraph, polymorphous.

polyp (pol'ip). A projection of hypertrophied mucous membrane in a body cavity such as the nose, the paranasal sinuses, and urinary bladder; a polypus.

popliteal (pop-lit'e-al). Of or pertaining to the part of the knee behind the joint.

porus (pō'rus). Latin for pore or opening; meatus; as, the porus acusticus internus, the internal auditory meatus.

post-. A prefix meaning behind, after, later; as, postnasal, postpartum, postdiastolic.

post cibum (post-sī'bum). Latin for after food. Abbreviation, p.c.

posterior (pos-ter'i-er). Pertaining to, designating, or situated in, the back part of the body or of an organ.

posteroanterior (pos''ter-o-an-ter'i-er). Directed or extending from back to front.

pre- (prē-). A prefix signifying before in time or place; as, prenatal, prevertebral.

primigravida (pri''mi-grav'i-dah). A woman pregnant for the first time

primipara (pri-mip'ah-rah). A woman who is bearing or has borne her first child.

pro- (prō-). A prefix signifying forward, to the front, according to; as, project, progress, prolapse, proportion.

procto- (prok'to-), **proct-**. A prefix denoting relation to the anus and rectum; as, proctopolypus, proctoscope, proctitis.

prognosis (prog-no'sis). A forecast of the course and probable outcome of a disease.

pronation (pro-nā'shun). Medial rotation of the hand so that it faces downward or backward; the act of lying face downward; opposite of supination.

prone (prōn). Lying face downward; having the palm of the hand facing downward or backward.

prophylaxis (pro''fi-lak'sis). The protection from, or prevention of, disease; protective or preventive treatment.

prostato- (pros'tah-to-), **prostat-**. A prefix denoting relation to the prostate gland; as, prostatocystitis, prostatitis.

prostatography (pros''tah-tog'ra-fe). The roentgenographic examination of the prostate gland.

protuberance (pro-tū'ber-ans). Any projecting part; a swelling; a general term for a process or projection.

proximal (prok'si-mal). Toward the beginning or source of a part; toward the head end of the body; opposed to distal.

pseudo- (sū'do-), **pseud-**. A prefix meaning false; illusory;

having a deceptive resemblance to; as, pseudoankylosis, pseudoparalysis, pseudarthrosis.

P.S.P. The abbreviation commonly used for a kidney function test with the use of either phenolsulfonphthalein or indigo carmine.

psychiatry (sī'kī'ah-tre). The science that treats of mental disorders, psychoses, and neurosis.

psycho- (sī'ko-), **psych-.** A prefix denoting relation to the mind or mental processes, as in psychogenic, psychoneurosis, psychosis.

psychology (sī-kol'o-je). The science that deals with the mind in all its aspects; the study of mental activity and behavior.

ptosis (tō'sis). The prolapse, or dropping, of an organ from its normal position; usually used as a suffix, as in enteroptosis, gastroptosis, viseroptosis.

puerile (pū'er-il). Of or pertaining to a child or children, or to childhood; immature; juvenile.

puerperal (pū-er'per-al). Of or pertaining to childbirth; as, puerperal sepsis, puerperal fever.

pulmonary, pulmonic (pul'mo-ner-e; pul-mon'ik). [L. *pulmo,* lung.] Of or pertaining to the lungs.

purgative (pur'gah-tiv). A purging or cathartic medicine, causing extensive evacuations. These agents are more drastic in action than the laxative or cathartic groups, which stimulate peristaltic activity and increase the tendency to evacuate the bowels with a minimum of irritation.

purulent (pū'rōō-lent). Consisting of, or of the nature of, pus or matter; associated with suppuration; as, a purulent lesion or wound.

pus (pŭs). The yellowish, greenish, or brownish matter generated by suppuration as a result of bacterial infection.

putrefaction (pū''tre-fak'shun). The decomposition of organic (animal or vegetable) matter, with the formation of various foul-smelling products; decay.

putrescent (pū-tres'ent). Undergoing decomposition or decay; pertaining to putrefaction; as, an offensive or putrescent odor.

pyelo- (pī'e-lo-), **pyel-.** A prefix denoting relation to the pelvis of the kidney, as in pyelogram, pyelitis.

pyo- (pī'o-.), **py-.** A prefix signifying the presence of pus; as, pyogenesis, pyonephrosis, pyuria.

Q

quadrant (qwod'rant). A fourth; a quarter; any one of four equal parts or divisions, as of the orbit or of the abdomen.

quadrate (kwod'rāt). Square or almost square in form; cubical.

quickening (kwik'en-ing). The first movement of the fetus in utero felt by the mother, usually occurring about midterm.

R

racemose (ras'e-mōs). [L. *racemosus,* having clusters like a bunch of grapes.] A compound saccular gland (such as the pancreas) having numerous branching ducts ending in acini arranged like grapes on a stalk.

rachio- (rā'ki-o-), **rachi-.** [G. *rachis,* spine.] A prefix denoting relation to the spine, as in rachiocentesis, rachioplegia, rachitis.

radio- (ra'di-o-). [L. *radius,* ray.] A prefix denoting (1) radial or radially, as lines radiating from a center, (2) radial, as in radiomuscular, (3) relation to the lateral and larger of the bones of the forearm, as in radioulnar, radiohumeral, and (4) relation to radiant energy, especially to roentgen and radium radiation, as in radioactive, radiosensitive, radionecrosis.

radiodontia (ra''di-o-don'shi-ah). The roentgenographic examination of the teeth and their supporting structures.

radiolucent (ra''di-o-lū'sent). Materials offering little resistance to the passage of x-radiation; those which have insufficient physical density to cast an appreciable image on the film when exposed to kilovoltages used in radiography of the body. Cf. radioparent.

radiopaque (ra''di-o-pāk'). Materials that are impenetrable to x-radiation generated by the kilovoltages usually employed in medical radiography.

radioparent (ra''di-o-păr'ent). Materials wholly transparent to x-radiation. Cf. radiolucent.

radius (ra'di-us). A line extending from the center to the periphery of a circle; the semidiameter; also, the lateral and larger bone of the forearm.

ramus (ra'mus). A branch or branchlike process, as one of the primary divisions of a nerve or blood vessel, or a projecting part of an irregularly shaped bone.

rarefaction (rar''e-fak'shun). The state of being, or the process of becoming, thin and porous or less dense without a diminution in size or volume; loss of substance; opposed to condensation and destruction.

recumbent (re-kum'bent). Reclining; lying down.

reflux (re'fluks). A flowing back, as the return or reflux of a fluid.

regurgitation (re-gur''ji-ta'shun). To flow or be cast backward, as blood from a heart chamber in insufficiency of a valve; also, the egestion, or casting up, of incompletely digested food.

Reid's base line (rēdz). (Robert William Reid, Scottish anatomist, 1851-1938.) *See* anthropologic base line.

renal (re'nal). [L. *ren,* kidney.] Of or pertaining to the kidney or kidneys.

resorption (re-sorp'shun). The process of absorbing again; the removal by absorption of an exudate or of bone.

respiratory (re-spīr'ah-tō''re; res'pi-rah-to''re). Of or pertaining to respiration or the respiratory organs.

retro- (rē'tro-; ret'ro-). A prefix signifying backward, as in retroflexion; behind, as in retrosternal; reversed, or against the natural course, as in retrostalsis.

retrograde (rē'tro-grad). Directed against the natural course; specifically, retrograde pyelography, in which the contrast solution is injected in a direction contrary to the natural flow of the urinary secretions.

rhinal (rī'nal). Of or pertaining to the nose; nasal.

ruga (rōō'gah); pl. **rugae** (rōō'jē). A wrinkle or fold of mucous membrane; specifically, the rugae or folds of gastric mucosa in the empty or nearly empty stomach.

S

š. Symbol for Latin *sine,* without.

sac (săk). A soft-walled bag or pouch; any bladderlike organ.

sacculated (săk'u-lāt''ed). Having the form of a sac or sacs; characterized by a series of pouched expansions or saccules.

sacralization (sa''kral-i-za'shun). Overdevelopment of one or both of the transverse processes of the last lumbar segment, with encroachment upon, or fusion with, the first sacral segment.

sagittal (saj'i-tal). Of or pertaining to the sagittal suture of the cranium, which lies in the median sagittal plane of the body; pertaining to any plane parallel with the midsagittal or median sagittal plane.

sal (sal). Latin for salt.

saline (sā'līn). Consisting of or containing a salt or salts; salty; a saline solution, especially a physiologic, or so-called normal, salt solution.

salpingo- (sal-ping'go-), **salping-.** A prefix denoting some relation to an oviduct or, less commonly, to a eustachian tube.

salpinx (sal'pingks); pl. **salpinges** (salpin'jēz). [G. *salpinx,* tube.] An oviduct; less commonly, a eustachian tube.

sarcoma (sar-ko'mah). A malignant tumor derived from tissue developed from the mesoderm (connective and lymphoid tissue, bone, cartilage, muscle, and part of the urogenital organs) and characterized by a fleshy consistency.

sclero- (skler'o-), **scler-.** A prefix meaning hard, indurated, fibrous; also used to denote relation to the sclera.

sclerosis (skle-ro'sis). Hardening, or induration, of tissue, especially of interstitial connective tissue.

scoliosis (sko''li-o'sis). [G. *skolios,* crooked.] Abnormal lateral curvature of the spinal column.

secreta (se-krē'tah). Any product of secretion; the secretions.

secrete (se-krēt'). To separate substances from the blood and emit as a secretion.

secretion (se-krē'shun). The process of secreting; also, the material secreted.

sedative (sed'ah-tiv). A soothing medicine.

semi- (sem'i-). A prefix meaning partly; half or approximately half; as, semiflexion, semiprone, semicoma.

sepsis (sep'sis). Poisoning due to the absorption of pathogenic bacteria and their products from a putrefactive process.

septic (sep'tik). Putrefactive; produced by or due to pathogenic bacteria.

septum (sep'tum). Any dividing wall or partition.

sequestrum (se-kwes'trum); pl. **sequestra** (se-kwes'trah). A piece of bone that has become detached as a result of trauma or necrosis.

shadowgram, shadowgraph (shad'o-gram, shad'o-graf). A radiograph; a roentgenogram.

sialaden (sī-al'ad-en). [G. *sialon*, saliva + *aden*, gland.] A salivary gland.

sialography (sī''al-og'ra-fe). The roentgenographic examination of a salivary gland or duct after the injection of a radiopaque contrast medium.

silicosis (sil'i-ko'sis). A condition of the lungs caused by prolonged inhalation of dust particles of stone or silica; pneumonoconiosis.

Sims' position (simz). A position in which the body is semiprone, lying on the left side, with the right knee drawn up.

sinciput (sin'si-put). The forehead; the anterior part of the cranium.

sine (sī'ne). Latin for without; symbol s̄.

sinistrad (sin'is-trad). Directed toward the left; opposite of dextrad.

sinistro- (sin'is-tro-), **sinistr-**. A prefix meaning left, as in sinistrocardia, sinistrocerebral.

sinus (sī'nus). A cavity or hollow space in bone or other tissue; a dilated channel for the passage of venous blood; a suppurating tract.

skiagraph, skiagram (ski'ah-graf, ski'ah-gram). An old term for a radiograph or roentgenogram.

solution (so-lū'shun). A homogeneous body (typically liquid, but may be gaseous or solid) consisting of two parts, (1) the *solvent*, or dissolving substance, and (2) the *solute*, or dissolved substance. The molecules of the solute, or dissolved substance, are dispersed among those of the solvent, and cannot be filtered out, nor will they settle out upon standing. The composition or concentration of a solution can be varied within certain limits. A solution is similar to a compound in that it is homogeneous, and similar to a mixture in that its composition is variable.

spasm (spaz'm). An involuntary, convulsive contraction of a muscle or muscles.

specific gravity (spe-sif'ik grav'i-te). Abbreviation, sp. gr. The relative density or weight of any volume of a substance compared with that of an equal volume of water at the same temperature and pressure.

sphincter (sfingk'ter). A circular muscle structure that serves to close one of the orifices of the body; as, the sphincter ani, the sphincter of Oddi, and the pyloric sphincter.

spicule (spik'ūl). A minute, needlelike fragment, especially of bone.

spina bifida (spi'nah bif'i-dah). A congenital malformation of the vertebral arch in which there is a cleft in a lamina, with hernial protrusion of the spinal cord and meninges.

spina bifida occulta (o-kul'tah). A cleft in the vertebral arch without herniation of the spinal cord and meninges.

spondylitis (spon''di-li'tis). Inflammation of a vertebra or vertebrae.

spondylolisthesis (spon''di-lo-lis-the'sis). Forward displacement of a lumbar vertebra, most frequently of the last lumbar segment on the sacrum.

stasis (sta'sis). Defective circulation of the blood; a slackening or stoppage of the normal flow of the contents of the vessels or of any organ of the body.

stellate (stel'āt). Shaped or radiated like a star; as, a stellate fracture of the cranium.

stenosis (ste-no'sis). A stricture, or narrowing, of the lumen or the orifice of a passage.

sternal angle (ster'nal ang'l). The angle formed by the junction of the manubrium and the gladiolus, or body, of the sternum.

sthenic (sthen'ik). Strength; vigor; opposed to asthenia.

sthenic habitus. A bodily type characterized by strong build; a modification of the more massive hypersthenic type.

stoma (sto'mah). A minute, mouthlike aperture; the surgically established opening into the intestine through the abdominal wall; also, the opening established between two anastomosed portions of the intestine.

strangulated (strang'gu-lat''ed). Compressed or constricted so as to arrest or congest circulation in a part; as, a strangulated hernia, one in which the protruding viscus is so constricted as to stop circulation.

stria (stri'ah); pl. **striae** (stri'e). A strip or line; a streak, distinguished by color, elevation, or texture.

stricture (strik'tur). A circumscribed narrowing of a canal; a constriction.

stroma (stro'mah). The tissue that forms the supporting framework of an organ, as distinguished from its parenchyma, or essential functional elements.

sub- (sub-). A prefix meaning below, under, beneath; as, subnormal, sublingual, subdiaphragmatic.

subacute (sub'ah-kūt). Between acute and chronic; having some acute symptoms.

subcutaneous (sub''ku-ta'ne-us). Situated beneath the skin.

submentovertex (sub''men-to-ver'teks). Directed from below the chin to the vertex; pertaining to the region beneath the chin and the vertex; submentovertical.

subphrenic (sub-fren'ik). Situated or occurring below the diaphragm.

sulcus (sul'kus). A furrow; a groove; a fissure; especially one of the sulci on the surface of the brain.

super- (su'per-). A prefix meaning over, above, in excess; as, superimpose, supernumerary, supersaturate.

supero- (su'per-o-). A prefix meaning above; situated or directed from above.

superoinferior (su''per-o-in-fēr'i-er). Directed from above downward; craniocaudal.

supination (su''pi-na'shun). The rotation of the hand and arm so that the palm faces forward; the act or state of lying face upward; opposed to pronation.

supine (su-pin'). Lying on the back; opposite of prone.

suppuration (sup''u-ra'shun). The process of generating and discharging pus.

supra- (su'prah-). A prefix meaning above, higher in position; as, supraclavicular, suprarenal, supraorbital.

symphysis (sim'fi-sis). The joint, or the line of fusion, between paired bones; as, the symphysis pubis, the symphysis menti.

synarthrosis (sin'ar-thro'sis). An immovable joint (such as a cranial suture) in which only fibrous connective tissue intervenes between the bones.

syncope (sing'ko-pe). Temporary suspension of respiration and circulation with loss of consciousness; fainting.

systole (sis'to-le). The contraction phase of the heartbeat; also the contraction itself, by which the blood is kept in circulation; correlative to diastole.

T

tachy- (tak'e-). A prefix meaning fast, swift; as, tachycardia, rapidity of heart action.

tangent (tan'jent). Touching at a point; meeting a curve or surface at a point and then extending beyond without intersection; as, a line or plane tangent to a curve, or a curve tangent to a line or a surface.

tangential (tan-jen'shal). Directed along or arranged in a tangent, as in the adjustment of a structure or a mass so that one or more points of its surface will be tangent to the central ray.

tele- (tel'e-; te'le-) **teleo-**. A prefix meaning far, at a distance; as, telecardiography.

teleoroentgenogram (tel''e-o-rent'gen-o-gram''). A radiograph made at a distance of six feet.

theca (the'kah). A protective case or sheath; as, theca vertebralis, the dura mater of the spinal cord.

thoracentesis (tho''rah-sen-te'sis). The surgical puncturing of the chest wall for the removal of fluid in cases of pleural effusion; tapping; also called pleuracentesis.

thoracic (tho-ras'ik). Pertaining to, or situated in the region of, the chest.

thoracoplasty (tho'rah-ko-plas''te). Plastic surgery of the thorax; especially, the resection of a part of several ribs so as to collapse the lung in cases of advanced unilateral tuberculosis.

thrombus (throm'bus). A plug or clot formed in the heart or in a blood or lymphatic vessel and remaining at the site of formation. Cf. embolus.

tomography (to-mog'ra-fe). Same as body section radiography.

tone (tōn). Healthy function; resiliency; normal vigor and elasticity; especially the tension of involuntary muscles; tonus.

tonic (ton'ik). Pertaining to or characterized by normal tone or tension, particularly muscular tension; also, an agent that tends to produce or restore a healthy condition.

topical (top'i-kal). Of or pertaining to a specific spot; local, or for local application; as a topical anesthetic.

torsion (tor'shun). The act of turning or twisting, or the state of being full of turns and twists.

torticollis (tor''ti-kol'is). Irregular contraction of the cervical muscles, with twisting of the neck and an unnatural position of the head; commonly called wryneck.

tortuous (tor'tu-us). Winding; circuitous; full of curves or bends; twisted.

trabecula (trah-bek'u-lah); pl. **trabeculae** (trah-bek'u-lē). A little beam or crossbar; one of the septal membranes in the framework of various organs; one of the intersecting osseous plates, or cancelli, composing the spongy, or cancellous, portion of a bone.

tragus (trā'gus). The cartilaginous projection in front of the external acoustic meatus.

trans- (trans-; also tranz-). A prefix meaning across, through, over; to pass across or through; as, transabdominal, passing through or across the abdomen; transoral, passing through or across the mouth.

transverse (trans-verse'). Crosswise, from side to side; horizontal; opposed to lengthwise and longitudinal.

transverse plane. A plane that divides the body or any one of its parts horizontally at any level.

trauma (traw'mah). An injury; also, the condition resulting from an injury.

traumatic (traw-mat'ik). Of, pertaining to, or caused by, a trauma.

tremor (trem'er; tre'mor). Involuntary trembling or shaking as a result of undue strain, weakness, injury, or disease.

Trendelenburg position (tren-del'en-berg). A position in which the body is recumbent on a plane inclined 45 degrees cranially.

trephine (tre-fīn'). A circular saw or trepan for removing a disk of bone, used chiefly in brain surgery for perforating the cranium; also, to operate with a trephine or trepan.

trocar (tro'kar). A sharp-pointed, rodlike instrument that is fitted into, and used for the insertion of, a cannula or a catheter.

trochanteric (tro''kan-ter'ik). Pertaining to a trochanter or trochanters.

tubercle (tu'ber-k'l). A small nodule or prominence; a small rounded process on a bone, serving for the attachment of muscles or ligaments.

tuberculosis (tu-ber''ku-lo'sis). An infectious disease caused by the tubercle bacillus and marked by the production of tubercles, fever, night sweats, and progressive emaciation. The lungs are the most common seat of infection, but such organs as the intestines, lymph nodes, larynx, kidneys, and bones are frequently involved.

tuberosity (tu''ber-os'i-te). A broad, roughened process on a bone, serving for the attachment of muscles or ligaments.

tumor (tu'mor). A circumscribed swelling; any morbid growth, innocent or malignant; a neoplasm.

U

ulcer (ul'ser). An open, suppurating sore occurring on the surface of the skin or a mucous membrane, as distinguished from an abscess, which is a sore of deep-seated origin.

umbilical (um-bil'i-kal). Of or pertain to the navel, or umbilicus.

umbilicus (um-bil'i-kus; um''bi-lī'kus). The scar on the center of the abdomen, marking the site of attachment of the umbilical cord; the navel.

uni- (ū'ni-). A prefix meaning one, single, first, as in unilocular, unidirectional, unigravida.

unilateral (u''ni-lat'er-al). Affecting, or situated upon, only one side.

uresis (u-re'sis). The discharge of urine; urination.

ureteral (u-re'ter-al). Pertaining to the ureter.

ureterography (u-re''ter-og'ra-fe). The roentgenographic examination of the ureter after the injection of a radiopaque solution.

urethral (u-re'thral). Pertaining to the urethra.

urethrogram (u-re'thro-gram). A radiograph of the contrast filled urethra.

urethrography (u-re-throg'ra-fe). The roentgenographic examination of the urethra during the injection of a contrast medium, or during voiding.

-uria (-u'ri-ah). A suffix denoting some relation to urine; as, hematuria, dysuria, pyuria.

uro- (u'ro-), **ur-**. A prefix denoting some relation to urine or to the urinary tract, as in urinalysis, urodynia, urolithiasis.

urography (u-rog'ra-fe). The roentgenographic examination of the urinary tract, or of any of its parts, with a contrast medium.

urticaria (ur''ti-kā'ri-ah). An inflammatory skin disease characterized by transient, whitish wheals on a reddish base, causing intense stinging and itching; uredo; nettle rash; hives.

uterine (u'ter-in). Of or pertaining to the uterus.

utero- (u'ter-o-), **uter-**. A prefix denoting some relation to the uterus; as, uterocele, uteroscope, uteritis.

uterography (u''ter-og'ra-fe). The roentgenographic examination of the uterus after the injection of a contrast medium.

uterosalpingography (u''ter-o-sal''pin-gog'ra-fe). The roentgenographic examination of the uterus and oviducts after the injection of a contrast medium.

V

Valsalva maneuver (văl-săl'vă). (Antonio Mario Valsalva, Italian anatomist, 1666-1723.) The act of forcing a deep breath against the closed glottis. This is achieved by a straining action, as if trying to move the bowels, without blowing out the cheeks or filling the pharynx.

varices (văr'i-sēz); pl. of varix (văr'iks). Permanently dilated and tortuous veins; varicosities.

varicose (văr'i-kōs). Irregularly dilated; enlarged and tortuous; pertaining to a venous varix or varices.

vas (văs); pl. **vasa** (vā'sah). A vessel or duct; specifically, a blood or lymph vessel.

vascular (vas'ku-lar). Pertaining to, or composed of, vessels; specifically, pertaining to the blood or lymph vessels.

vena (vē'nah); pl. **venae** (vē'nē). A vein.

venogram (ven'o-gram). A radiograph of veins filled with contrast medium; a phlebogram.

venography (ve-nog'ra-fe). The radiologic examination of veins during the injection of a radiopaque solution.

ventrad (ven'trad). [L. *venter*, belly.] Situated or directed toward the abdomen or the anterior aspect of the body; ventrally.

ventral (ven'tral). Pertaining to the abdomen or to the anterior aspect of the body or a part; designating, or situated near, the anterior aspect.

ventricle (ven'tri-k'l). A cavity of an organ, such as the ventricles of the brain or of the heart.

ventriculography (ven-trik''u-log'ra-fe). The roentgenographic examination of the brain following the injection of a radioparent medium into the ventricles; pneumoventriculography.

vermiform (ver'mi-form). Resembling a worm; as, the vermiform appendix of the cecum.

vertex (ver'teks). The top or highest part of the head.

verticomental (ver''ti-ko-men'tal). Pertaining to the vertex and the chin; as, a verticomental projection of the facial bones.

verticosubmental (ver''ti-ko-sub-men'tal). Pertaining to the vertex and the region of the throat below the chin; as, a verticosubmental projection of the petrosae.

vesicle (ves'i-k'l). A fluid-containing cavity or sac; a blister.

villi (vil'ī); sing. villus (vil'us). The minute, threadlike vascular processes that project from specialized mucous membrane, as from the mucosa of the small intestine.

Virchow's plane (fēr'chō). (Rudolf Virchow, German pathologist, 1821-1902.) See infraorbitomeatal line.

virulent (vir'u-lent). Extremely poisonous or noxious; violent; malignant.

visceral (vis'er-al). Pertaining to a viscus or viscera.

visceroptosis (vis''er-op-to'sis). A falling or downward displacement of the abdominal organs.

viscid (vis'id). Having a gelatinous or sticky consistency; adherent; viscous.

viscosity (vis-kos'i-te). The state or quality of being thick and sticky; viscid; gluey; glutinous.

viscus (vis'kus). An internal organ, such as the heart, kidney, or stomach.

vitiate (vish'i-āt). To render faulty or defective; to impair the quality of; contaminate; to make impure, as the air by electrical corona or by the products of respiration.

voluntary (vol'-un-ter"e). Proceeding in obedience to the will; acting according to choice.

vomit (vom'it). The spontaneous expulsion of the contents of the stomach by the mouth; also, the vomited matter.

vomitus (vom'i-tus). Matter ejected from the stomach through the mouth; vomiting.

Z

zoster (zos'ter). An acute inflammatory skin disease of nervous origin, causing tenderness, itching, and neuralgic pains; it is characterized by clusters of small vesicles on a reddish base following along the course of a peripheral nerve; herpes zoster; zona; shingles.

zygapophysial (zīg"ap-of-iz'e-al). Of or pertaining to a zygapophysis or to zygapophyses.

zygapophysis (zīg"ah-pof'i-sis). [G. *zygon*, yoke + *apophysis*, process.] A yokelike articular process; specifically, one of the articular processes of the neural arch of a vertebra.

zygion (zig'i-on; zij'i-on). The point at either end of the bregmatic diameter of the skull.

zygoma (zī-go'mah). The arch formed by the union of the malar bone of the face and the zygomatic process of the temporal bone of the cranium; also, the malar bone.

zygomatic (zī"go-mat'ik). Of or pertaining to the zygomatic arch or to the malar bone.

Volume I
Bibliography

HISTORY

1895   Röntgen, Wilhelm Conrad: Ueber eine neue Art von Strahlen. Part I, Sitzungsber. phys.-med. Gesellsch. Würzburg, pp. 132-141, 1895, English translation in Science 3:Feb. 14, 1896.

1896   Röntgen, Wilhelm Conrad: Ueber eine neue Art von Strahlen. Part II, Sitzungsber. phys.-med. Gesellsch. Würzburg, pp. 11-19, 1896, English translation in Science 3:May 15, 1896.

1897   Röntgen, W. C.: Weitere Beobachtungen über X-strahlen, Mitt. Sitzungsberichte Preuss. Akad. Wess., Physik. Math. K1., p. 392, 1897.

1905   Albers-Schönberg, H. E.: The development and present state of radiology, Arch. Roentgen Ray 10:105, 1905.

1909   Pfahler, G. E.: Notes from some of the roentgen laboratories in Europe, Amer. Quart. Roentgen. 2:15-22, 1909-1910.

1923   Grashey, R.: Wilhelm Conrad Röntgen, Fortschr. Roentgenstr. 30:409, 1923.

1929   Memenov, M. I.: Das Staatsinstitut für Röntgenologie, Radiologie und Krebsforschung in Leningrad, Fortschr. Roentgenstr. 40:1069-1087, 1929.

1931   Brown, P.: Early American roentgenology; manners and men, Radiogr. Clin. Photogr. 7:2-6, 1931.

Glasser, Otto: Dr. W. C. Roentgen and the discovery of the roentgen ray, Amer. J. Roentgen. 25:437-450, 1931.

Hickey, Preston M.: The Caldwell lecture, 1928, Amer. J. Roentgen. 25:177-195, 1931.

1932   Glasser, Otto: Reception of Roentgen's discovery in America, Radiogr. Clin. Photogr. 8:2-6, 1932.

O'Hara, F. S.: Looking backward, Radiogr. Clin. Photogr. 8:3-9, 1932.

1934   Crane, A. W.: The research trail of the x-ray, Radiology 23:131-148, 1934.

Curie, Marie Sklodowska: An editorial by E. W. Hall, Amer. J. Roentgen. 32:395, 1934.

Donaghey, J. P.: Reminiscences of Röntgen, Radiogr. Clin. Photogr. 10:2-7, 1934.

Forssell, Gösta: Marie Curie—in memoriam, Acta Radiol. 15:685-688, 1934.

Glasser, Otto: Wilhelm Conrad Röntgen and the early history of roentgen rays, Springfield, Ill., 1934, Charles C Thomas, Publisher.

Schinz, Hans R.: Röntgen und Zürich, Acta Radiol. 15:562-575, 1934.

1936   Brown, Percy: American martyrs to science through the roentgen ray, Springfield, Ill., 1936, Charles C Thomas, Publisher.

1937   Glasser, Otto: The life of Röntgen as revealed in his letters, Scient. Monthly 45:193-206, 1937.

1938   Pancoast, H. K.: Reminiscences of a radiologist, Amer. J. Roentgen. 39:169-186, 1938.

1939   Casey, Frances S.: Early scientists in the field of radiology, Xray Techn. 11:88-92, 1939.

1944   Glasser, O., Quimby, E. H., Taylor, L. S., and Weatherwax, J. L.: Physical foundations of radiology, New York, 1944, Paul B. Hoeber, Inc.

1945   Case, James T.: Fifty years of roentgen rays in gastroenterology, Amer. J. Roentgen. 54:607-625, 1945.

Davidoff, Leo M.: The development of modern neuroroentgenology, Amer. J. Roentgen. 54:640-642, 1945.

Glasser, Otto: Fifty years of roentgen rays, Radiogr. Clin. Photogr. 21:58-66, 1945.

Glasser, Otto: Scientific forefathers of Röntgen, Amer. J. Roentgen. 54:545-546, 1945.

Glasser, Otto: Chronology of Röntgen's life, Amer. J. Roentgen. 54:541-544, 1945.

Glasser, Otto: W. C. Röntgen, Springfield, Ill., 1945, Charles C Thomas, Publisher.

Hodges, Paul C.: Development of diagnostic x-ray apparatus during the first fifty years, Radiology 45:438-448, 1945.

Kirklin, B. R.: Background and beginning of cholecystography, Amer. J. Roentgen. 54:637-639, 1945.

Lough, Thomas W.: Commemorating a great discovery and half a century of its development, Xray Techn. 17:325-330, 1945.

Reynolds, Lawrence: The history of the use of the roentgen ray in warfare, Amer. J. Roentgen. 54:649-672, 1945.

Rigler, Leo G.: The development of roentgen diagnosis, Radiology 45:467-502, 1945.

Roesler, Hugo: History of the roentgen ray in the study of the heart, Amer. J. Roentgen. 54:647-648, 1945.

Röntgen, Wilhelm Conrad: On a new kind of rays, Reprint from Röntgen's original papers, Radiology 45:428-435, 1945.

Shields, David G.: Fashion parade of x-ray apparatus 1895-1945, Xray Techn. 17:348-360, 1945.

Spillman, Ramsay: Early history of roentgenology of the sinuses, Amer. J. Roentgen. 54:643-646, 1945.

Wolcott, Roy E.: X-ray horizons, Xray Techn. 17:337-347, 377, 1945.

1946   Chevalier, Jean: Vie et travaux de Roentgen, J. Radiol. Electr. 27:107-110, 1946.

Dariaux, A.: Hommage aux victimes des rayons X, J. Radiol. Electr. 27:101-104, 1946.

Delherm, L.: Première communication en France, sur les applications médicales de la découverte de Roentgen, J. Radiol. Electr. 27:105-106, 1946.

Lacharite, H.: The healing and lethal rays, Xray Techn. 18:111-115, 138, 1946.

Ledoux-Lebard, R.: Les rayons X dans le diagnostic médical, J. Radiol. Electr. 27:116-125, 1946.

Pilon, H.: Cinquante ans de construction radiologique, J. Radiol. Electr. 27:111-115, 1946.

Stolz, Sister Mary Fides: Contributions of some of Röntgen's predecessors, Xray Techn. 18:1-4, 1946.

1947   Fuchs, Arthur W.: Edison and roentgenology, Amer. J. Roentgen. 57:145-156, 1947.

1951   Scott, W. G.: The development of angiocardiography and aortography, Radiology 56:485-518, 1951.

1952   Leucutia, T.: Pneumoperitoneum and pneumoretroperitoneum (editorial), Amer. J. Roentgen. 68:655-658, 1952.

1954   Diehl, K. L.: Bronchography; study of its techniques and presentations of improved modification, Arch. Otolaryng. 60:277-290, 1954.

Stevenson, C. A.: Development of colon examination, Amer. J. Roentgen. 71:385-397, 1954.

1955   Olson, L. G.: Roentgen's scientific forefathers, Xray Techn. 27:184-189, 1955.

1956   Caffey, John: The first sixty years of pediatric roentgenology in the United States, Amer. J. Roentgen. 76:437-454, 1956.

Maluf, N. S. R.: Role of roentgenology in the development of urology, Amer. J. Roentgen. 75:847-854, 1956.

1958   Glasser, Otto: W. C. Röntgen, Springfield, Ill., 1958, Charles C Thomas, Publisher.

Kincaid, O. W., and Davis, G. D.: Abdominal aortography, New England J. Med. 259:1017-1024, 1958.

1960   Scott, John: Ancient and modern, Radiography 26:97-107, 1960.

1961   Bull, J. W. D.: History of neuroradiology, Brit. J. Radiol. 34:69-84, 1961.

Cole, W. H.: Historical features of cholecystography, Radiology 76:354-375, 1961.

Gershon-Cohen, J.: Breast roentgenology; a historical review, Amer. J. Roentgen. 86:879-883, 1961.

Watson, W.: 1895 and all that, Radiography 27:305-315, 1961.

1964   Bruwer, A. J., editor: Classic descriptions in diagnostic roentgenology, Springfield, Ill., 1964, Charles C Thomas, Publisher.

Strain, W. H., Rogoff, S. M., Greenlaw, R. H., Johnston, R. M., Huegin, F., and Berliner, W. P.: Radiologic diagnostic agents: a compilation, Med. Radiogr. Photogr. 40(supp.):1-110, 1964.

1965   Grigg, E. R. N.: The trail of the invisible light, Springfield, Ill., 1965, Charles C Thomas, Publisher.

Grigg, E. R. N.: The new history of radiology, Radiol. Techn. 36:229-257, 1965.

Schatzki, R.: Esophagus; progress and problems; the Caldwell lecture, Amer. J. Roentgen. 94:523-540, 1965.

JOURNALS

Acta Radiologica, Stockholm, Sweden, 1921-

American Atlas of Stereo-roentgenology, Troy, 1916-1920.

American Journal of Roentgenology, Pittsburgh, Pa., 1913-1923, and continued as
American Journal of Roentgenology and Radium Therapy, Pittsburgh, Pa., 1923-
American Journal of Surgery, New York, 1890-
American Quarterly of Roentgenology, Pittsburgh, Pa., 1906-1913.
American X-ray Journal, St. Louis, Mo., 1897-1904.
Anales del Instituto Municipal de Radiologia y Fisioterapia, Buenos Aires, 1934-
Anales de Radiologia . . . órgano oficial de la Sociedad cubana de radiología y fisioterapía, Havana, 1929-
Annales de Roentgenologie et Radiologie; Journal de l'Institut d'état de Radiologie à Pétersbourg, Pétersbourg, 1922-
Annali di Radiologia e Fisica Medica, Bologna, 1934-
Annals of Otology, Rhinology and Laryngology, St. Louis, Mo., 1897-
Annals of Surgery, Philadelphia, Pa., 1885-
Archives of Electrology and Radiology, Chicago, 1904-
Archives of Radiology and Electrotherapy, London, 1915-
Archivio di Radiologia, Naples, 1925-
Archivos del Instituto Municipal de Radiología y Fisioterapía, Buenos Aires, 1934-
Archivos Uruguayos de Medicina, Cirugía y Especialidades, Montevideo, Uruguay, 1932-
Atti del Congresso Italiano di Radiologia Medica, Pavia, Italy, 1914-
British Journal of Radiology, London, 1928-
Bulletins et Mémoirs de la Société d'électroradiologie Médicale de France, Paris, 1938-
Clinical Orthopaedics, Philadelphia, Pa., 1958-
Fortschritte auf dem Gebiet der Röntgenstrahlen, Hamburg, 1897-
Journal of the American Medical Association, Chicago, Ill., 1883-
Journal of Bone & Joint Surgery, Boston, 1922-
Journal of Radiology, Iowa City; Omaha, 1920-1925.
Journal of the Faculty of Radiologists, 1949-1959, and continued as
Clinical Radiology, Bristol, England, 1959-
Journal of the Röntgen Society, London, 1904-1923.
Journal of Thoracic Surgery, St. Louis, Mo., 1931-
Journal of Urology, Baltimore, Md., 1917-
Klinische Wochenschrift, Berlin, 1922-
Laryngoscope, St. Louis, Mo., 1896-
Medical Journal of Australia, Sydney, Australia, 1914-
Presse Médicale, Paris, France, 1893-
Quaderni di Radiologia, Belluno, Italy, 1937-
Quarterly Bulletin of Sea View Hospital, New York, 1935-
Radiography . . . Society of Radiographers, London, 1935-
Radiography and Clinical Photography; Eastman Kodak Co., Rochester, N. Y., 1930-
Radiologe (Der), Berlin, 1961-
Radiología . . . órgano oficial de la Sociedad argentina de radiología, Buenos Aires, 1942-
Radiologia Diagnostica, Berlin, 1960-
Radiologia Medica . . . organo della Società italiana di radiologia medica, Pavia and Milano, 1914-
Radiologic Clinics of North America, Philadelphia, Pa., 1963-
Radiologica, Berlin and Leipzig, 1937-
Radiology; Radiological Society of North America, Syracuse, N. Y., 1923-
Radiology, section 14 of Excerpta Medica, L. Paul, M. D., sub-editor, Amsterdam, C., The Netherlands, International, 1948.
Revista de Radiología y Fisioterapía; General Electric X-ray Corp., Chicago, 1934-
Röntgenpraxis, Leipzig, 1929-
Scritti Italiani di Radiobiologia Medica, Feltre, Italy, 1934-
Southern Medical Journal, Birmingham, Ala., 1908-
Surgery, St. Louis, 1935-
Surgery, Gynecology and Obstetrics, Chicago, Ill., 1905-
Vestnik rentgenologii i radiologii, Leningrad and Moskva, 1921-
X-ray Technician; American association of radiological technicians, St. Paul, Minn., 1929-1963, and continued as
Radiologic Technology, St. Paul, Minn., 1963-
X-ray Bulletin; Eastman Kodak Co., Rochester, N. Y., 1925-1930.
Year Book of Radiology; The Year Book Medical Publishers, Inc., Chicago, 1932-

GENERAL TEXTBOOKS ON ROENTGENOGRAPHY

1901 Williams, Francis H.: The roentgen rays in medicine and surgery, New York, 1901, The Macmillan Co.

1903 Albers-Schönberg, H. E.: Die Röntgentechnik, Hamburg, 1903 Gräfe & Sillem.

1917 Christie, Arthur C.: A manual of x-ray technic, ed. 2, Philadelphia, 1917, J. B. Lippincott Co.

1919 Albers-Schönberg, H. E.: Die Röntgentechnik, ed. 5, Hamburg, 1919, Gräfe & Sillem.

1920 Hirsch, I. Seth: The principles and practice of roentgenological technique, New York, 1920, American X-ray Publishing Co.

1924 Robertson, John K.: X-rays and x-ray apparatus; an elementary course, New York, 1924, The Macmillan Co.

1926 Grashey, Rudolf: Allegemeine Aufnahmetechnik und Deutung der Röntgenbilder, Berlin, 1926, Urban & Schwarzenberg.

1927 Fürstenau, R., Immelman, M., and Schutze, J.: Leitfaden des Röntgenverfahrens, ed. 5, Stuttgart, 1927, Ferdinand Enke.
Lilienfeld, Leon: In Mayer, E. G., and Pardes, F., editors: Anordnung der normalisierten Röntgenaufnahmen des menschlichen Körpers, ed. 4, Berlin, 1927, Urban & Schwarzenberg.

1928 Jerman, E. C.: Modern x-ray technic, St. Paul, Minn., 1928, The Bruce Publishing Co.

1931 Jerman, E. C., and others: X-ray studies in advanced radiographic technic, no. 1, Chicago, 1931, General Electric X-ray Corp.

1932 Pillsbury, H. C., editor: United States Army x-ray manual, ed. 2, New York, 1932, Paul B. Hoeber, Inc.

1934 Palazzi, Silvio: Roentgengrafia, 1934, Milano, Ulrico Hoepli.

1936 Files, Glenn W., and others: X-ray studies in advanced radiographic technic, no. 2, Chicago, 1936, General Electric X-ray Corp.

1938 Porcher, P., and de Juguelier, A.: Précis de technique radiographique, Paris, 1938, Gauthier-Villars.

1939 Delherm, Louis, and Kahn, H. L. M.: Les principals positions utilisées en radiographie, ed. 2, Paris, 1939, Norbert Maloine.

1940 Bauer, Karl: A B C der Röntgentechnik, Leipzig, 1940, Georg Thieme.
Davies, Nancy, and Isenburg, U.: Standard radiographic positions, London, 1940, Bailliere, Tindall & Cox.

1941 McNeill, Clyde: Roentgen technique, ed. 2, Springfield, Ill., 1941, Charles C Thomas, Publisher.
Russell, John J.: Outline of modern x-ray technic, ed. 3, New York, 1941, Picker X-ray Corp.

1942 Letterman General Hospital, San Francisco: Special service school; Instructions in the use of roentgen rays and roentgen ray apparatus, San Francisco, 1942.

1943 Files, Glenn W., and others: Medical radiographic technic, Springfield, Ill., 1943, Charles C Thomas, Publisher.
Rhinehardt, Darmon A.: Roentgenographic technique, ed. 3, Philadelphia, 1943, Lea & Febiger.
Sante, L. R.: Manual of roentgenological technique, ed. 10, Ann Arbor, Mich., 1943, Edwards Brothers, Inc.

1944 Castillo, E.: Técnica de la exploración roentgenscopica roentgenografíca, Barcelona, Madrid, 1944, Editorial Labora, S. A., vol. 1, p. 745.
Military Roentgenology: War Department technical manual, TM 8-280, Washington, D. C., 1944.
Naval Medical School: Fundamentals of x-ray physics and technique, National Naval Medical Center, Bethesda, Md., 1944.

1945 Janker, R.: Röntgenaufnahmetechnik, II. Leipzig, 1945, Johann Ambrosius Barth, vol. 1.

1947 Hardman, G. L.: Guide to positioning, Radiography, 13:42-43, 1947.

1948 Davies, N., and Isenburg, V.: Standard radiographic positions, ed. 2, Baltimore, 1948, The Williams & Wilkins Co.

1950 Porcher, P.: Précis de technique radiographique, ed. 3, Paris, 1950, Gauthier-Villars.

1955 Castillo, E.: Técnica de la Exploración roentgenoscópia y roentgenográfica, Madrid, 1955, Instituto Radiologico Del Dr. Castillo.

1956 LeDoux-LeBard, R., and Garcia-Calderon, J.: Technique du radiodiagnostique, ed. 2, Paris, 1956, Masson & Cie.

Sante, L. R.: Manual of roentgenological technique, ed. 18, Ann Arbor, Mich., 1956, Edward Brothers.

Schlosshauer, B.: Röntgenaufnahmetechnik in der Hals-Nasen-Ohren-Heilkunde, Stuttgart, 1956, Georg Thieme.

Schoen, H.: Medizinische Röntgentechnik, ed. 2, Stuttgart, 1956, Georg Thieme.

1962 Schurtleff, F. E.: Children's radiographic technic, ed. 2, Philadelphia, 1962, Lea & Febiger.

1964 Bloom, W. L., Jr., and others: Medical radiographic technic, ed. 3, Springfield, Ill., 1964, Charles C Thomas, Publisher.

Clark, K. C.: Positioning in radiography, ed. 8, New York and London, 1964, Grune & Stratton.

Jacobi, C. A., and Paris, D. Q.: X-ray technology, ed. 3, St. Louis, 1964, The C. V. Mosby Co.

Vennes, C. H., and Watson, J. C.: Patient care and special procedures in x-ray technology, ed. 2, St. Louis, 1964, The C. V. Mosby Co.

1965 Bauer, D. deF.: A textbook of elementary radiography for students and technicians, Springfield, Ill., 1965, Charles C Thomas, Publisher.

MEDICAL TEXTBOOKS CONTAINING POSITION INSTRUCTIONS

1905 Brühl, Gustav: Grundriss und Atlas der Ohrenheilkunde, ed. 2, München, 1905, J. F. Lehman.

Grashey, Rudolf: Atlas typischer Röntgenbilder vom normalen Menschen, 1905, München, J. F. Lehman.

Schüller, Arthur: Die Schädelbasis im Röntgenbilde, Hamburg, 1905, Gräfe & Sillem.

1910 Köhler, Alban: Grenzen des Normalen und Anfänge des Pathologischen im Röntgenbilde, Hamburg, 1910, Gräfe & Sillem.

1912 Denker and Brünings: Die Krankheiten des Ohres und der Luftwege, Jena, 1912, Gustav Fischer.

Grashey, Rudolf: Atlas typischer Röntgenbilder vom normalen Menschen, ed. 2, München, 1912, J. F. Lehman.

1914 Sonnenkalb, Victor: Die Röntgendiagnostik des Hals-, Nasen-, Ohrenarztes, Jena, 1914, Gustav Fischer.

1918 Holzknecht, Guido: Rontgenologie, ed. 2, Berlin, 1918, Urban & Schwarzenberg.

Rhese, Hans: Die Kriegsverletzungen und Kriegserkrankungen von Ohr, Nase und Hals, 1918, Wiesbaden, J. F. Bergmann.

1920 Law, Frederick M.: Mastoids roentgenologically considered, Ann. Roentgen. 1:1920.

Schaeffer, J. Parsons: The nose, paranasal, sinuses, nasolacrimal passages, and olfactory organ in man, Philadelphia, 1920, P. Blakiston's Son & Co.

1923 Sonnenkalb, V., and Beyer, E.: Die Röntgendiagnostik von Ohr, Nase und Nebenhöhlen, Rachen, Kehlkopf, Mund und Zähne, Leipzig, 1923, Dr. Werner Klinkhardt, Handbuch Röntgendiagnostik, III, no. 3.

1924 Schüller, Arthur: Röntgen Diagnostik der Erkrankungen des Köpfes, Berlin, 1924, Urban & Schwarzenberg.

1928 Grashey, Rudolf: Typische Röntgenbilder vom normalen Menschen. In Lehmann's medizinische Atlanten, ed. 5, v. 5, 1928.

1929 Assmann, Herbert: Clinical roentgendiagnosis of internal diseases (Die klinische Röntgendiagnostik der inneren Erkrankungen), translated by New York Academy of Medicine Library, Bibliographic Department, March, 1929.

Köhler, Alban: Roentgenology, New York, 1929, William Wood & Co.

1930 Mayer, E. G., and Eisinger, Karl: Otologische Röntgendiagnostik, Wien, 1930, Julius Springer, pp. 283-304.

1933 Busi, A.: Tecnica e diagnostica radiologica nelle malattie chirurgiche, Cl. T.E.T., 1933.

Davis, Loyal: Intracranial tumors, Ann. Roentgen., 1933.

Engel, S., and Schall, L.: Handbuch der Röntgendiagnostik und Therapie im Kindesalter, Leipzig, 1933, Georg Thieme.

1934 Codman, A. E.: The shoulder, Boston, 1934, Little, Brown & Co.

1936 Harrison, B. J. M.: A textbook of roentgenology, Baltimore, 1936, William Wood & Co.

Hartman, Edward: La radiographie en ophthalmologie, Paris, 1936, Masson & Cie.

1939 Ferguson, Albert B.: Roentgen diagnosis of the extremities and spine, Ann. Roentgen., 1939.

1940 Pancoast, H. K., Pendergrass, E. P., and Schaeffer, J. P.: The head and neck in roentgen diagnosis, Springfield, Ill., 1940, Charles C Thomas, Publisher.

1941 Golden, Ross, and others: Diagnostic roentgenology, ed. 3, New York, 1941, Thomas Nelson & Sons.

1945 Archer, Vincent W.: The osseous system, Chicago, 1945, Year Book Medical Publishers, Inc.

1947 Pillmore, George U., and others: Clinical radiology, Philadelphia, 1947, F. A. Davis Co.

1948 Young, Barton R.: The skull, sinuses, and mastoids; a handbook of roentgen diagnosis, Chicago, 1948, Year Book Medical Publishers, Inc.

1950 Chaumet, G.: Traité de radiodiagnostic, ed 2, Paris, 1950, Vigot Frères.

Chaussé, C.: Premiers elements de radio-otologie, Paris, 1950, Masson & Cie.

1955 Bateman, J. E.: The shoulder and environs, St. Louis, 1955, The C. V. Mosby Co.

1956 Pendergrass, E. P., Schaeffer, J. P., and Hodes, P. J.: The head and neck in roentgen diagnosis, ed. 2, Springfield, Ill., 1956, Charles C Thomas, Publisher.

1957 Gamble, F. O.: Applied foot roentgenology, Baltimore, 1957, The Williams & Wilkins Co.

1961 Abrams, H., editor: Angiography, Boston, 1961, Little, Brown & Co.

1962 Bull, J. W., McKissock, W., Bloom, W., Chynn, K. Y., and Potts, D. G.: Atlas of myelography, New York, 1962, Grune & Stratton, Inc.

Darling, D. B.: Radiography of infants and children, Springfield, Ill., 1962, Charles C Thomas, Publisher.

1963 Stafne, E. C.: Oral roentgenographic diagnosis including an appendix on roentgenographic technic, ed. 2, Philadelphia, 1963, W. B. Saunders Co.

1964 Egan, Robert L.: Mammography, Springfield, Ill., 1964, Charles C Thomas, Publisher.

Etter, Lewis E., and others: Roentgenography and roentgenology of the middle ear and mastoid process, Springfield, Ill., 1964, Charles C Thomas, Publisher.

Taveras, J. M., and Wood, E. H.: Diagnostic neuroradiology, Baltimore, 1964, The Williams & Wilkins Co.

NURSING PROCEDURES AND PATIENT CARE

1957 Furushiro, Tamako: Handling the handicapped patient, Xray Techn. 28:246-249, 1957.

1960 Chesney, M. O.: Emergency radiography, Radiography 26:277-286, 1960.

1961 Bentley, H. B.: Nursing points for students and radiographers, Radiology 27:75-84, 1961.

Reinhart, M. J.: Cross infection; the significance of efficient aseptic technique in the department of radiology, Xray Techn. 32:487-495, 1961.

1962 Chesney, D. N., and Chesney, M. O.: Care of the patient in diagnostic radiography, Philadelphia, 1962, F. A. Davis Co.

Howell, H. B.: Hospital practice and the care of the patient in x-ray departments, Radiology 28:2-10, 1962.

1964 Vennes, C. H., and Watson, J. C.: Patient care and special procedures in x-ray technology, ed. 2, St. Louis, 1964, The C. V. Mosby Co.

1965 Brinkbok, G. C. F.: Pathology for radiographers, London, 1965, Butterworth & Co., Ltd.

1966 Nelson, S. W.: Some important diagnostic and technical fundamentals in the radiology of trauma; with particular emphasis on skeletal trauma, Radiol. Clin. N. Amer. 4:241-259, 1966.

ANATOMY

Textbooks and special articles

1884 Kollman, J., Ranke, T., and Virchow, R.: Verständingung über ein gemeinsames craniometrisches Verfahren, Arch. Anthrop. 15:1-8, 1884.

Reid, Robert W.: Relation of the principal fissures and convolutions of the cerebrum to the outer surface of the scalp, Lancet 2:539-540, 1884.

1901 Zuckerkandl, Emil: Atlas der topographischen Anatomie, München, 1901, J. F. Lehman.

1906 Addison, Christopher. In Ellis: Demonstrations of anatomy, ed. 12, New York, 1906, William Wood & Co.

1914 Knox, Robert, and Salmond, R. W.: A system of topography for use in the radiography of the head, Arch. Roentgen. Ray 19:393-398, 1914-1915.

1917 Mills, Walter R.: The relation of bodily habitus to visceral form, position, tonus, and motility, Amer. J. Roentgen. 4:155-169, 1917.

1925 Goldhamer, Karl, and Schüller, Arthur: Die Vertikal- und die Horizontalebene des Kopfes, Fortschr. Roentgenstr. 33:183-190, 1925.

1926 Goldhamer, Karl, and Schüller, Arthur: Varietäten im Bereich der hinteren Schädelgrube, Fortschr. Roentgenstr. 35:1163-1189, 1926.

Hasselwander, Albert: Anatomie des menschlichen Körpers in Röntgenbild, München, 1926, J. F. Bergmann.

1927 Mosher, H. P.: X-ray study of movements of tongue, epiglottis, and hyoid bone in swallowing, Laryngoscope 37:235, 1927.

1929 Ralph, S., Jr.: Radiographic appearance of anatomical landmarks, Xray Bull. 6:4-7, 11, 1929.

1930 Goldhamer, Karl: Normal anatomy of the head, Radiologische Paraktika 12-13:1930-1931.

1931 Camp, John D., and Cilley, Earl I. L.: Diagrammatic chart showing time of appearance of the various centers of ossification and period of union, Amer. J. Roentgen. 26:905, 1931.

1934 Reese, Mildred: The physiology of respiration—its relation to radiography, Xray Techn. 5:165-168, 1934.

Weski, Oskar: Röntgenanatomie des Schädels, der Kiefer und der Zähne, Berlin, 1934, Berlinische Verlag Anstalt.

1937 Benner, Fritz: Das Röntgenschnittaufnahmeverfahren und seine Bedeutung für die Röntgendiagnostik des Kopfes, Berlin theses, 1937.

1939 McNeill, Clyde: Planos corrientes del craneo, Rev. Rad. Fis. 6:297-302, 1939.

Sobotta, J.: Atlas of human anatomy, edited from 9th German ed. by McMurrich, J. P., New York, 1939, G. E. Stechert & Co.

1940 Cunningham, D. J.: In Brash, J. C., and Jameson, E. B., editors: Manual of practical anatomy, ed. 10, New York, 1940, Oxford University Press.

1942 Gray, Henry: Anatomy of the human body, ed. 24, Edited by Lewis, W. H., Philadelphia, 1942, Lea & Febiger.

Greisheimer, Esther M.: Physiology and anatomy, ed. 4, Philadelphia, 1942, J. B. Lippincott Co.

1943 Williams, J. F.: A textbook of anatomy and physiology, ed. 7, Philadelphia, 1943, W. B. Saunders Co.

1945 Denley, K. C.: Importance of anatomical study in radiographic positioning, Radiography 11:82-84, 1945.

Vickers, A. A.: Radiographical investigation of diaphragmatic movements, Brit. J. Radiol. 18:229-230, 1945.

1946 Appleton, A., Hamilton, W. J., and Tchaperoff, Ivan C. C.: Surface and radiological anatomy, ed. 2, Baltimore, 1946, The Williams & Wilkins Co.

Bishop, Paul A., and Lindskog, G. E.: The diaphragm in relation to the thorax. In Pillmore, G. U.: Clinical radiology, Philadelphia, 1946, F. A. Davis Co., vol. 1, pp. 442-451.

Esposito, Joseph J.: The diaphragm in relation to the abdomen. In Pillmore, G. U.: Clinical radiology, Philadelphia, 1946, F. A. Davis Co., vol. 1, pp. 486-495.

Henderson, S. G., and Sherman, S. L.: Roentgen anatomy of the skull in the newborn infant, Radiology 46:107-118, 1946.

Mahoney, H. O., Anson, B. J., and Dent, R. F.: Roentgenographic preparations from gross anatomic sections, Amer. J. Roentgen. 56:49-54, 1946.

Sussman, Marcy L.: Cardiac roentgenography and anatomy. In Pillmore, G. U.: Clinical radiology, Philadelphia, 1946, F. A. Davis Co., vol. 1, pp. 3-27.

1947 Chalton, P., and Malcki, A.: Anatomie radiologique du poumon, J. Radiol. Electrol. 28:285-310, 1947.

1948 Brown, S., and Fine, A.: The diaphragm, Radiology 51:157-166, 1948.

1952 Girdany, B. R., and Golden, Ross: Centers of ossification of the skeleton, Amer. J. Roentgen. 68:922-924, 1952.

1959 Meschan, I., and Farrer-Meschan, R. M. F.: An atlas of normal radiographic anatomy, ed. 2, Philadelphia, 1959, W. B. Saunders Co.

1960 Blewett, J. E., and Rackow, A. M.: Anatomy and physiology for radiographers, London & Washington, D. C., 1960, Butterworth & Co., Ltd.

1962 Mallett, M.: A handbook of anatomy and physiology for student x-ray technicians, Fond du Lac, Wis., 1962, American Society of Xray Technicians.

Upper extremity

1916 Masmonteil, F.: Examen radiologique des fractures diaphysaires de l'avant-bras-position de choix, J. Radiol. Electr. 2:704-709, 1916-1917.

1918 Laquerrière, and Pierquin: De la nécessité d'employer une technique radiographique spéciale pour obtenir certains détails squelettiques, J. Radiol. Electr. 3:145-148, 1918.

1921 Arcelin, F.: L'exploration radiologique du carpe, J. Radiol. Electr. 5:349-361, 1921.

Staunig, Konrad: Die Darstellung der Hand in der Zitherspielerstellung, Fortschr. Roentgenstr. 28:464, 1921-1922.

1924 Buxton, Dudley: A radiographic survey of normal joints: the elbow joint, Brit. J. Radiol. 29:395-410, 1924.

1925 Dress, Louis C., and Payne, W. F.: Suggestions in making lateral roentgenograms of the hand, Amer. J. Roentgen. 13:292, 1925.

1926 McBride, Earl: Wrist joint injuries: a plea for greater accuracy in treatment, J. Okla. Med. Ass. 19:67-70, 1926.

1927 Buxton, Dudley: A radiographic survey of normal joints; the wrist joint and hand, Brit. J. Radiol. 32:199-213, 1927.

1928 Belot, J., Lepennetier, F., and Pellizza, J.: Radiodiagnostic de quelques alterations osseuses de l'articulations due coude, J. Radiol. Electr. 12:457-500, 1928.

1930 Schneider, Cathryn C.: Mechanical devices for immobilizing the head and hand, Xray Techn. 1:70-71, 1930.

1931 Fiolle, J.: Le "carpe bossu," Bull. Soc. Chir. Paris 57:1687, 1931.

1932 Fiolle, J., and Alland: Nouvelle observation de "carpe bossu," Bull. Soc. Chir. Paris 58:187-188, 1932.

Mills, R. E.: Some common errors in posturing, Radiogr. Clin. Photogr. 8:16-17, 1932.

1933 Archer, Vincent W., and Rawles, Benjamin W.: Roentgenologic examination of injuries of the wrist joint, Southern Med. J. 26:211-214, 1933.

1935 Hill, Thomas, Farmer, and Winkler: Radiography of the wrist and ankle, Radiogr. Clin. Photogr. 11:14-15, 1935.

1937 Stecher, William R.: Roentgenography of the carpal-navicular bone, Amer. J. Roentgen. 37:704-705, 1937.

1938 Alexander, O. M.: Radiography of the wrist, Radiology 4:181-183, 1938.

Persnal, A.: Zur röntgenologischen Diagnostik der frischen Kahnbeinbrüche der Hand, Röntgenpraxis 10:11-16, 1938.

1939 Schmitt, H.: Die röntgenologische Darstellung des Radiusköpfchens, Röntgenpraxis 11:33-36, 1939.

1940 Graziani, Aldo: L'esame radiologico del carpo, Radiol. Med. 27:382-392, 1940.

1941 Carter, R. M.: Carpal boss: A commonly overlooked deformity of the carpus, J. Bone Joint Surg. 23:935-940, 1941.

Hart, Vernon L., and Gaynor, Valeria: Roentgenographic study of the carpal canal, J. Bone Joint Surg. **23**:382-383, 1941.

1942 Hart, Vernon L., and Gaynor, Valeria: Radiography of the carpal canal, Radiogr. Clin. Photogr. **18**:23-24, 1942.

Whitehead, J.: Technique for obtaining a true postero-anterior and true lateral view of the carpal scaphoid bone, Radiology **8**:105, 1942.

1943 Lewis, Raymond W.: Oblique views in roentgenography of the wrist, Amer. J. Roentgen. **50**:119-121, 1943.

Shefferin, A. J.: An axial view of the head of the radius, Radiography **9**:202-221, 1943.

1944 Burman, Michael S., and others: Fractures of the radial and ulnar axes, Amer. J. Roentgen. **51**:455-480, 1944.

1945 Evans, Mervyn E.: Rotational deformity in the treatment of fractures of both bones of the forearm, J. Bone Joint Surg. **27**:373-382, 1945.

Holly, E. W.: Radiography of the pisiform bone, Radiogr. Clin. Photogr. **21**:69-70, 1945.

1946 Roderick, J. F.: The roentgenographic examination of the carpus, Xray Techn. **18**:8-11, 1946.

1947 Cleveland, Mather: Fracture of the carpal scaphoid, Surg. Gynec. Obstet. **84**:769-771, 1947.

Perkins, B.: Radiography of the carpus, Radiography **13**:8-10, 1947.

1948 Jacobs, Lewis G.: Isolated fracture of the pisiform bone, Radiology **50**:529-531, 1948.

1949 Bridgman, C. F.: Radiography of the carpal navicular bone, Med. Radiogr. Photogr. **25**:104-105, 1949.

1951 Alexander, O. M.: Radiography of the carpal scaphoid bone in inclined planes, Radiography **17**:14-15, 1951.

1954 Wilson, J. N.: Profiles of the carpal canal, J. Bone Joint Surg. **36-A**:127-132, 1954.

1956 Dorosin, N., and Davis, J. G.: Carpal boss, Radiology **66**:234-236, 1956.

Holly, E. W.: Radiography of the radial head, Med. Radiogr. Photogr. **32**:13-14, 1956.

1957 Lentino, W., and others: The carpal-bridge view: a position for the roentgenographic diagnosis of abnormalities in the dorsum of the wrist, J. Bone Joint Surg. **39-A**:88-90, 1957.

Viehweger, G.: Zum Problem der Deutung der knöchernen Gebilde distal des Epikondylus medialis humeri, Fortschritte **86**:643-652, 1957.

1958 Burman, M.: Anteroposterior projection of the carpometacarpal joint of the thumb by radial shift of the carpal tunnel view, J. Bone Joint Surg. **40-A**:1156-1157, 1958.

Stripp, W. J.: Radiography of the ulnar groove and of the carpal tunnel, Radiography **24**:277-280, 1958.

1960 Bing, B.: Radiographic demonstration of the scaphoid fracture, Xray Techn. **31**:380-381, 1960.

Russe, O.: Fracture of the carpal navicular, J. Bone Joint Surg. **42-A**:759-768, 1960.

Vasilas, A., and others: Roentgen aspects of injuries to the pisiform bone and pisotriquetral joint, J. Bone Joint Surg. **42-A**:1317-1328, 1960.

1964 Templeton, A. W., and Zim, I. D.: The carpal tunnel view, Missouri Med. **61**:443-444, 1964.

1965 Nørgaard, F.: Earliest roentgenological changes in polyarthritis of the rheumatoid type: rheumatoid arthritis, Radiology **85**:325-329, 1965.

1966 Gramiak, R.: Oblique radiography of the hands, Med. Radiogr. Photogr. **42**:28-29, 1966.

Lower extremity

1907 Haenisch, H.: Diskussionsbemerkung, Verhandl. Deutsch. Röentgengesell. **3**:54, 1907.

1909 Settegast, H.: Fraktur des calcaneus und röntgenographische Diagnose derselben, Verhandl. Deutsch. Röentgengesell. **5**:114-117, 1909.

1910 Kuchendorf: Drei Fälle von Längsbrüchen der Kniescheibe mittels schräger Durchleuchtung festgestellt, Fortschr. Roentgenstr. **15**:368-369, 1910.

1922 Walters, Ray A.: Radiography of the os calcis, J. Radiol. **3**:493-494, 1922.

1923 Scott, E.: Technique radiography of the knee joint, Arch. Radiol. Electr. **28**:57-58, 1923.

1924 Béclère, H.: La radiographie des films courbes, Paris, 1924, Amédée Legrand.

Marchand, Joseph-Henri: La radiographie sur films courbes, Paris theses, 1924.

Schütze, T.: Die isolierte Darstellung der distalen Fusswurzel und der Mittelfussknochen bei der Röntgenaufnahme, Fortschr. Roentgenstr. **32**:121, 1924.

1925 Belot, J., Talon, and Nadal: A propos des films courbes, J. Radiol. Electr. **9**:454, 1925.

1926 Conn, A. R.: Fractures of the os calcis, Radiology **6**:228-235, 1926.

Slomann, H. C.: On the demonstration and analysis of calcaneonavicular coalition by roentgen examination, Acta Radiol. **5**:304-312, 1926.

1927 Altschul, Walter: Some new methods in roentgenography, Amer. J. Roentgen. **17**:659-666, 1927.

Badgley, C. E.: Coalition of the calcaneus and the navicular, Arch. Surg. **15**:75-88, 1927.

Lillienfeld, Leon: Anordnung der normalisierten Röntgenaufnahmen des menschlichen Körpers, ed. 4, Berlin, 1927, Urban & Schwarzenberg, p. 36.

1929 Hülten, O.: Ueber die indirekten Brüche des Tibiakopfes nebst Beiträgen zur Röntgenologie des Kniegelenks, Acta Chir. Scandinav. **15** (supp.):66, 1929.

1930 Petrignani, Roger: Étude radiologique de la maladie de Pellegrini-Stieda, J. Radiol. **14**:544, 1930.

1931 Doub, Howard P.: A useful position for examining the foot, Radiology **16**:764-766, 1931.

1932 Colaneri and Laguiere: Les fractures du scaphoide tarsien, J. Radiol. Electr. **16**:68, 1932.

Dittmar, Otto: Der Kniegelenks-Meniskus im Röntgenbilde, Röntgenpraxis **4**:442-445, 1932.

Frik, K.: Neue Röntgenuntersuchungen am Kniegelenk, Verhandl. Deutsch. Röntgengesell. **24-25**:155, 1932.

Grasman: Die exacte Messung der Malleolengabelverbreitung, München. Med. Woch. **79**:1721, 1932.

Popovic, L., and Doric, L.: Beitrag zur Röntgenuntersuchung des Kniegelenks, Röntgenpraxis **4**:905-910, 1932.

Regele-Bozen, H.: Die Verletzungen des inneren Seitenbandes des Kniegelenkes, München. Med. Woch. **79**:1474-1476, 1932.

Stankiewics, Zygmunt: Àpropos d'un cas d'ostéochondrite de l'os sésamoide du gros orteil, J. Radiol. **16**:65, 1932.

1935 Danelius, Gerhard, and Miller, F. L.: Roentgen examination of the intercondyloid fossa of the knee joint, Radiology **25**:605-608, 1935.

Felsenreich, Fritz: Darstellung des verletzten Meniscus medialis im Röntgenbild bei veralterter Kreuzband- und Seitenbandverletzung, Röntgenpraxis **7**:331-333, 1935.

Hellmer, Hans: Röntgenologische Beobachtungen über die Ossifikationen der Patella, Acta Radiol. **27** (supp.): 112-114, 1935.

Hill, Thomas, Farmer, and Winkler: Radiography of wrist and ankle, Radiogr. Clin. Photogr. **11**:14-15, 1935.

Kaiser, R.: Die röntgenologische Darstellung der Fossa intercondyloidea und ihre Bedeutung für die Kniegelenkediagnostik (Frik's method), Bruns' Beitr. Klin. Chir. **161**:528, 1935.

1936 Allen, Norman S.: Radiography of the os calcis, Radiology **2**:145-146, 1936.

Laarman, A.: Darstellung des Knieinnern im Röntgenbild, Arch. Klin. Chir. **187**:234-251, 1936-1937.

Thomsen, Wilhelm: Vorrichtung für Aufnahme des Fussskelettes unter Belastung zum Messen der Weichteile, Röntgenpraxis **8**:241-242, 1936.

Widmann, Bernard P., and Stecher, William R.: Roentgenographic demonstration of the true articular space, Radiology **27**:541-544, 1936.

1937 Holmblad, Edward C.: Postero-anterior x-ray view of the knee in flexion, J.A.M.A. **109**:1196, 1937.

Lachman, Ernst: Roentgen anatomy of the knee joint, Radiology **29**:455, 1937.

Scott, V. M.: Radiography of the os calcis, Radiology **3**:28-30, 1937.

Zweifel, C.: Zur Röntgendiagnostik der Patella, Röntgenpraxis **9**:313-318, 1937.

1938 Guntz, Eduard: Ein Gerät für sämtliche Röntgenaufnahmen der Füsse mit und ohne Belastung in genauer Einstellung, Röntgenpraxis 10:17-23, 1938.

Holmgreen, Bengt S.: Variationem im Röntgenbild des normalen ersten Metatarsophalangealgelenks bedingt durch kleine Underungen in der Richtung des Zentralstrahls, Acta Radiol. 19:67-71, 1938.

Lewis, R. W.: Non-routine views in roentgen examination of the extremities, Surg. Gynec. Obstet. 69:38-45, 1938.

Löhr, R., and Hellpap, W.: Der Kniegelenkspalt im Röntgenbild, Fortschr. Roentgenstr. 58:45-56, 1938.

Piotrowski, Brother Dominic: Oblique view of the ankle joint and foot, Amer. J. Roentgen. 45:127-128, 1938.

Wordhein, Yngve: Eine neue Methode, den Gelenkknorpel besonders die Kniegelenks-Menisken, roentgenologisch darzustellen, Fortschr. Roentgenstr. 57: 479-495, 1938.

1939   Alexander, O. M.: The utility of the curved cassette, Radiography 5:57, 1939.

Genders, Richard A.: The os calcis, Xray Techn. 11:60, 1939.

Holmblad, Edward C.: Improved x-ray technic in studying knee joints, Southern Med. J. 32:240-243, 1939.

Kite, J. H.: Principles involved in the treatment of congenital clubfoot, J. Bone Joint Surg. 21:595-606, 1939.

1940   Evans, William A.: Roentgenological demonstration of true articular space, Amer. J. Roentgen. 43:860, 1940.

Lindblom, Knut: Roentgenographic symptoms of meniscal lesion in the knee joint, Acta Radiol. 21:274-285, 1940.

Piotrowski, Brother Dominic: The knee joint, Xray Techn. 12:45-46, 1940.

1941   Knutsson, Folke: Ueber die Röntgenologie des Femoropatellargelenks sowie eine gute Projection für das Kniegelenk, Acta Radiol. 22:371-376, 1941.

Santora, P. J.: Anteroposterior view of the ankle joint and foot, Amer. J. Roentgen. 45:127-128, 1941.

1942   Marique, P.: La réintégration non saglante de l'astragale, Rev. Orthop. 28:37-50, 1942.

1943   Anthonsen, W.: An oblique projection for roentgen examination of the talocalcaneal joint, particularly in intra-articular fracture of calcaneus, Acta Radiol. 24:306-310, 1943.

Ball, R. P., and Egbert, E. W.: Ruptured ligaments of the ankle, Amer. J. Roentgen. 50:770-771, 1943.

Cahoon, John B.: Radiography of the foot, Xray Techn. 15:13, 15, 1943.

Causton, J.: Projection of sesamoid bones in the region of the first metatarsophalangeal joint, Radiology 9:39, 1943.

Gamble, Felton O.: A special approach to foot radiography, Radiogr. Clin. Photogr. 19:78-80, 1943.

Knish, Mary: The knee, Xray Techn. 14:200-201, 1943.

1944   Berridge, F. R., and Bonnin, J. B.: The radiographic examination of the ankle joint including arthrography, Surg. Gynec. Obstet. 79:383-389, 1944.

Camp, John D., and Coventry, M. B.: Use of special views in roentgenography of the knee joint, U. S. Nav. M. Bull. 42:56-58, 1944.

Long, Leonard: Non-injection method for roentgenographic visualization of the internal semilunar cartilage, Amer. J. Roentgen. 52:269-280, 1944.

Mohr, Seth: Special consideration in radiography of the knee and ankle, Xray Techn. 16:7-12, 1944.

Piotrowski, Brother Dominic: An instrument to facilitate the making of oblique views of the ankle joint, Xray Techn. 16:62-65, 1944.

1945   Gershon-Cohen, J.: Internal derangements of the knee joint; the diagnostic scope of the soft tissue roentgen examinations and the vacuum technique demonstration of the menisci, Amer. J. Roentgen. 54:337-347, 1945.

Grossman, J. D., and Minor, H. H.: Roentgen demonstration of the semilunar cartilages of the knee, Amer. J. Roentgen. 53:454-465, 1945.

Marique, Pierre: L'examen radiographique du pied bot, (Roentgenographic examination of club foot), Presse Méd. 53:633-634, 1945.

Pendergrass, Eugene P., and Lafferty, John O.: Roent-

gen study of the ankle in severe sprains and dislocations, Radiology 45:40-45, 1945.

Simor, R. S.: A third routine x-ray exposure of the ankle joint, J. Bone Joint Surg. 27:520, 1945.

1946   Bonnet, William L., and Baker, D. R.: Diagnosis of pes planus by x-ray, Radiology 46:36-45, 1946.

Cahoon, John B.: Radiography of the foot, Radiogr. Clin. Photogr. 22:2-9, 1946.

Hendelberg, Thorsten: Roentgenographic examination of ankle joint in malleolar fractures, Acta Radiol. 27:23-42, 1946.

Jones Henry: Radiography of the knee for internal derangement, Xray Techn. 17:390-393, 408, 1946.

Moreau, H. M., Bertani, Guido Costa, and Moreau, G. E.: Mediciones angulares en el estudio radiologico del valguismo y varismo del pie, Radiologica 9:65-75, 1946.

Runge, Roy K.: The roentgenographic examination of the knee joint, Xray Techn. 18:97-100, 1946.

Wilner, Daniel: Diagnostic problems in fractures of the foot and ankle, Amer. J. Roentgen. 55:594-616, 1946.

1947   Carter, D. R.: Radiographic examination of the knee joint, Xray Techn. 19:77, 82, 1947.

Crawford, Henry B., and Bridgman, C. F.: Radiography of injured lower extremities, Med. Radiogr. Photogr. 23:31-33, 1947.

Weismann, J. C.: An improved technique for the roentgen demonstration of the semilunar cartilages of the knee, Amer. J. Roentgen. 58:255-256, 1947.

1948   Harris, R. I., and Beath, T.: Etiology of peroneal spastic flatfoot, J. Bone Joint Surg. 30-B:624-634, 1948.

Kestler, O. C.: Traumatic instability of the ankle joint, Amer. J. Roentgen. 60:498-504, 1948.

Palmer, I.: The mechanism and treatment of fractures of the calcaneus, J. Bone Joint Surg. 30-A:2-8, 1948.

1949   Broden, Bror: Roentgen examination of the subtaloid joint in fractures of the calcaneus, Arch. Radiol. 31:85-91, 1949.

Odell, O. C.: Lateral knee technique, Xray Techn. 20:274, 1949.

1950   Chambers, C. H.: Congenital anomalies of the tarsal navicular, Brit. J. Radiol. 23:580-586, 1950.

Coventry, M. B.: Flatfoot with special consideration of tarsal coalition, Minnesota Med. 33:1091-1097, 1950.

Vaughan, F. M. A.: Lateral knees, Radiography 16:75-77, 1950.

Wilson, G. E.: Fractures of the calcaneus, J. Bone Joint Surg. 32-A:59-70, 1950.

1951   Alexander, O. M.: Routine lateral radiography of the knee and ankle joints, Radiography 17:10-11, 1951.

1952   Burdick, A. V.: Calcaneus, Xray Techn. 23:276-277, 1952.

Kancel, B.: The suroplantar projection in the congenital clubfoot of the infant, Acta Orthop. Scand. 22:161-173, 1952.

1953   Vaughan, W. H., and Segal, G.: Tarsal coalition with special reference to roentgenographic interpretation, Radiology 60:855-863, 1953.

1954   Lauge-Hansen, N.: Fractures of the ankle, Amer. J. Roentgen. 71:456-471, 1954.

Sonnenschein, A.: Roentgenographic visualization of the patella, J. Bone Joint Surg. 36-A:109-112, 1954.

1955   Davis, L. A., and Hatt, W. S.: Congenital abnormalities of the feet, Radiology 64:818-825, 1955.

Denny, J. C., and and Lyons, N. J.: Radiography of the talocalcaneal articulations, Xray Techn. 26:245-248, 1955.

Holly, E. W.: Radiography of the tarsal sesamoid bones, Med. Radiogr. Photogr. 31:73, 1955.

1956   March, H. C., and London, R. I.: The os sustentaculi, Amer. J. Roentgen. 76:114-1118, 1956.

Wenzlik, G.: Zur Einstelltechnik des oberen Sprunggelenkes, Fortschr. Roentgenstr. 84:362-365, 1956.

1958   Denny, J. C., and Lyons, N. J.: Radiography of the knee, Xray Techn. 30:87-91, 1958.

Kreppert, L. C.: A modified axial view of the patella, Xray Techn. 29:375-377, 1958.

1960   Funke, Thomas: Radiography of the knee joint, Med. Radiogr. Photogr. 36:1-37, 1960.

Scheller, Sven: Roentgenographic studies on epiphyseal

growth and ossification in the knee, Acta Radiol. **195**(supp.):12-16, 1960.

1961 Isherwood, Ian: A radiological approach to the subtalar joint, J. Bone Joint Surg. **43-B**:566-574, 1961.

Kleiger, B., and Mankin, H. J.: A roentgenographic study of the development of the calcaneous by means of posterior tangential view, J. Bone Joint Surg. **43-A**:961-969, 1961.

1962 Feist, J. H., and Mankin, H. J.: The tarsus: basic relationships and motions in the adult and definition of optimal recumbent oblique projection, Radiology **79**:250-263, 1962.

Graham, D., and Rorrison, J.: Radiography of the tarsal bones, Radiography **28**:156-163, 1962.

1964 Kite, J. Hiram: The clubfoot, New York, 1964, Grune & Stratton, Inc.

Willets, C., and Gerdes, R. A.: Radiographic improvement through application of anatomical stress, Radiol. Techn. **36**:176-178, 1964.

1965 Harris, J.: Radiography of the lower limb, Radiography **31**:235-248, 1965.

Templeton, A. W., and others: Standardization of terminology and evaluation of osseous relationships in congenitally abnormal feet, Amer. J. Roentgen. **93**:374-381, 1965.

Extremities—general

1915 Case, James T.: Bone and joint lesions; necessity for constant technique in roentgenography, Interstate Med. J. **22**:584-597, 1915.

McKendrick, A.: Radiography of normal parts, Arch. Radiol. Electrol. **20**:243-259, 285-295, 1915-1916.

1918 Lacquerrière and Pierquin: De la nécessité d'employer une technique radiographique spéciale pour obtenir certains détails squelettiques, J. Radiol. Electrol. **3**:145-148, 1918.

1924 Marchand, J. H.: Technique de l'examen des articulations sur film courbe, Paris thèses 102, chap. 2, Paris, 1924, Amédée Legrand.

1927 Altschul, Walter: Some new methods in roentgenography, Amer. J. Roentgen. **17**:659-666, 1927.

1930 Dittmar, Otto: Weitere Mitteilungen über Schrägaufnahmen von Knochen und Gelenken, Röntgenpraxis **2**:1022, 1930.

1932 Leman, R. M.: General technique for radiography of the joints, Brit. J. Radiol. **5**:501-512, 1932.

Thompson, Mary: Variations of standard positions in taking radiographs, Xray Techn. **4**:18-20, 1932.

1933 Longervy, T., and Stecher, W. R.: Useful procedures in radiologic practice, Radiology **20**:225-230, 1933.

1935 Baer, Aubrey: Cast problem in radiography, Xray Techn. **7**:66-67, 93, 1935.

1936 Eller, Virginia H.: Extremities, Xray Techn. **7**:114-117, 135, 1936.

Thompson, Mary: Technic and position in radiography of the skeleton, Xray Techn. **8**:9-10, 31, 1936.

1937 Thomas, M. A.: The importance of a thorough examination in radiographic diagnosis, Xray Techn. **8**:103-106, 1937.

Wolcott, Roy: Technics for unusual cases, Xray Techn. **9**:38-42, 1937.

1938 Garland, H. L.: The roentgen diagnosis of fractures and dislocations, Diagn. Roentgen. **2**:827-854, 1938.

Leman, Ralph M.: Some radiographic techniques, Radiology **4**:41-44, 1938.

Lewis, Raymond W.: Nonroutine views in roentgen examination of the extremities, Surg. Gynec. Obstet. **67**:38-45, 1938.

Nordhein, Y.: Eine neue Methode, den Gelenkknorpel, besonders die Kniegelenks-Menisken, roentgenologisch darzustellen, Fortschr. Roentgenstr. **57**:479-495, 1938.

Potter, C. F.: Roentgenologic considerations of certain joint injuries, Amer. J. Surg. **42**:785-790, 1938.

1939 Rubin, E. L.: The delineation of articular cartilage by x-rays without the aid of contrast media, Brit. J. Radiol. **12**:649-657, 1939.

1940 Kahle, Laura M.: Solutions to some problems in x-ray technique, Xray Techn. **11**:172-174, 206, 1940.

1941 Larsen, Ruth M.: Radiography of extremities, Xray Techn. **12**:215-216, 1941.

Thvelkeld, Ann: Routine for fracture clinics, Xray Techn. **13**:110-111, 141, 1941.

1942 Ashwin, C.: Economy in radiography, Radiology **8**:121, 1942.

Colson, Douglas H.: Inventive radiographic positions, Xray Techn. **14**:59-61, 1942.

1943 Eller, Virginia H.: Special multiple views as diagnostic aid to the radiologist, Xray Techn. **15**:51-54, 1943.

Lewis, Raymond W.: El estudio roentgenográfico de tejidos blandos en un hospital para ortopedia, Rev. Rad. Fis. **10**:147-155, 1943.

1944 Zintheo, Clarence J.: Extremity radiography with no-screen film, Xray Techn. **16**:115, 1944.

1945 Champness, Lillian J.: Variations of routine techniques, Radiography **11**:17-20, 1945.

1947 Garland, Henry L.: The roentgen diagnosis of fractures and dislocations. In Golden, Ross, editor: Diagnostic roentgenology, ed. 3, New York, 1947, Thomas Nelson & Sons, vol. 2, pp. 827-854.

Hodges, Paul C., Phemister, D. B., and Brunschwig, Alexander: The roentgen-ray diagnosis of diseases of bones, In Golden, Ross, editor: Diagnostic roentgenology, ed. 3, New York, 1947, Thomas Nelson & Sons, vol. 1, pp. 351-560T.

1949 Forsyth, H. H.: Some clinical examples of the value o. supplemental radiographs, Med. Radiogr. Photogrf **25**:34-40, 1949.

1964 Willets, C., and Gerdes, R. A.: Radiographic improvement through application of anatomical stress, Radiol. Techn. **36**:176-178, 1964.

Long bone measurement

1924 Hickey, P. M.: Teleoroentgenography as an aid in orthopedic measurements, Amer. J. Roentgen. **11**:232-233, 1924.

1937 Millwee, Robert H.: Slit scanography, Radiology **28**:483-486, 1937.

1942 Gill, G. G., and Abbott, L. C.: Practical method of predicting growth of femur and tibia in the child, Arch. Surg. **45**:286-315, 1942.

Merrill, O. E.: A method for the roentgen measurement of the long bones, Amer. J. Roentgen. **48**:405-406, 1942.

1944 Gill, G. G.: A simple roentgenographic method for the measurement of bone growth; modification of Millwee's method of slit scanography, J. Bone Joint Surg. **26**:767-769, 1944.

1946 Green, W. T., Wyatt, G. M., and Anderson, M.: Orthoroentgenography as a method of measuring the bones of the lower extremities, J. Bone Joint Surg. **28**:60-65, 1946.

Rush, W. A., and Steiner, H. A.: A study of lower extremity length inequality, Amer. J. Roentgen. **56**:616-623, 1946.

1949 Cartwright, L. J.: Orthoroentgenography as applied to the lower extremities of children, Radiography **15**:234-235, 1949.

Mueller, W. K., and Higganson, J. M.: Spot scanography; a method of determining bone measurement, Amer. J. Roentgen. **61**:402-403, 1949.

1950 Bell, J. S., and Thomson, W. A. L.: Modified spot scanography, Amer. J. Roentgen. **63**:915-916, 1950.

Goldstein, L. A., and Dreisinger, F.: Spot orthoroentgenography; a method for measuring the length of the bones of the lower extremity, J. Bone Joint Surg. **32-A**:449-452, 1950.

1952 Sandaa, E.: Orthoroentgenographic measurement of long bones, Acta Orthop. Scand. **22**:76-79, 1952.

Sevastikoglou, J.: A simple application of orthoroentgenography, Acta Orthop. Scand. **22**:80-84, 1952.

1953 Farill, J.: Orthoradiographic measurement of shortening of the lower extremity, Med. Radiogr. Photogr. **29**:32-38, 1953.

1954 Kumpel, K.: Bone length radiography, Xray Techn. **25**:265-267, 1954.

Kunkle, H. M., and Carpenter, E. B.: A simple technique for x-ray measurement of limb-length discrepancies, J. Bone Joint Surg. **36-A**:152-154, 1954.

1955 Lewis, M. G.: Investigation of scanography, Xray Techn. **26**:327-333, 1955.
1961 Holohan, F.: Modified spot scanography, Xray Techn. **33**:106-112, 1961.
1966 Woodruff, J. H., Jr., and Lane, G.: A technique for slit scanography, Amer. J. Roentgen. **96**:907-912, 1966.

Contrast arthrography

1905 Robinsohn, and Werndorff: Ueber eine neue röntgenologische Methode (Sauerstoffinsufflation) zur Untersuchung der Gelenke und Weichteile, Verhandl. Deutsch. Röntgengesell. **1**:161, 1905.
1907 Kaisin: Emploi du gaz oxygène pour la radiographie des articulations, J. Belg. Radiol. **1**:61-69, 1907.
1931 Bircher, E.: Pneumoradiographie des Knies und der anderen Gelenke, Schweiz. Med. Wchnschr. **61**:1210-1211, 1931.
1933 Bircher, E.: Ueber Binnenverletzungen des Kniegelenkes, Arch. Clin. Chir. **177**:290-359, 1933.
1936 Simon, T., Hamilton, S. A., and Farrington, L. C.: Pneumography of the knee, Radiology **27**:533-539, 1936.
1937 Leveuf, J., and Bertrand, P.: L'arthrographie dans la luxation congénitale de la haunche, Presse Méd. **23**:437-440, 1937.
1938 Lindblom, Knut: Arthrographic appearance of the ligaments of the knee joint, Acta Radiol. **19**:582-600, 1938.
 Oberholzer, J.: Röntgendiagnostic des Gelenkes mittels Doppelkontrast-méthode, Leipzig, 1938, Georg Thieme.
1939 Lindblom, Knut: Arthrography and roentgenography in ruptures of the tendons of the shoulder joint, Acta Radiol. **20**:548-562, 1939.
1941 Axen, Oliver: Ueber den Wert des Arthrographie des Schultergelenkes, Acta Radiol. **22**:269, 1941.
 Hansson, C. J.: Arthrographic studies of the ankle joint, Acta Radiol. **22**:281-287, 1941.
1944 Andersen, J.: Some experiences with a new method for arthrography, Acta Radiol. **25**:33-39, 1944.
 Berridge, F. R., and Bonnin, J. B.: The radiographic examination of the ankle joint including arthrography, Surg. Gynec. Obstet. **79**:383-387, 1944.
 Glazebrook, L.: Air arthrography of the knee joint, Radiography **10**:43-44, 1944.
 Hauch, Paul P.: Pneumoroentgenography of the knee joint, Brit. J. Radiol. **17**:70-74, 1944.
 Nørgaard, F.: Arthrography of the mandible joint, Acta Radiol. **25**:679-685, 1944.
1945 Brooke, H. W., Mackenzie, W. C., and Smith, J. R.: Pneumoroentgenography with oxygen in the diagnosis of internal derangements of the knee joint, Amer. J. Roentgen. **54**:462-469, 1945.
 McGaw, W. H., and Weckesser, E. C.: Pneumoarthrograms of the knee, J. Bone Joint Surg. **27**:432-445, 1945.
1946 Jacobsen, H. H.: On the normal arthrogram of the mandibular joint, Acta Radiol. **27**:93-97, 1946.
 Somerville, E. W.: Air arthrography as an aid to the diagnosis of lesions of the menisci of the knee joint, J. Bone Joint Surg. **28**:451-465, 1946.
1947 Meschan, I., and McGaw, W. H.: New methods of pneumoarthrography of the knee with an evaluation of the procedure in 315 operated cases, Radiology **49**:675-711, 1947.
 Nørgaard, F.: Temporomandibular arthrography, Copenhagen, 1947, E. Munksgaard Publishing Co.
1948 Andersen, K.: Pneumoarthrography of the knee joint with particular reference to the semilunar cartilages, Acta Orthop. Scand. 4 (supp.):3-108, 1948.
 Lindblom, Knut: Arthrography of the knee; roentgenographic and anatomic study, Acta Radiol. **74** (supp.):1-112, 1948.
1949 Kelikian, H., and Lewis, E. K.: Arthrograms, Radiology **52**:465-487, 1949.
1950 Sachs, M. D., McGaw, W. H., and Rizzo, R. P.: Studies in the scope of pneumoarthrography of the knee as a diagnostic aid, Radiology **54**:10-31, 1950.
1951 Leroux, G. F.: L'examen des arthculations au moyen des produits de contraste, J. Radiol. Electr. **32**:210-224, 1951.
1953 Archimbaud, J.: L'arthrographie du genou, J. Radiol. Electr. **34**:623-633, 1953.
 Candardjis, G., and Saegesser, F.: L'arthrographie du genu par la methode du double contraste, Radiol. Clin. **22**:521, 1953.
 Kelly, F.: The technique of pneumoarthrography, Xray Techn. **24**:399-401, 1953.
1955 Wolfe, T. F.: Fundamentals and technique of arthrography, Xray Techn. **27**:171-174, 1955.
1957 Kerwein, G. A., Roseberg, B., and Sneed, W. R.: Arthrographic studies of the shoulder joint, J. Bone Joint Surg. **39-A**:1267-1279, 1957.
1959 Philippon, J.: Étude des malformations congénitales méniscales par arthropneumographie, J. Radiol. **40**:1-6, 1959.
1960 Andrén, L., and Wehlin, L.: Double-contrast arthrography of knee with horizontal roentgen ray beam, Acta Orthop. Scand. **29**:307-314, 1960.
1961 Kessler, L, Silberman, Z., and Nissim, F.: Arthrography of the knee; a critical study of errors and their sources, Amer. J. Roentgen. **86**:359-365, 1961.
 Samilson, R. L., Raphael, R. L., Post, L., Noonan, C., Sirés, E., and Raney, F. L., Jr.: Shoulder arthrography, J.A.M.A. **175**:773-778, 1961.
 Wadi, H.: Ueber die Anwendung eines einfachen Gerätes bei der Kniegelenksarthrographie, Fortschr. Roentgenstr. **95**:407-409, 1961.
1962 Heiser, S., Labriola, J. H., and Meyers, M. H.: Arthrography of the knee, Radiology **79**:822-828, 1962.
1963 Aye, R. C., Dorr, T. W., and Drewry, G. R.: Arthrography of the knee in office practice, Radiology **80**:829-836, 1963.
1965 Fleischer, H.: Die Arthrographie des Daumengrundgelenks, Röntgen. Blätter **18**:64-66, 1965.
1966 Freiberger, R. H., Killoran, P. J., and Cardona, G.: Arthrography of the knee by double contrast method, Amer. J. Roentgen. **97**:736-747, 1966.

Shoulder

1915 Iselin, Hans: Die Röntgenuntersuchung der Schulter in zwei zueinander senkrechten Richtungen, Bruns' Beiträge **97**:473, 1915.
 Lawrence, W. S.: New position in radiographing the shoulder joint, Amer. J. Roentgen. **2**:728-730, 1915.
1917 Lorenz: Die röntgenographische Darstellung des subskapularen Raumes und des Schenkelhalses im Querschnitt, Fortschr. Roentgenstr. **25**:342-343, 1917-1918.
1918 Bailleul, L. C., and Dubois-Roquebert: Le decalage dans les fractures de l'humérus, J. Radiol. Electr. **3**:251-256, 1918.
 George, Frank D.: Importance of the upper arm in the detection of roentgenological shadows in the region of the shoulder joint, Amer. J. Roentgen. **5**:187-188, 1918.
 Laquerrière and Pierquin: De la nécessite d'employer une technique radiographique spéciale pour obtenir certains details squelettiques, J. Radiol. Electr. **3**:145-148, 1918.
 Lawrence, W. S.: Method of obtaining accurate lateral roentgenogram of the shoulder joint, Amer. J. Roentgen. **5**:193-194, 1918.
1920 Arcelin, F.: L'exploration radiologique des grandes articulations, Lyon Chir. **17**:669-686, 1920.
 Chassard, M.: Résultats de l'exploration radiologique de l'articulation scapulo-humérale, J. Radiog. Electr. **4**:68-70, 1920.
1922 Béclère, H.: Radiographie de profil de l'omoplate, Bull. Soc. Radiol. Med. Paris **10**:53-55, 1922.
1924 Behn, Otto: Schulter-und Hüftaufnahmen in der Frontalebene, Fortschr. Roentgenstr. **32**:123, 1924.
 Buxton, Dudley, and Knox, Robert: A radiographic survey of normal joints, Part I: the shoulder, Brit. J. Radiol. **29**:115-134, 1924.
 Marko, D.: Isolierte Schlüsselbeinaufnahme, Fortschr. Roentgenstr. **32**:442, 1924.
1925 Pilz, W.: Zur Röntgenuntersuchung der habituellen Schulterverrenkung, Arch. Klin. Chir. **135**:1-22, 1925.

1926 Quesada, Fortunato: Technique for the roentgen diagnosis of fractures of the clavicle, Surg. Gynec. Obstet. **42**:424, 1926.

1927 King, J. M., and Homes, G. W.: Review of 450 roentgen ray examinations of the shoulder, Amer. J. Roentgen. **17**:214-218, 1927.

Mauclaire: Radiographies de profil et radiographies a pic de la hanche et de l'épaule, Arch. Prov. Chir. **30**:677-694, 1927.

1928 Dittrich, Rudolf: Eine neue Stellung zur röntgenologischen Erfassung der Schultergegend, Fortschr. Roentgenstr. **37**:526-529, 1928.

1929 Cohoon, Carl W.: Lateral transthoracic roentgenogram as a diagnostic aid in fractures of the upper end of the humerus, Amer. J. Roentgen. **21**:174-175, 1929.

Didiée, J.: Une position nouvelle pour la radiographie de la tête humérale: son intérét dans l'étude de la luxation récidivante de l'épaule, Bull. Soc. Radiol. Med. Paris **17**:150-154, 1929.

William, H. H.: Oblique views of the clavicle, Radiogr. Clin. Photogr. **5**:191-192, 1929.

1930 Didiée, J.: Le radiodiagnostic dans la luxation récidivante de l'épaule, J. Radiol. Electr. **14**:209-218, 1930.

Wahl, Rudolf: Ueber eine neue Scapulaaufnahme, Röntgenpraxis **2**:652-657, 1930.

1933 Berent, F., and von Hecker, H.: Zur axialen Aufnahmetechnik des Schultergelenks, Der Chir. **5**:210, 1933.

Wijnbladh, H.: Zur Röntgendiagnose von Schulterluxationen, Der Chir. **5**:702-704, 1933.

1934 Fergusson, N. J.: An improved technique for the examination of the shoulder, Brit. J. Radiol. **7**:33-42, 1934.

Freedman, Eugene: Radiography of the shoulder, Radiogr. Clin. Photogr. **10**:8-9, 1934.

Timpano, Mario: Aspetti radiografici dell'articolazione coraco-clavicolare, Ann. Radiol. Fis. Med. **8**:491, 1934.

1935 Henry, Lucas S.: Roentgenographic evidence in the tuberosity of the humerus of recent and old injuries to the supraspinatus tendon attachment, Amer. J. Roentgen. **33**:486, 1935.

Jordan, H.: New technic for the roentgen examination of the shoulder joint, Radiology **25**:480-484, 1935.

Philips, Herman B.: A lateral view of the clavicle, J. Bone Joint Surg. **17**:202-203, 1935.

Schoen, H.: Zur Technik der axialen Schulterfernaufnahme, Röntgenpraxis **7**:264, 1935.

1936 Jones, Myrtle L.: Radiographic examination of the shoulder, Xray Techn. **7**:104-105, 134-135, 1936.

Pearson, Gertrude R.: Radiographic technic for acromioclavicular dislocation, Radiology **27**:239, 1936.

1937 Blackett, Charles W., and Healy, Thomas R.: Roentgen studies of the shoulder, Amer. J. Roentgen. **37**:760-766, 1937.

Fray, Walter W.: Effect of position on the production of cystlike shadows around the shoulder joints, Radiology **28**:673-682, 1937.

Liberson, F.: The value and limitation of the oblique view as compared with the ordinary anteroposterior exposure of the shoulder, Amer. J. Roentgen. **37**:498-509, 1937.

Moreau, L.: Remarks on certain profile radiographs of the bone, Bull. Soc. Radiol. Med. Paris **25**:49-50, 1937.

Moreau, L.: Remarques sur quelques radiographies osseuses de profil, Bull. Soc. Radiol. Med. Paris **25**:49-50, 1937.

1938 Codman, E. A.: Rupture of the supraspinatus, Amer. J. Surg. **42**:603, 1938.

Holmblad, Edward C.: X-ray examination of the clavicles and acromioclavicular joints, Amer. J. Surg. **42**:791-797, 1938.

Massa, J.: Une nouvelle position pour l'examen radiologique de l'épaule de profil, Gaz. Méd. France (supp. Cah. Radiol.) **45**:363, 1938.

Mullins, S. A.: Technique for radiography of the luxations of joints, Radiology **4**:94-96, 1938.

Scaglietti, O.: The obstetrical shoulder trauma, Surg. Gynec. Obstet. **66**:868-877, 1938.

Wehl, Grace F.: A useful and easily obtained view of the scapula, Radiography **4**:174-175, 1938.

1939 Pinelli, I.: Frattura della spina della scapola; sua proiezione e immagine radiografica, Quad. Radiol. **4**:92-97, 1939.

Williams, H. H.: An oblique view of the clavicle, Radiography **5**:191-192, 1939.

1940 Gunson, Edward F.: Technical procedure in the x-ray examination of the scapula, Xray Techn. **11**:165-167, 203, 1940.

Hill, H. A., and Sachs, M. D.: Grooved defect of the humeral head, Radiology **35**:690-700, 1940.

Perry, Esther C.: Radiography of the shoulders, Xray Techn. **11**:168-169, 193, 1940.

Watson, W.: An abnormal view of the shoulder, Radiography **6**:76-77, 1940.

1941 Alexander, O. M.: Simple technique for obtaining a lateral view of the upper end of the humerus, Radiology **7**:31-32, 1941.

Bosworth, B. M.: Examination of the shoulder for calcium deposits, J. Bone Joint Surg. **23**:567-577, 1941.

Cleaves, Edwin N.: A new film holder for roentgen examination of the shoulder, Amer. J. Roentgen. **45**:288-290, 1941.

Devvis et Proux, Ch.: Sur une technique de radiographie de l'épaule de profil, J. Radiol. Electr. **24**:111-112, 1941.

Rendich, Richard H., and Poppel, M. H.: Roentgen diagnosis of the posterior dislocation of the shoulder, Radiology **36**:42-45, 1941.

Sachs, Maurice D., Hill, H. A., and Chuinard, Eldon L.: Further studies of the shoulder joint with special reference to the bicipital groove, Radiology **36**:731-735, 1941.

1942 Johnson, Dora Rhodes: Lateral projection of the scapula, Radiogr. Clin. Photogr. **18**:47-48, 1942.

Jones, Laurence: The shoulder joint; observations on the anatomy and physiology, Surg. Gynec. Obstet. **75**:433-444, 1942.

1943 Alexander, Sidney: Study of the shoulder with special reference to the humerus, Xray Techn. **14**:147-150, 1943.

1944 Oppenheimer, Albert: Lesions of the acromioclavicular joint causing pain and disability of the shoulder, Amer. J. Roentgen. **51**:699-706, 1944.

1945 Howorth, Beckett M.: Calcification of tendon cuff of shoulder, Surg. Gynec. Obstet. **80**:337-345, 1945.

1946 Soule, A. B.: Ossification of the coraco-clavicular ligament following dislocation of the acromioclavicular articulation, Amer. J. Roentgen. **56**:607-615, 1946.

1947 Lane, R. G.: A technique for radiography of the humerus in the lateral view, Xray Techn. **19**:129, 168, 1947.

1948 Fengler, Kaethe: Special projections for the coracoid process and clavicle, Amer. J. Roentgen. **59**:435-438, 1948.

Alexander, O. M.: Radiography of the acromioclavicular joint, Radiography **14**:139-141, 1948.

Bosworth, B. M.: Acromioclavicular dislocations, Ann. Surg. **127**:98-111, 1948.

Howes, W. E., and Alicandri, B. B.: A method of roentgenologic examination of the shoulder, Radiology **50**:569-580, 1948.

Knutsson, F.: An axial projection of the shoulder joint, Acta Radiol. **30**:214-216, 1948.

Porcher, Pierre: Précise de Technique Radiographique, ed. 2, Paris, 1948, Gauthier-Villars.

Warrick, C. K.: Posterior dislocation of the shoulder joint, J. Bone Joint Surg. **30-B**:651-655, 1948.

1950 Tarrant, R. M.: The axial view of the clavicle, Xray Techn. **21**:358-359, 1950.

1952 McLaughlin, H. L.: Posterior dislocation of the shoulder, J. Bone Joint Surg. **34-A**:584-590, 1952.

1953 Mazujian, M.: Lateral profile view of the scapula, Xray Techn. **25**:24-25, 1953.

1954 Alexander, O. M.: Radiography of the acromioclavicular articulation, Med. Radiogr. Photogr. **30**:34-39, 1954.

1956 O'Connor, S. J., and Jacknow, A. S.: Posterior dislocation of the shoulder, Arch. Surg. **72**:479-491, 1956.

1957 Brown, W. H., and others: Posterior dislocation of the shoulder, Radiology **69**:815-822, 1957.

Schönbauer, H. R.: Zur Röntgentechnik des Schlüsselbeinbruches, Fortschr. Roentgenstr. **86**:349-351, 1957.

1958 Barraco, N. R.: A lateral projection of the shoulder joint to permit an evaluation of the degree of dislocation, Xray Techn. **29**:221-224, 1958.

Funke, Thomas: Tangential view of the scapular spine, Med. Radiogr. Photogr. **34**:41-43, 1958.

1959 Conklin, W. A., and Atwill, J. H., Jr.: Lateral radiography of the scapula with the patient supine, Med. Radiogr. Photogr. **35**:46-47, 1959.

Seyss, R.: Zur Röntgentechnik des Schlüsselbeinbruches, Fortschr. Roentgenstr. **90**:768-769, 1959.

1960 Berens, D. L., and Lockie, L. M.: Ossification of the coracoacromial ligament, Radiology **74**:802-805, 1960.

1961 Künlen, H.: Beitrag zur Darstellung der Klavikel in der 2. Ebene, Fortschr. Roentgenstr. **94**:739-750, 1961. Abst.: Radiology **78**:848, 1962.

1962 Golding, F. C.: The shoulder—the forgotten joint, Brit. J. Radiol. **35**:149-158, 1962.

Nobel, W.: Posterior traumatic dislocation of the shoulder, J. Bone Joint Surg. **44-A**:523-538, 1962.

1963 Stripp, W. J.: Radiographs of the scapulothoracic region, Xray Focus **4**:8-12, 1963.

Stripp, W. J.: The clavicle and the acromioclavicular joint, Xray Focus **4**:21-26, 1963.

1964 Stripp, W. J.: Sternoclavicular joint and the bicipital groove, Xray Focus **5**:11-13, 1964.

1965 Fisk, Charles: Adaptation of the technique for radiography of the bicipital groove, Radiol. Techn. **37**:47-50, 1965.

Warrick, C. K.: Posterior dislocation of the shoulder joint, Brit. J. Radiol. **38**:758-761, 1965.

Bony thorax
Sternum

1919 Drüner, L.: Ueber die Röntgenologie des Brustbeins, Fortschr. Roentgenstr. **27**:54, 1919-1921.

1920 Delherm and Chaperon: Radiographie du sternum en position oblique antérieure droite, J. Radiol. Elect. **4**:227-228, 1920.

1924 Pfahler, G. E.: Study of the sternum by roentgen rays, Amer. J. Roentgen. **9**:311, 1924.

1929 Pendergrass, R. C.: Roentgenographic demonstration of sternal injury, Radiology **13**:451-455, 1929.

1936 Blumensaat, Carl: Zur Röntgendarstellung des Brustbeins, Bruns' Beitr. Klin. Chir. **163**:120, 1936.

Holman, Cranston, and Stober, Eugene: Technic for radiography of the sternum, Radiology **26**:757-758, 1936.

1937 Jönsson, Gunnar: Method of obtaining structural pictures of the sternum, Acta Radiol. **18**:336-339, 1937.

1939 Zimmer, E. A.: Das Brustbein und seine Gelenke, Fortschr. Roentgenstr. **58**:1939.

1940 Dixon, F. L.: Technic for roentgenography of the sternum, Xray Techn. **12**:8-12, 1940.

Kraft, E.: Respiratory blurring in routine roentgenography, Quart. Bull. Sea View Hosp. **5**:167-174, 1940

Mullans, S. A.: Technique for radiography of the sternum, Radiography **6**:12-13, 1940.

Weinbren, M.: Tomography of the spine and the sternum, Brit. J. Radiol. **8**:325-336, 1940.

1942 Holly, E. W.: Some radiographic techniques in which movement is utilized, Radiogr. Clin. Photogr. **18**:78-83, 1942.

Runge, R. K.: A technique for roentgenography of the sternum, Xray Techn. **13**:153-154, 175, 1942.

1946 Jensen, Christina: Radiographic examination of the sternum—posterior-anterior position, Xray Techn. **18**:18, 41, 1946.

1953 Benmussa, M.: Technique d'examen radiographique du sternum, J. Radiol. Electr. **34**:646-648, 1953.

1955 Russell, D. A., and Albrecht, L.: A new technic for radiology of the bony thorax and sternum, Radiology **64**:721-723, 1955.

1956 Balzarini, E., and Pompili, G.: Tecnica e anatomia radiografica normale dello sterno, Radiol. Med. **42**:625-637, 1956.

1959 Saudan, Yves: Aspects radiologiques de quelques lésions sternales, Radiol. Clin. **28**:313-319, 1959.

Sternoclavicular articulation

1937 Schnarr, A.: Die Darstellung des Sternum und der Sternoklavikulargelenke im Tomogramm, Röntgenpraxis **9**:622-629, 1937.

1938 Leman, R. M.: Some radiographic techniques, Radiography **4**:41-44, 1938.

1939 Zimmer, E. A.: Das Brustbein und seine Gelenke, Fortschr. Roentgenstr. **58**:1939.

1943 Gunson, E. F.: Radiography of the sternoclavicular articulation, Radiogr. Clin. Photogr. **19**:20-24, 1943.

1946 Kurzbauer, Robert: The lateral projection in roentgenography of the sternoclavicular articulation, Amer. J. Roentgen. **56**:104-105, 1946.

1947 Ritvo, Max, and Ritvo, Meyer: Roentgen study of the sternoclavicular region, Amer. J. Roentgen. **58**:644-650, 1947.

1949 Blocklage, M. H.: A comparison of roentgenographic examinations of the sternum and sternoclavicular joints, Xray Techn. **21**:19-27, 1949.

1964 Pretorius, R.: Radiography of the sternoclavicular joints—a new technique, Radiography **30**:26-27, 1964.

Stripp, W. J.: Sternoclavicular joint and the bicipital groove, Xray Focus **5**:11-13, 1964.

Ribs

1920 Knox, Robert: Special points in technique for the radiograph of the clavicle and lateral aspect of the ribs for detection of injuries, Arch. Radiol. Elect. **24**:248-252, 1920.

1931 Perry, L. M., and Newton, E. S.: Rib position and radiographic technic of mid-axillary and mid-clavicular lines, Xray Techn. **2**:74-75, 1931.

1933 Ernst, George: Einfache Einstellungstechnik zur Darstellung zeitlicher Rippenbrüche im Bereich der unteren Brusthälfte, Röntgenpraxis **5**:154, 1933.

1939 Bloom, Arthur R.: A new technic of taking roentgenographs of the upper ribs, Radiology **33**:648-649, 1939.

1942 Bartsch G. W.: Radiographic examination of the ribs, Xray Techn. **14**:18-22, 29, 1942.

1943 Rogers, N. J. S.: A technique of x-ray examination of the ribs, Radiography **9**:7, 1943.

Sanborn, R. L.: Radiography of the ribs, Xray Techn. **14**:202-203, 1943.

1945 Kalsbeek, Ann: Tube angle rib technique, Xray Techn. **16**:147-148, 1945.

1947 Liberson, F.: Fractures of the ribs (with comparison of the standard and the one-film two-exposure technic), Amer. J. Roentgen. **57**:349-354, 1947.

1956 Bridgeman, C. F., Holly, E. W., and Zariquiey, M. O.: Radiography of the ribs and costovertebral joints, Med. Radiogr. Photogr. **32**:38-60, 1956.

1963 Agnesia, Sr. Mary: A wide-angle rib technique, Xray Techn. **34**:289-290, 1963.

Berlin, H. S., Unger, S. M., Corbin, L. J., Jacobson, E. G., and Poppel, M. H.: Wide angle roentgenography, Amer. J. Roentgen. **90**:189-197, 1963.

1966 Reynolds, J., and Davis, J. T.: Injuries of the chest wall, pleura, pericardium, lungs, bronchi, and esophagus, Radiol. Clin. N. Amer. **4**:383-401, 1966.

Pelvic bones and upper femora

1897 Cowl: Ein Sagittal nebst Frontalbild eines anomalen coxalen Femurendes, Fortschr. Roentgenstr. **1**:136, 1897-1898.

1900 Lauenstein, Carl: Das Röntgenbild einer Luxato femoris infraglenoidalis, Fortschr. Roentgenstr. **3**:186, 1900-1901.

1916 Arcelin, F.: Rapport mensuel des services d'électroradiologie de la XIV region, Dec., 1916.

Hickey, P. M.: Value of the lateral view of the hip, Amer. J. Roentgen **3**:308-309, 1916.

1917 Lilienfeld, Leon: Die seitliche Aufnahme des Hüftgelenkes, Deutsche Med. Wschr. **43**:294-296, 1917.

Salmond, A. W. R.: Technique for the lateral view of the upper end of the femur, Arch. Radiol. Electr. **22**:297-300, 1917-1918.

Lorenz: Die röntgenographische Darstellung des subskapularen Raumes und des Schenkelhalses im Querschnitt, Fortschr. Roentgenstr. 25:342-343, 1917-1918.

1918 Prentiss, H. J.: Standardization of roentgenography of the shoulder and hip joint, J. Roentgen. 1:145-150, 1918.

1919 Lilienfeld, Leon: Die axiale Aufnahme der Regio pubica, Fortschr. Roentgenstr. 26:285-290, 1919.

Staunig, Konrad: Die axiale Aufnahme der Regio pubica, Fortschr. Roentgenstr. 27:514-517, 1919-1921.

1920 Arcelin, F.: Technique et résultats de l'exploration radiographique de profil de l'extremité supérieure du fémur, J. Radiol. Electr. 4:12-18, 1920.

Kisch, Eugen: Eine neue Methode für röntgenologische Darstellung des Hüftgelenks in frontaler Ebene, Fortschr. Roentgenstr. 27:309, 1920.

1921 Arcelin, F., and Duchene Marullaz, Lyon: L'exploration radiologique de profil de la hanche, Bull. Soc. Radiol. Méd. Paris 9:40-45, 1921.

Bouchacourt: Des avantages et des inconvenients respectifs des radiographies de la hanche en position de profil et en position de trois quarts obliques, Bull. Soc. Radiol. Méd. Paris 9:90, 1921.

1927 Béclère, H., and Porcher, Pierre: La radiographie latérale de la hanche, J. Radiol. Electr. 10:97-105, 1926. Abst.: Amer. J. Roentgen. 17:132, 1927.

Regner, and LeFloch: Radiographie du profil de la hanche dans les luxations congénitales, J. Radiol. Electr. 11:167-170, 1927.

1928 Philips, Herman B.: New roentgenographic demonstration of the fractured neck of the femur, Amer. J. Surg. 5:392-393, 1928.

1929 Schertlein, A.: Die Bestimmung des Schenkelhalstorsionswinkels mit Hilfe der Röntgenstrahlen, Fortschr. Roentgenstr. 39:304-318, 1929.

1930 Paschetta, Vincent: La méthode des radiographies en trois positions dans les fractures du col du femur, Arch. Électr. Méd. 38:12-17, 1930.

1931 Kniper, E.: Röntgenaufnahmen des Oberschenkelhalses bei seitlicher Strahlenrichtung, Röntgenpraxis 3:909-911, 1931.

1932 Johansson, Sven: Zur Technik der Osteosynthese der Fract. colli femoris, Zbl. Chir. 59:2019, 1932.

Johnson, C. R.: A new method for roentgenographic examination of the upper end of the femur, J. Bone Joint Surg. 30:859-866, 1932.

Leonard, R. D., and George, A. W.: Cassette with convex curve, Amer. J. Roentgen. 28:261-263, 1932.

Wittek-Saltzberg, R.: Ueber seitliche Aufnahmen des Schenkelhalses und Trochanterregion, Röntgenpraxis 4:965-968, 1932.

1933 Jones, Laurence: Intracapsular fracture of the neck of the femur, Ann. Surg. 97:237-246, 1933.

1934 George, A. W., and Leonard, R. D.: Ununited intracapsular fractures of the femoral neck roentgenologically considered, Amer. J. Roentgen. 31:433, 1934.

1935 Erlacher, J.: Eine zweite Röntgenaufnahme des Hüftgelenkes, Zbl. Chir. 62:731-734, 1935.

Jones, Laurence: Lateral roentgenography of the neck of the femur, Amer. J. Roentgen. 33:504-510, 1935.

Manfredi, Morris, and Swenson, Paul C.: Lateral roentgenography of the hip, Amer. J. Roentgen. 34:404-405, 1935.

1936 Danelius, G., and Miller, L.: Lateral view of the hip, Amer. J. Roentgen. 35:282-284, 1936.

Friedman, Lewis J.: Lateral roentgen ray study of the hip joint, Radiology 27:240-241, 1936.

Gaenslen, F. J.: Fracture of the neck of the femur, J.A.M.A. 107:105-114, 1936.

Hsieh, C. K.: Posterior dislocation of the hip, Radiology 27:450-455, 1936.

Pletz, Flora: Lateral roentgenography of the hip, Xray Techn. 8:60-61, 1936.

1937 Kewesch, E. L.: De l'examen radiologique de l'articulation de la hanche et du col du femur dans la projection latérale, Vestnik Rentgen. Radiol. 18:71-73, 1937.

Polgar, F.: Die Incisura acetabuli im Röntgenbilde des Hüftgelenkes, Fortschr. Roentgenstr. 56:521, 1937.

1938 Cleaves, Edwin N.: Observations on lateral views of the hips, Amer. J. Roentgen. 34:964-966, 1938.

Danelius, G., and Miller, L.: Lateral view of the hip, Xray Techn. 9:176-178, 1938.

Dooley, E. A., Caldwell, C. W., and Glass, G. A.: Roentgenography of the femoral neck, Amer. J. Roentgen. 39:834, 1938.

Douglas, John J.: Modified lateral hip technique, Xray Techn. 10:77-78, 1938.

Douglas, John J.: Further notes on hip technique, Xray Techn. 10:134, 138, 1938.

Grasser, C. H.: Hilfsmethoden zur Darstellung des Hüftgelenkes und des Schenkelhalses, Röntgenpraxis 10:544-551, 1938.

Teufel, Siegfried: Eine gezielte Aufsichtsaufnahme der Hüftgelenkpfanne, Röntgenpraxis 10:398-402, 1938.

1940 Dooley, E. A., Caldwell, C. W., and Glass, G. A.: Roentgenografía del cuello del femur; técnica para obtener vistas lateral y anteroposterior verdaderas, Rev. Rad. Fis. 7-8:49, 1940.

Hovious, Catherine: X-ray technic for fractures of the hip, Xray Techn. 12:90-91, 1940.

1941 Taylor, Robert: Modified anteroposterior projection of the anterior bones of the pelvis, Radiogr. Clin. Photogr. 17:67-69, 1941.

1942 Wolcott, Roy E.: Technique for securing lateral roentgenograms of the femoral neck in the operating room, Xray Techn. 13:155-158, 181, 1942.

1943 Barnard, V. L.: A new surgical table top and cassette holder for surgical roentgenographic examinations of the hip, Radiology 40:599-602, 1943.

1945 Lane, Robert G.: Radiographic technique for lateral hip position with the Potter-Bucky diaphragm, Xray Techn. 16:175-176, 1945.

Massa, J.: Contribution à l'étude de la radiographie de la hanche de profit, chez les traumatisés du col fémoral, J. Radiol. Electr. 26:288-291, 1944-1945.

Wood, F. G., Camb, M. B., and Wilkinson, M. C.: The x-ray examination of the hip in tuberculous disease, Brit. J. Radiol. 18:332-334, 1945.

1948 Donaldson, S. W., Badgley, C. E., and Hunsberger, W. G.: Lateral view of the pelvis in examination for hip dislocation, J. Bone Joint Surg. 30-A:512-514, 1948.

Urist, M. R.: Fracture-dislocation of the hip joint, J. Bone Joint Surg. 30-A:699-727, 1948.

1950 Bridgman, C. F.: Radiography of the hip joint, Med. Radiogr. Photogr. 26:2-17, 70-83, 1950.

1951 Bridgman, C. F.: Radiography of the hip joint, Med. Radiogr. Photogr. 27:2-13, 34-38, 70-80, 1951.

de Cuveland, E., and Hueck, F.: Osteochondropathie der Spina iliaca anterior inferior unter Berücksichtigung der Ossifikationsvorgänge der Apophyse des lateralen Pfannenrandes, Fortschr. Roentgenstr. 75:430-445, 1951.

Mitton, K. L., and Auringer, E. M.: Roentgenological study of the femoral neck, Amer. J. Roentgen. 66:639-641, 1951.

Williams, A. Justin: Roentgenographic study of the hip joint in the lateral projection, Amer. J. Roentgen. 66:459-460, 1951.

1952 Bridgman, C. F.: Radiography of the hip bone, Med. Radiogr. Photogr. 28:38-46, 1952.

1953 Colonna, Paul C.: A diagnostic roentgen view of the acetabulum, S. Clin. N. Amer. 33:1565-1569, 1953.

Dunlap, K., Swanson, A. B., and Penner, R. S.: A new method for determination of torsion of the femur, J. Bone Joint Surg. 35-A:289-311, 1953.

Laage, H., Barnett, J. C., Brady, J. M., and Dulligan, P. J.: Horizontal lateral roentgenography of the hip in children, J. Bone Joint Surg. 35-A:387-398, 1953.

1954 Marz, C. D., and Taylor, C. C.: The 45-degree angle roentgenographic study of the pelvis in congenital dislocation of the hip, J. Bone Joint Surg. 36-A:528-532, 1954.

1955 Broderick, Thomas F.: Complementary roentgenographic view of the hip, J. Bone Joint Surg. 37-A:295-298, 1955.

1956 Dunlap, K., Swanson, A. B., and Penner, R. S.: Studies of the hip joint by means of lateral acetabular roentgenograms, J. Bone Joint Surg. **38-A**:1218-1230, 1956.

Magilligan, D. J.: Calculation of the angle of anteversion by means of horizontal lateral roentgenography, J. Bone Joint Surg. **38-A**:1231-1246, 1956.

1958 Fisk, C., and Fry, M. J.: Femoral torsion and the Shands technique, Xray Techn. **29**:225, 1958.

Shands, A. R., and Steele, M. K.: Torsion of the femur; a follow-up report on the use of the Dunlap method for its determination, J. Bone Joint Surg. **40-A**:803-816, 1958.

1962 Fisk, Charles: A review of the clinical and radiographic studies of dislocated hips, Xray Techn. **34**:66-69, 1962.

Voorhis, C. C.: A cassette holder to be used in pinning hips, Surg. Gynec. Obstet. **115**:359-360, 1962.

1964 Fisk, Charles: Actabular fractures—where? Radiol. Techn. **35**:330-333, 1964.

1965 Berkebile, R. D., Fischer, D. L., and Albrecht, L. F.: The gull wing sign; value of the lateral view of the pelvis in fracture dislocation of the acetabular rim and posterior dislocation of the femoral head, Radiology **84**:937-939, 1965.

1966 Mounts, R. J., and Schloss, C. D.: Injuries to the bony pelvis and hip, Radiol. Clin. N. Amer. **4**:307-322, 1966.

Vertebral column
Occipitocervical articulations

1920 Massimo, Lupo: Contributo allo studio dell'anatomia radiografica delle prime vertebre cervicali e del cranio, Rad. Med. **7**:393-407, 1920.

1926 Goldhamer, Karl: Beitrag zur röntgenographischen Darstellung des Atlas und der Pars lateralis occipitis, Fortschr. Roentgenstr. **35**:627-629, 1926-1927.

1942 Englander, O.: Non-traumatic occipito-atlanto-axial dislocation; a contribution to the radiology of the atlas, Brit. J. Radiol. **15**:341-345, 1942.

1961 Lombardi, G.: The occipital vertebra, Amer. J. Roentgen. **86**:260-269, 1961.

Atlas and axis

1910 Albers-Schönberg, H. E.: Die Röntgentechnik, ed. 3, Hamburg, 1910, Grafe & Sillem.

1919 George, A. W.: Method for more accurate study of injuries to the atlas and axis, Boston Med. Surg. J. **181**:395-398, 1919.

1931 Fuchs, Arthur W.: Regional radiographic technique Radiogr. Clin. Photogr. **7**:12-13, 1931.

1937 Kulka, Z.: Transkranielle Aufnahme des ersten Halswirbels, Röntgenpraxis **9**:128-129, 1937.

1938 Plaut, H. F.: Fractures of the atlas resulting from automobile accidents, Amer. J. Roentgen. **40**:867, 1938.

1939 Kasabach, H. H.: A roentgenographic method for the study of the second cervical vertebra, Amer. J. Roentgen. **42**:782-785, 1939.

1942 Dariaux: Radiographie de face de la colonne cervicale en incidence anterieure, J. Radiol. Electr. **25**:28, 1942.

1943 Judd, George: A useful view of the odontoid process of the axis vertebra, Radiography **9**:46, 1943.

1950 Schunk, F.: Radiography of the first cervical ring (atlas), Xray Techn. **21**:219-220, 1950.

Walters, B.: An additional technique for the roentgen demonstration of the first cervical vertebra, Amer. J. Roentgen. **63**:739-740, 1950.

1951 Buetti, C.: Zur Darstellung der Atlanto-epistropheal Gelenke bzw. der Procc. transversi atlantis und epistrophei, Radiol. Clin. **20**:168-172, 1951.

1956 Jacobson, G., and Adler, D. C.: Examination of the atlanto-axial joint following injury, Amer. J. Roentgen. **76**:1081-1094, 1956.

1962 Herrmann, E., and Stender, H. S.: Eine einfache Aufnahmetechnik zur Darstellung der Dens axis, Fortschr. Roentgenstr. **96**:115-119, 1962.

Cervical vertebrae

1916 Hobbs, Austin L.: A method of showing the lower cervical vertebrae, Amer. J. Roentgen. **3**:233, 1916.

1923 Feil, André: Comment doit-on radiographier la colonne cervicale quand on soupçonne l'existence d'une anomalie, J. Radiol. Electr. **7**:125-133, 1923.

1925 Grandy, C. C.: A new method for making radiographs of the cervical vertebrae in lateral position, Radiology **4**:128-129, 1925.

1926 Barsóny, Theodor, and Koppenstein, Ernst: Eine neue Methode zur Untersuchung der Halswirbelsäule, Fortschr. Roentgenstr. **35**:593-594, 1926-1927.

1929 Barsóny Theodor, and Koppenstein, Ernst: Beitrag sur Aufnahmetechnik der Halswirbelsäule; Darstellung der Foramina intervertebralia, Röntgenpraxis **1**:245-249, 1929.

Erdélyi, Joseph: Neues Verfahren zur seitlichen Aufnahme der Halswirbel, Röntgenpraxis **1**:138-140, 1929.

Gally and Bernard: Technique particulière pour la radiographie de profil de la colonne cervicale, Bull. Mém. Soc. Rad. Méd. Paris **17**:288-289, 1929.

Ottonello, Pietro: Nuevo método para la radiografía de la columna cervicale completa en proyección sagital ventrodorsal, Anal. Radiol. (Havana) **1**:57-58, 1929.

1930 Ottonello, Pietro: New method for roentgenography of the entire cervical spine in ventrodorsal projection, Rev. Rad. Fis. Med **2**:291-294, 1930.

Schneider, Cathryn C.: Mechanical devices for immobilizing the head and hand, Xray Techn. **1**:70-71, 1930.

1931 Arskussky, J.: Eine vereinfachte Methode der Röntgenaufnahme des oberen Halswirbel, Röntgenpraxis **3**:953-957, 1931.

Pélissier, G.: Radiographie de face de la colonne cervicale dans son ensemble technique nouvelle, Bull. Mém. Soc. Rad. Méd. Paris **19**:360-361, 1931.

1935 Lupacciolu, Giovanni Fratture del rachide cervicale all'indagine radiologica, Rad. Med. **22**:529-562, 1935. Abst.: Am. J. Roentgen. **37**:135, 1937.

1938 Gaudentia, Sister M.: The cervical vertebrae, Xray Techn. **10**:74-75, 86, 1938.

Jacobs, Lewis: Roentgenography of the cervical second vertebra by Ottonello's method, Radiology **31**:412-413, 1938.

Kovács Ákos: Röntgendarstellung und Diagnostik der zervicalen Zwischenwirbellöcher, Röntgenpraxis **10**:478-484, 1938.

Oppenheimer, Albert: The swollen atrophic hand, Surg. Gynec. Obstet. **67**:446-454, 1938.

1940 Fuchs, Arthur W.: Cervical vertebrae, Radiogr. Clin. Photogr. **16**:2-17, 34-41, 1940.

1942 Beatrice, Sister M.: Roentgenography of the cervical spine, Xray Techn. **13**:147-149, 1942.

Belot, J.: À propos de la radiographie de la colonne vertebrale, J. Radiol. Electr. **25**:135-136, 1942-1943.

1943 Garthright, E. G.: Technique for roentgenography of the upper cervical vertebrae, Xray Techn. **14**:241-242, 1943.

1944 Hadley, Lee A.: Roentgenographic studies of the cervical spine, Amer. J. Roentgen. **52**:173-195, 1944.

1946 Polino, W. William: Method for obtaining optimum visualization of the seventh cervical vertebra in lateral projections, Roentgenography **1**:10-11, 1946.

1948 Marchand, J. H., Djian, A., and Fétiveau: Radiographie de la colonne cervicale en double obliquite, J. Radiol. Electr. **29**:291-295, 1948.

1950 Marks, J. L., and Parks, S. L.: A simplified position for demonstrating the cervical intervertebral foramina, Amer. J. Roentgen. **63**:575-577, 1950.

1954 Albers, D.: Eine Studie über die Funktion der Halswirbelsüle bie dorsaler und vertraler Flexion, Fortschr. Roentgenstr. **81**:605-615, 1954.

1955 Bumstead, H. D.: Routine examination of the cervical spine, Xray Techn. **27**:247-250, 1955.

1957 Boylston, B. F.: Oblique roentgenographic views of the cervical spine in flexion and extension; an aid in the diagnosis of cervical subluxations and obscure dislocations, J. Bone Joint Surg. **39-A**:1302-1309, 1957.

Dorlard, P., and Frémont, J.: Aspect radiologique normale du rachis postérieur cervicodorsal (vue postérieure ascendante), Semaine Hôpit., 1457-1464, 1957.

Gersh, M., and Vincent, P. J.: Anteroposterior projection of the cervical vertebrae on one film, Med. Radiogr. Photogr. **33**:2-3, 1957.

1958 Abel, M. S.: Moderately severe whiplash injuries of the cervical spine and their roentgenologic diagnosis, Clin. Orthop. **12**:189-208, 1958.

Dorland, P., Frémont, J., Parer, and Perez: Technique d'examen radiologique de l'arc postérieur des vertèbres cervico-dorsales, J. Radiol. Electr. **39**:509-519, 1958.

Hartley, Joel: Modern concepts of whiplash injury, New York J. Med. **58**:3306-3310, 1958.

1961 Conklin, W. A.: Radiographic studies of the cervical spine, Xray Techn. **33**:181-185, 1961.

1962 Coupe, C. W.: Cervicodorsal region: lateral projection, Xray Techn. **33**:256-257, 1962.

1963 Beatson, T. R.: Fractures and dislocations of the cervical spine, J. Bone Joint Surg. **45-B**:21-35, 1963.

1964 Cahoon, J. B., Jr.: All in one, C-1 and you see seven, Radiol. Techn. **35**:252-258, 1964.

Hagen, D. E.: Introduction to the pillar projection of the cervical spine, Radiol. Techn. **35**:239-242, 1964.

Thoracic vertebrae

1925 Badolle, M.: La radiographie de la colonne dorsale chez l'adulte en positions obliques, Lyon Méd. **135**:224-232, 1925.

1926 Alberti, Olindo: Tecnica radiografica per la proiezione esattamente laterale delle prime vertebre dorsali, Rad. Med. **13**:212-214, 1926.

1927 Barsóny, Theodor, and Koppenstein, Ernst: Eine neue Methode zur Röntgenuntersuchung der oberen Brustwirbelsäule, Fortschr. Roentgenstr. **36**:338-341, 1927.

1928 Alberti, Olindo: Tecnica radiografica per la proiezione esattamente laterale delle prime vertebre dorsali, Atti Congresso Ital. Rad. Med. **8**:340-345, 1928.

Dall'Acqua, Virgilio: Nuovo metodo per la proiezione laterale delle ultime vertebre cervicali e delle prime dorsali, Rad. Med. **15**:843-845, 1928.

Gutzeit: Aufnahmetechnik der oberen Brustwirbelsäule in frontaler Richtung, Fortschr. Roentgenstr. **37**:400, 1928.

1929 Pawlov, M. K.: Zur Frage über die seitliche Strahlenrichtung bei den Aufnahmen der unteren und oberen Brustwirbel, Röntgenpraxis **1**:285-288, 1929.

Sgalitzer, Max: Zur Technik der Röntgenuntersuchung der 4 obersten Brustwirbel in seitlicher Richtung, Fortschr. Roentgenstr. **40**:267-271, 1929.

1933 Corlay, Georges: Contribution à l'étude radiologique de la region cervico-dorsale, Paris theses, 1933.

1937 Twining, E. W.: Lateral view of the lung apices, Brit. J. Radiol. **10**:123-131, 1937.

Barsóny, Theodor, and Winkler, K.: Beiträge zur Röntgenologie der Wirbelsäule; die "elektive" Profil-Röntgenaufnahme der Brustwirbelsäul, Röntgenpraxis **9**:601-608, 1937.

1938 Bartsch, Gerald W.: Radiography of the upper dorsal spine, Xray Techn. **10**:135-138, 1938.

Fletcher, James: Radiography of the upper vertebrae, Radiogr. Clin. Photogr. **14**:10-12, 1938.

Oppenheimer, Albert: The apophyseal intervertebral articulations roentgenologically considered, Radiology **30**:724-740, 1938.

1940 Clarke, E. K.: Visualization of the first and second dorsal and the fifth lumbar vertebrae in lateral or slightly semilateral positions, Xray Techn. **12**:5-7, 1940.

Horwitz, T., and Smith, R. M.: An anatomical, pathological and roentgenological study of the intervertebral joints of the lumbar spine and of the sacroiliac joints, Amer. J. Roentgen. **43**:173-186, 1940.

1941 Eller, Virginia H.: Radiography of the thoracic spine, Xray Techn. **13**:18-20, 36, 1941.

Fuchs, Arthur W.: Thoracic vertebrae, Radiogr. Clin. Photogr. **17**:2-13, 42-51, 1941.

1944 Desgrez and Pioux: Contribution à l'étude des premières vertèbres dorsales en profil vrai, J. Radiol. Electr. **26**:29, 1944-1945.

1946 Orgeron, Eddie A.: An additional technique for the demonstration of the cervical and upper thoracic spine in a lateral position, Xray Techn. **17**:385-386, 1946.

1950 Guerreiro, G.: Lateral roentgenographic examination of the thoracic spine, J. Bone Joint Surg. **32-A**:192, 1950.

Lumbar vertebrae

1917 Hammes, J.: Ueber die Technik und den Wert seitlicher Wirbelaufnahmen, Fortschr. Roentgenstr. **25**:1, 1917-1918.

Hickey, Preston M.: Lateral roentgenology of the spine, Amer. J. Roentgen. **4**:101-106, 1917.

1919 Gage, H. C.: La radiographie de lésions suspectés de la colonne vertébrale par la methode latérale, J. Radiol. Electr. **3**:219-221, 1918-1919.

1924 Magnuson, Paul B.: Reasons for lack of positive roentgen findings in many cases of low back pain, Amer. J. Roentgen. **12**:15-23, 1924.

1929 Dittmar, Otto: Die sagittal und lateral flexorische Bewegung der menschlichen Lendenivirbelsaule im Rontgenbild, Ztschr. Ges. Anat. (Abt. I) **92**:644-667, 1929.

Samuel, Max: Ueber Ausbau und Bedeutung einer röntgenologischen Darstellung der Bechengelenke, Röntgenpraxis **1**:944-947, 1929.

1931 Bell, Mary E.: Lateral spine technic, Xray Techn. **2**:91-96, 1931.

Hibbs, R. A., Risser, J. C., and Ferguson, A. B.: Scoliosis treated by the fusion operation; an end result study of 360 cases, J. Bone Joint Surg. **13**:91-104, 1931.

Hubney, M. J.: The oblique projection in examination of the lumbar spine, Radiology **16**:720-724, 1931.

Meyer-Burgdorff, H.: Untersuchungen über das Wirbelgleiten, Leipzig, 1931, Georg Thieme.

1933 Ghormley, Ralph K.: Low back pain with special reference to articular facets with presentation of an operative precedure, J.A.M.A. **101**:1773-1777, 1933.

1935 Files, Glenn: La radiografía de la espina lumbar, Rev. Rad. Fis. **4**:22-37, 1935.

1937 Hodges, Fred J., and Peck, Willis S.: Clinical and roentgenological study of low back pain with sciatic radiation, Amer. J. Roentgen. **37**:461, 1937.

Jordan, H.: Roentgen analysis of the spine, Radiology **28**:714-724, 1937.

Morton, S. A.: Value of the oblique view in radiographic examination of lumbar spine, Radiology **29**:568-573, 1937.

1939 Eller, Virginia H.: Various positions for the x-ray examination of the lumbar spine, Xray Techn. **11**:57-59, 1939.

Elward, J. F.: Motion in the vertebral column, Amer. J. Roentgen. **42**:91-99, 1939.

1940 Horwitz, Thomas, and Smith, Manges R.: An anatomical, pathological and roentgenological study of the intervertebral joints of the lumbar spine and of the sacroiliac joints, Amer. J. Roentgen. **43**:173, 1940.

1941 Doub, H. P., and Camp, John D.: Oblique radiography of the spine, Radiology **37**:232-233, 1941.

Gibson, Mervin: The use of diaphragms in radiography of the lumbar spine, Xray Techn. **12**:128-129, 145, 1941.

1942 Cornwell, William S.: Lumbar vertebrae, Radiogr. Clin. Photogr. **18**:2-11, 30-35, 54-61, 1942.

Cornwell, William S.: Some aspects of radiography of the lumbar vertebrae, Xray Techn. **14**:77-83, 88, 1942.

Duncan, William, and Hoen, Thomas: A new approach to the diagnosis of herniation of the intervertebral disc, Surg. Gynec. Obstet. **75**:257-267, 1942.

Morgan, Forrest E.: Technical considerations in x-raying the lumbar and sacral spine, Xray Techn. **13**:228-230, 245, 1942.

Scott, Wendell G.: Low back pain resulting from arthritis and subluxations of the apophyseal joints and fractures of the articular facets of the lumbar spine, Amer. J. Roentgen. **48**:491-509, 1942.

1943 Gunson, Edward F.: Technique for oblique radiography of the spine, Xray Techn. **14**:188-193, 210, 1943.

Maltson, Segred: Technique for spot radiography, Xray Techn. **14**:233-235, 247, 1943.

Scott, Wendell G.: Dolor en la parte inferior de la espalda debido a artritis y a subluxaciones de las articulaciones apofisarias y fracturas de las facetas articulares de la columna lumbar, Rev. Rad. Fis. **10**:55-72, 1943.

1944 Copleman, Benjamin: The roentgenographic diagnosis of the small central protruded intervertebral disc,

Amer. J. Roentgen. **52**:245-260, 1944.

Gianturco, C.: A roentgen analysis of the motion of the lower lumbar vertebrae in normal individuals and in patients with low back pain, Amer. J. Roentgen. **52**:261-268, 1944.

Knutsson, F.: The instability associated with disk degeneration in the lumbar spine, Acta Radiol. **25**:593-609, 1944.

1945 Slauson, D. B.: A new principle in the roentgenography of the lateral lumbar spine, Radiography **44**:280-282, 1945.

1946 Meschan, Isadore: A radiographic study of spondylolisthesis with special reference to stability determination, Radiology **47**:249-262, 1946.

Slauson, D. B.: A new principle in roentgenography of the lateral lumbar spine, Xray Techn. **17**:383-384, 400, 1946.

1947 Boyland, Kathleen G.: True lateral positioning of lumbar spine and pelvis, Radiography **13**:44, 1947.

Melamed, Abraham, and Ansfield, David J.: Posterior displacement of lumbar vertebrae, Amer. J. Roentgen. **58**:307-328, 1947.

1949 Etter, L. E., and Carabello, N. C.: Roentgen anatomy of oblique views of the lumbar spine, Amer. J. Roentgen **61**:699-705, 1949.

1950 Kovács, A.: X-ray examination of the exit of the lowermost lumbar root, Radiol. Clin. **19**:6-13, 1950.

1951 Kröker, P.: Ueber die Röntgenuntersuchung beim lumbalem Bandscheibenvorfall mit Hilfe der lumboinguinalen Einstellung von Kovács, Fortschr. Roentgenstr. **74**:519, 1951.

1952 Hasner, E., Schalimtzek, M., and Snorrason, E.: Roentgenological examination of the function of the lumbar spine, Acta Radiol. **37**:141-149, 1952.

1953 Lyons, N. J.: Dynamic views of the lumbar spine, Xray Techn. **24**:402-407, 1953.

1961 Stevens, R., and Bauer, D.: Posteroanterior view of the lumbar spine, Xray Techn. **32**:603-608, 1961.

1963 Holohan, F.: Simplified positioning of the scoliotic spine, Xray Techn. **34**:347-351, 1963.

Lumbosacral region

1905 Ludloff, Karl: Verletzungen der Lendenwirbelsäule und des Kreuzbeins, Fortschr. Roentgenstr. **9**:175, 1905.

1920 Marcel, Galland, and de Berck: La radiographie de face de la Ve vertèbre lombaire, Rev. Méd. Française, Oct., 1920.

1921 Garcin, J.: Radiographie de la Ve vertèbre lombaire, J. Radiol. Electr. **5**:410-412, 1921.

1924 LeWald, Leon T.: Lateral roentgenography of the lumbosacral region, Amer. J. Roentgen. **12**:362-367, 1924.

1929 Dittmar, Otto: Halbseitliche Aufnahme des Lendenwirbel-kreuzbeinabschnittes, Fortschr. Roentgenstr. **39**:864-865; 1929; **40**:99-107, 1929.

Galland, Marcel, and Las Casas, H.: La dynamique lombo-sacrée, J. Radiol. Electr. **13**:529-547, 1929.

Samuel, Max: Ueber Ausbau und Bedeutung einer röntgenologischen Darstellung der Beckengelenke, Röntgenpraxis **1**:944-947, 1929.

Warner, F.: Studien zur Pathologie des Lumbosakralgebietes, Verhandl. Deutsch. Ges. Unfallheilkunde, Sept., 1929.

1931 Belden, Webster W.: Fifth lumbar vertebra roentgenologically demonstrated, Radiology **16**:905-932, 1931.

Harttung, Heinrich: Technisches zur Röntgenaufnahme des Lenden-Kreuzbeinwinkels, Zbl. Chir. **58**:453, 1931.

Reisner, A.: Unterscheidungs-merkmale normaler, ertzündlicher und post-traumalischer Zustände an der Wirbelsäule, Fortschr. Roentgenstr. **44**:726-751, 1931.

1932 Barsóny, T., and Schulhoff, O.: Die Aufnahmetechnik zur Sagitallen. Darstullung des lumbo-sakro-iliakalen Gebietes im Röntgenbilde, Röntgenpraxis **4**:594-598, 1932.

Samuel, M.: Technisches zur Röntgenaufnahme des Lenden-Kreuzbeinwinkels, Zbl. Chir. **59**:661, 1932.

1933 Warner, F.: Der 5. Lendenwirbel, Arch. Orthop. Unfall-Chir. **33**:279-306, 1933.

1934 Ferguson, Albert B.: The clinical and roentgenographic interpretation of lumbosacral anomalies, Radiology **22**:548, 1934.

Ghormley, Ralph K., and Kirklin, B. R.: The oblique view for demonstration of the articular facets in lumbosacral backache and sciatic pain, Amer. J. Roentgen. **31**:173-176, 1934.

1935 Williams, Paul C., and Wigby, Palmer E.: Technique for the roentgen examination of the lumbosacral articulation, Amer. J. Roentgen. **33**:511-515, 1935.

1937 Gage, Clement: A new position for the examination of the lumbosacral area, Radiology **28**:495, 1937.

Chamberlain, W. Edward: Low back pain, J. Proc. Calif. Acad. Med., 1937-1938.

1938 Petsing, Harold C.: The fifth lumbar body and lumbosacral junction, Xray Techn. **9**:187-190, 1938.

1939 Geissenberger, Hans: Roentgenography of the lumbar and lumbosacral spine, Xray Techn. **10**:174-176, 196, 1939.

1943 Cornwell, W. S.: The lumbosacral junction, Radiogr. Clin. Photogr. **19**:30-39; 58-69, 1943.

1944 Cornwell, W. S.: The lumbosacral junction, Radiogr. Clin. Photogr. **20**:2-11, 1944.

1945 Wilsey, R. B., Holly, E. W., and Cornwell, W. S.: Special problems in lateral radiography of the lumbar and lumbosacral region, Radiogr. Clin. Photogr. **21**:2-8, 1945.

1946 Bonfilia, Sister Mary: Some aspects of radiography of the lumbosacral region, Xray Techn. **17**:381-382, 1946.

1949 Kovács, Ákos: Vertebral ligaments on native roentgenograms, Acta Radiol. **32**:287-303, 1949.

1953 Holly, E. W., and Weingartner, G.: Oblique lateroposterior radiography of the lumbosacral junction, Med. Radiogr. Photogr. **29**:91-92, 1953.

1961 Sparks, O. J.: Lumbosacral oblique: Improvement by longitudinal deviation, Xray Techn. **33**:93-99, 1961.

Sacroiliac joints

1911 Fischer, Wilhelm: Der letzte Lendenwirbel; eine Röntgenstudie, Fortschr. Roentgenstr. **8**:346-359, 1911-1912.

1923 Allen, H. R.: The iliosacral joint, Indianapolis Med. J. **26**:151-155, 1923.

1924 Darling, B. C.: The sacro-iliac joint; its diagnosis as determined by x-ray, Radiology **3**:486-491, 1924.

1927 Pincherle, Pino: La sacro-ileite, Radiol. Med. **14**:153-167, 1927.

1930 Chamberlain, W. Edward: The symphysis pubis in the roentgen examination of the sacro-iliac joint, Amer. J. Roentgen. **24**:621-625, 1930.

1932 Chamberlain, W. Edward: The x-ray examination of the sacro-iliac joint, Delaware State Med. J. **4**:195-200, 1932.

1934 Ghormley, R. K., and Kirklin, B. R.: The oblique view for demonstration of the articular facets in lumbosacral backache and sciatic pain, Amer. J. Roentgen. **31**:173-176, 1934.

1935 Kovács, Ákos: Die sakroiliale Spaltenaufnahme, Röntgenpraxis **7**:763-768, 1935.

1936 Legròscino, D.: L'anca e la sacro-illiaca in una nuova proiezione radiografica, Boll. Ass. Med. Trieste **27**:82-89, 1936; Röntgenpraxis **8**:433-445, 1936.

Legròscino, D.: Das Hüftgelenk und das Sakroiliakalgelenk in günstiger röntgenographischer Projektion, Röntgenpraxis **8**:433-445, 1936.

1937 Collez, R.: La radiographie de l'articulation sacroiliaque, Bull. Soc. Radiol. Méd. Paris **25**:263, 1937.

Nemcurs-Auguste: À propos de la radiographie de l'articulation sacro-iliaque, Bull. Soc. Radiol. Méd. Paris **25**:181-183, 1937.

Tillier, H., and Coriat, P.: Anatomie radiographie de l'articulation sacro-iliaque dans les incidences de face et de trois quarts, Bull. Soc. Radiol. Méd. Paris **25**:449, 1937.

1940 Ruwett, L. H.: Technic in radiography of the sacro-iliac joint; an evaluation of the symphysis pubis method, Xray Techn. **11**:214-218, 1940.

Horowitz, T., and Smith, M. R.: An anatomical, pathological and roentgenological study of the intervertebral joints of the lumbar spine and of the sacroiliac joints, Amer. J. Roentgen. **43**:173-186, 1940.

1953 Bridgman, C. F., and Cornwell, W. S.: Radiography of the sacroiliac articulation, Med. Radiogr. Photogr. **29**:78-90, 1953.

1957 Kamieth, H.: What do spot films of the sacroiliac joint accomplish? Pathology of the sacroiliac joint, Radiol. Clin. **26**:139-157, 1957.

Sacrum and coccyx

1917 Lilienfeld, Leon: Die seitliche Kreuzbeinaufnahme, München. Med. Wschr. **64**:211-214, 1917.

1930 Nölke, Wilhelm: Axiale Aufnahmen zur Darstellung des Sakralkanalquerschnittes und des Beckens, Röntgenpraxis **2**:742-748, 1930.

1933 Zochert, R. W.: The sacrum and coccyx; location and technic for radiography, Xray Techn. **4**:118-120, 1933.

1935 Hoing, Margaret: A new technic of coccyxography, Xray Techn. **7**:68-72, 89, 1935.

1936 Sabat, Bronislaw: Intrarectal radiography, Fortschr. Roentgenstr. **53**:143-165, 1936. Abst.: Yearbook Radiol., 354, 1936.

1937 Guarini, Carlo: La radiografia del coccige, Arch. Radiol. **13**:228-235, 1937.

1957 Ruttimann, A.: Eine einfache Methode zur Verbesserung der Steissbeinaufnahmen, Fortschr. Roentgenstr. **86**:511-514, 1957.

Vertebral column—entire

1909 Simon, M.: Ueber die Röntgenanatomie der Wirbelsäule, und die Röntgendiagnose von Wirbelverletzungen, Fortschr. Roentgenstr. **14**:353-419, 1909.

1910 Putti, V.: Die angeborenen Deformitäten der Wirbelsäule, Fortschr. Roentgenstr. **15**:65-92, 1910.

1921 Suggars, H. J.: Thesis upon the subject of radiographing the spine and the pelvis, Arch. Radiol. Electr. **26**:382-396, 1921-1922.

1924 George, Arial W., and Leonard, Ralph D.: Fundamental facts relative to the study of the vertebrae in industrial accident cases, Radiology **2**:197-213, 1924.

1926 Kloiber: Fehlerquelle bei Röntgenaufnahmen der Wirbelsäule, Fortschr. Roentgenstr. **35**:451-454, 1926.

1929 George, Arial W., and Leonard, R. D.: The vertebrae roentgenologically considered, Ann. Roentgen. **8**: 1929.

1930 Ferguson, A. B.: The study and treatment of scoliosis, Southern Med. J. **23**:116-120, 1930.

1931 Jaeger, Walter: Ueber Fernaufnahmen der Wirbelsäule, Verhandl. Deutsch. Röntgengesell. **23**:1931; Röntgenpraxis **4**:193-209, 1932.

Meyer-Burgdorff, Hermann: Untersuchungen über das Wirbelgleiten, Leipzig, 1931, Georg Thieme.

Thoma, E.: Die Zwischenwirbellöcher im Röntgenbild, ihre normale und pathologische Anatomie, Ztschr. Orthop. Chir. **55**:55-115, 1931.

1932 Dittmar, Otto: Die Wirbelsäule, Fortschr. Roentgenstr. **43**:1932.

Jaeger, W.: Distant roentgenography of the spinal column, Röntgenpraxis **4**:193-209, 1932. Abst.: Yearbook, 327, 1932.

Schmorl, G.: Die gesunde und die kranke Wirbelsäule im Röntgenbild, Leipzig, 1932, Dr. Werner Klinkhardt.

1933 Jaeger, Walter: Beobachtungen über den Achsenverlauf der Wirbelsäule, Fortschr. Roentgenstr. **47**:299, 1933.

Joyner, T. H.: Radiography of the spine, Xray Techn. **5**:11-14, 1933.

1934 Lange, M.: Die Wirbelgelenke, (supp. 61): Ztschr. Orthop. Chir., 1934.

Lapenna, Marino: La radiologia delle affezioni e delle lesion; traumatiche vertebrale, Atti Congresso Ital. Rad. Med. **11**:1-22, 1934.

1935 Lewis, Raymond W.: Certain aspects of roentgenology of the spine from the orthopedic viewpoint, Amer. J. Roentgen. **33**:491-503, 1935.

Pearson, Gertrude R.: Technic for the use of a small cone in check radiographs of the spine, Radiology **24**:601-606, 1935.

Storck, Hans: Die Röntgenraumbildmessung in der Orthopädie, Fortschr. Roentgenstr. **51**:369-379, 1935.

1936 Fuchs, Arthur W.: Radiography of the spine—a new method, Radiogr. Clin. Photogr. **12**:2-7, 1936.

Hadley, Lee A.: Apophyseal subluxation, J. Bone Joint Surg. **34**:428, 1936.

Perry, Esther C.: Spinal radiography, Xray Techn. **7**:108-109, 1936.

1937 Jordan, H.: Roentgen analysis of the spine, Radiology **28**:714-724, 1937.

Mensor, M. C.: Injuries to the accessory processes of the spinal vertebrae, J. Bone Joint Surg. **35**:381, 1937.

Oppenheimer, A.: Diseases affecting the intervertebral foramina, Radiology **28**:582-592, 1937.

1938 Brocher, J. E. W.: Der Kreutzschmerz in seiner Beziehung zur Wirbelsäule, Fortschr. Roentgenstr. **57**: 1938.

Oppenheimer, Albert: The apophyseal intervertebral articulations roentgenologically considered, Radiology **30**:724-740, 1938.

Palmer, P. E.: Fractures of the spine with injuries to the cord, Southwestern Med. **22**:360, 1938.

1940 Krogdahl, Trygve, and Torgersen, Olav: Die "Unco-Vertebralgelenke" und die "Arthrosis deformans unco-vertebralis," Acta Radiol. **21**:234-235, 1940.

Oppenheimer, Albert: The apophyseal intervertebral joints, Surgery **8**:699-712, 1940.

Stinchfield, F. E.: Fractures of the vertebrae, Surg. Gynec. Obstet. **70**:378, 1940.

1941 McElvenny, Robert T.: Principles underlying treatment of scoliosis, Surg. Gynec. Obstet. **72**:228-236, 1941.

1943 Albu, Zylpha: Synopsis of spine radiography, Xray Techn. **14**:241-242, 1943.

Carey, Eben: Anatomical and physiological considerations prerequisite to diagnosis of back trauma, Radiology **41**:554-559, 1943.

Gianturco, Cesare: Lateral roentgenography of the spine, Amer. J. Roentgen. **50**:695, 1943.

1946 Davis, Arthur G.: Fractures and dislocations of the spine. In Pillmore, G. U., editor: Clinical radiology, Philadelphia, 1946, F. A. Davis Co., vol. 2, pp. 167-168, 171, 173, 182, 185.

1966 Hanafee, W., and Crandall, P.: Trauma of the spine and its contents, Radiol. Clin. N. Amer. **4**:365-382, 1966.

1967 Board, R. F.: Radiography of the scoliotic spine, Radiol. Techn. **38**:219-224, 1967.

INFANTS AND CHILDREN

1912 Benjamin, E., and Goett, T.: Interpretation of chest roentgenogram in the nursling, Deutsch. Arch. Klin. Med. **107**:508-517, 1912.

1915 Waldron, Carl W.: Roentgenology of the accessory nasal sinuses with special reference to sinusitis in children, Interstate Med. J. **22**:1031, 1915.

1921 Blackfan, K. D., and Little, K.: Clinical and radiographic study of thymus in infants, Amer. J. Dis. Child. **22**:459-470, 1921.

Gerstenberger, H. J.: Factor of position of diaphragm in roentgen-ray diagnosis of enlarged thymus, Amer. J. Dis. Child. **21**:534-545, 1921.

Noback, G. I.: A contribution to the topographical anatomy of the thymus glands, Amer. J. Dis. Child. **22**:120, 1921.

1922 Wimberger, Hans: Technische Erfahrungen aus der Kinderröntgenologie, Fortschr. Roentgenstr. **29**:98, 1922.

1923 Evans, W. A.: The value of the roentgen study of mastoid disease in children under five, Amer. J. Roentgen. **10**:382, 1923.

1924 Allen, B.: Nasal accessory sinuses in infants and children, Radiology **3**:136-138, 1924.

Schultz, J.: Die Darstellung der Torsionswinkels vom Femur mit Helfe von Röntgenstrahlen, Ztschr. Orthop. Chir. **44**:325-334, 1924.

1925 Wasson, W. W.: Radiography of the infant chest, Radiology **5**:365-396, 1925.

1926 Carter, Thomas M.: Technique and devices used in radiographic study of wrist bones of children, J. Educ. Psychol. **17**:237-247, 1926.

Noback, G. I.: The thymus in the newborn and early infancy, Radiology **7**:416, 1926.

Wasson, Walter D.: The thymus gland, Arch. Otolaryng. 4:495-511, 1926.

1928 Bonar, B. E.: Thymus in childhood, Northwest Med. 27:178-182, 1928.

1929 Martin, Charles L.: Roentgenologic studies of mastoid in infants, Amer. J. Roentgen. 22:431-439, 1929.

1930 Pancoast, H. K., and Pendergrass, E. P.: Roentgenologic diagnosis of diseases of the upper respiratory tract in children, Amer. J. Roentgen. 23:241-264, 1930.

Stoloff, Gordon: The thymus. In: The chest in children, Ann. Roentgen. 12:345-356, 1930.

1931 Allison, R. G.: Non-opaque foreign bodies in the air passages of infants, Xray Techn. 3:53-55, 1931.

1932 Bowen, David R.: Roentgen examination of the infant thorax, Amer. J. Roentgen. 27:610-615, 1932.

Eley, Cannon R., and Vogt, Edward C.: Encephalography in children, Amer. J. Roentgen. 27:686-696, 1932.

Granger, Amédee: Infant mastoid. In Radiological study of the para-nasal sinuses and mastoid, Philadelphia, 1932, Lea & Febiger, pp. 118-122.

1933 Anderson, Walter S.: The thymus and its radiographic technic, Xray Techn. 4:116-117, 1933.

Freund, Leopold: Ueber die Zurichtung des Kleinkindes für das Röntgenverfahren, Röntgenpraxis 5:112-121, 1933.

Herpel, F. K.: Roentgenologic examination of the nasal accessory sinuses in infants and children, Radiology 20:181-185, 1933.

1934 Pottenger, F. M.: Tuberculosis in the child and in the adult, St. Louis, 1934, The C. V. Mosby Co., pp. 275-291.

Stunz, I. Dorothy: X-ray technic for children, Radiology 22:694-700, 1934.

1935 Hanner, Dorothy D.: Chest radiography in infants and uncooperative children, Xray Techn. 7:62-65, 91, 1935.

1937 Shields, David G.: General roentgenologic technic for infants and children, Xray Techn. 9:10-18, 42, 1937.

1939 Hart, Cecilia: Intravenous pyelography in children, Xray Techn. 10:212-213, 1939.

Loew, Johana: Problems in mastoid radiography of infants, Xray Techn. 11:10-11, 1939.

1940 Batt, Cecilia C.: Technical procedure in the x-ray examination of the mastoids in children, Xray Techn. 11:175-176, 1940.

1941 Wyatt, George M.: Excretory urography for children, Radiology 36:664-671, 1941.

1942 Harvey, Roger Allen: Restraining device and technical factors for chest roentgenography of infants, Amer. J. Roentgen. 47:322-327, 1942.

1943 Shapiro, A. V., and Bell, Leo: Study of the widened mediastinum in children and pitfalls in diagnosis, Amer. J. Roentgen. 49:159-176, 1943.

1944 Alexander, O. M.: Radiographic techniques applicable to infants, Radiography 10:77-80, 1944.

Alexander, O. M.: Radiographic techniques applicable to infants, Radiography 10:81-84, 1944.

1945 Christiansen, Harold: Some practical hints on the performance of urography on infants, Acta Radiol. 26:46-48, 1945.

Freeth, D. H.: Dental radiography of children and some of its problems, Radiography 11:65-69, 1945.

Hrdlicker, Victor E., Watkins, Carlton G., and Robb, John A.: Cholecystography for children, Amer. J. Dis. Child. 70:325, 328, 1945.

1946 Eilert, Genevieve J.: The psychological and technical handling of children in the radiographic department, Xray Techn. 17:396-398, 1946.

Schaper, Marie: Intramuscular urography in children as carried out at the Children's Hospital of Pittsburgh, Xray Techn. 18:71, 1946.

Shields, David G.: Radiography of the mastoid portion of the temporal bone in infants and children, Xray Techn. 17:426-431, 433, 1946.

1947 Fletcher, Catherine: X-ray examination of the thymus of the newborn infant, Xray Techn. 18:172-174, 1947.

1948 Schoen, Cyrus P.: X-ray technique in pediatric cases, Xray Techn. 19:241-243, 1948.

Waldeier Sister Mary Armella: Child psychology in the x-ray room, Xray Techn. 19:191-194, 1948.

1949 Koiransky, H. G., and others: Radiologic study of the mastoid bone in infants in conjunction with anatomic and pathologic investigations, New York J. Med. 49:1291-1292, 1949.

Scatchard, G. N.: Orthopedic x-ray problems in children, New York J. Med. 49:2545-2547, 1949.

1951 Crooks, M. L.: Roentgen examination of the urinary tract in children, Xray Techn. 23:24-26, 1951.

1953 Dunlap, K., and Shands, A. R., Jr.: A new method for determination of torsion of the femur, J. Bone Joint Surg. 35-A:289-311, 1953.

Laage, H., and others: Horizontal lateral roentgenography of the hip in children, J. Bone Joint Surg. 35-A:387-389, 1953.

1954 Billings, Lars: Roentgen examination of the proximal femur end in children and adolescents; standardized technique also suitable for determination of collum-, anteversion-, and epiphyseal angles: study of slipped epiphysis and coxa plana, Acta Radiol. 110 (supp.):1-80, 1954.

Cleaver, H. W.: An apparatus for the measurement of femoral torsion, Xray Techn. 25:7-10, 1954.

Martz, C. D., and Taylor, C. C.: The 45-degree angle roentgenographic study of the pelvis in congenital dislocation of the hip, J. Bone Joint Surg. 36-A:528-532, 1954.

1955 Chumard, E. G.: Early weight-bearing and the correction of anteversion in the treatment of congenital dislocation of the hip, J. Bone Joint Surg. 37-A:229-244, 1955.

Hope, J. W., and Campoy, F.: The use of carbonated beverages in pediatric excretory urography, Radiology 64:66-71, 1955.

1956 Edgren, W., and Laurent, L. E.: A method of measuring the torsion of the femur in congenital dislocation of the hip in children, Acta Radiol. 45:371-376, 1956.

Magilligan, D. J.: Calculation of the angle of anteversion by means of horizontal lateral roentgenography, J. Bone Joint Surg. 38-A:1231-1246, 1956.

1957 Backman, Stig: The proximal end of the femur: investigations with special reference to the etiology of femoral neck fractures: anatomical studies: roentgen projections, Acta Radiol. 146 (supp.):35-42, 1957.

Budin, E., and Chandler, E.: Measurement of femoral neck anteversion, Radiology 69:209-213, 1957.

Hope, J. W., O'Hara, A. E., Tristan, T. A., and Lyon, J. A.: Pediatric radiography, Med. Radiogr. Photogr. 33:25-56, 1957.

Rossmann, B.: Einfache röntgenologische Aufnahmetechnik des Säuglingsohres, Fortschr. Roentgenstr. 86:741-748, 1957.

Wolf, H. G.: The roentgen examination of the gastrointestinal tract in the newborn, with particular reference to examination without the use of an oral contrast medium, Fortschr. Roentgenstr. 86:323-334, 1957. Abst.: Radiology 70:128, 1958.

1958 Andrén, L., and Rosen, S.: The diagnosis of dislocation of the hip in newborns and the primary results of immediate treatment, Acta Radiol. 49:89-95, 1958.

Antoine, M., Pierson, M., Lesure, J., and de Kersauson, M. C.: Le diagnostic radiologique des fractures du crane chez le nourrisson par la technique des incidences tangentielles, J. Radiol. Electr. 39:573-576, 1958.

Fisk, C., and Fry, M. J.: Femoral torsion and the Shands technique, Xray Techn. 29:225, 1958.

Hope, J. W., and O'Hara, A. E.: Use of air as a contrast medium in the diagnosis of intestinal obstruction of the newborn, Radiology 70:349-361, 1958.

1959 Billing L., and Severin, E.: Slipping epiphysis of the hip: a roentgenological and clinical study based on a new roentgen technique, Acta Radiol. 174 (supp.):15-18, 1959.

Darling, D. B.: A simple device for obtaining lateral acetabular views of the hip in infants, Radiology 73:432-433, 1959.

1960 Barrett, A. F., and Verney, G. I.: Tomography and other radiological methods in the management of congenital dislocation of the hip, Brit. J. Radiol. 33:684-690, 1960.

Pius, Sister M.: The pede-ply: restraining device for pediatric radiography, Xray Techn. 31:382-386, 1960.

1961 Andrén, Lars: Aetiology and diagnosis of congenital dislocation of the hip in newborns, Radiology 1:89-94, 1961.

Dunbar, J. S., and others: An automatic device for voiding urethrography in infants and small children, Radiology 76:467-471, 1961.

Green, R. I.: The radiology of speech defects, Radiology 27:331-338, 1961.

Gugliantini, P.: Utilità delle incidenze oblique caudo-craniali nello studio radiologico della stenosi congenita ipertrofica del piloro, Ann. Radiol. Diagn. 34:56-69, 1961.

1962 Altman, W. S., and Morace, V.: Laminagraphy, an aid in accurate localization in congenital hip dysplasia, Radiology 78:19-28, 1962.

Darling, D. B.: Radiography of infants and children, Springfield, Ill., 1962, Charles C Thomas, Publisher.

Hope, J. W., and Koop, C. E.: Abdominal tumors in infants and children, Med. Radiogr. Photogr. 38:2-51, 1962.

Lyons, C. D.: A new device for lateral radiography of the hip in children, Xray Techn. 33:251-255, 1962.

Owsley, W. C.: Palate and pharynx: roentgenographic evaluation in the management of cleft palate and related deformities, Amer. J. Roentgen. 87:811-821, 1962.

Rosen, S.: Diagnosis and treatment of congenital dislocation of the hip joint in the newborn, J. Bone Joint Surg. 44-B:284-291, 1962.

Shurtleff, F. E.: Children's radiographic technic, Philadelphia, 1962, Lea & Febiger.

1963 Anderson, M. L., and Zatz, L. M.: Voiding cystourethrography in children, Radiol. Techn. 35:171-175, 1963.

Brünner, S., and Buchmann, G.: Anesthesiologic problems in pediatric radiology, Amer. J. Roentgen. 89:1075-1079, 1963.

Pinck, R. L., and others: Congenital dislocation of the hip: determination of the anterior-posterior position of the femoral head on the Chassard-Lapiné view, Radiology 80:650-652, 1963.

1964 Franklyn, P. P.: Paediatric radiology, Radiography 30:243-251, 1964.

Kreel, L., and others: Pneumo-mediastinography by the transternal method, Clin. Radiol. 15:219-223, 1964.

1965 O'Hara, A. E., and others: Controlled pulmonary roentgenographic exposures in newborn infants, Amer. J. Roentgen. 95:99-103, 1965.

Tausend, M. E., and Stern, W. Z.: Thymic patterns in the newborn, Amer. J. Roentgen. 95:125-130, 1965.

BEDSIDE RADIOGRAPHY

1933 Bell, Mary E.: Bedside unit technic, Xray Techn. 4:75-79, 1933.

1935 Ottonello, Pietro: Technica radiografica ad ampolla mobile, Ann. Rad. Fis. Med. 9:22-25, 1935.

1937 Moser, Leonie: Schönende Aufnahmetechnik zur seitlichen Darstellung der unteren Hals- und Brustwirbelsäule, Röntgenpraxis 9:488-490, 1937.

1939 Baker, W. E.: Bedside radiography, Radiography 5:89-97, 1939.

1942 Estelle, Sister: Technique for radiographing the mandible at the bedside, Xray Techn. 14:118-120, 133, 1942.

Rigler, Leo G.: X-ray technique in emergency conditions (bedside technique), Xray Techn. 13:183-187, 220, 1942.

OPERATING ROOM RADIOGRAPHY

1931 Beer, Edwin: Roentgenological control of exposed kidneys in operations for nephrolithiasis with the use of special intensifying cassette, J. Urol. 25:159-164, 1931.

Benjamin, E. W.: Notes on the technique of x-ray control in the operating room, J. Urol. 25:165-171, 1931.

1942 Wolcott, Roy E.: Technique for securing lateral roent-

genogram of the femoral neck in the operating room, Xray Techn. 13:155-158, 181, 1942.

1945 Minear, W. L.: Rapid roentgenography in the operating room, J. Bone Joint Surg. 27:157-159, 1945.

Ritchie, David: Radiography in the operating theatre, Radiography 11:73-76, 1945.

1947 Judd, George: Radiography—an auxiliary in surgery, Radiography 13:49-50, 1947.

1948 Olsson, O.: Rubber cassette with intensifying screens designed for roentgen examination of operatively exposed organs, Acta Radiol. 30:91-96, 1948.

1950 Crawford, H. B., Merrill, E. F., and Bridgman, C. F.: Radiography of the hip joint. Part III, Radiographic procedures during hip-joint operations, Med. Radiogr. Photogr. 26:106-117, 1950.

1952 Bridgman, C. F.: Improving radiographic quality during hip-nailing operations, Xray Techn. 23:406-409, 1952.

1954 Young, B. R., and Scanlan, R. L.: New explosion-proof and shock-proof mobile roentgenographic equipment for the operating room, Amer. J. Roentgen. 71:873-877, 1954.

1957 Pyper, J. B.: An aid in the reduction of radiation hazard in the operating theatre, Lancet 2:1204-1205, 1957.

1959 Madsen, E. T.: An adjustable mobile cassette holder for orthopaedic operations, J. Bone Joint Surg. 41-B:774-775, 1959.

Nachlas, I. W., and Feldman, J. R.: X-ray control for operations on the hip, J. Bone Joint Surg. 41-A:1339-1341, 1959.

1962 Voorhis, Charles C.: A cassette holder to be used in pinning hips, Surg. Gynec. Obstet. 115:359-360, 1962.

1964 Leslie, C. G., and Deguire, F.: Helpful hint for operating room radiography, Radiol. Techn. 36:70, 1964.

ANESTHETICS IN X-RAY DEPARTMENTS

1944 Clark, L. H.: Some dangers involved in the use of anesthetics in x-ray departments, Radiography 10:25-27, 1944.

Hadfield, C. F.: The use of anesthetics in x-ray departments, Radiography 10:17-23, 1944.

FOREIGN BODY LOCALIZATION

1904 Poirier de Clisson, Henri: Sur un procéde simple de localisation des projectiles par la radioscopie, Paris, 1904.

1915 Coleschi, Lorenzo: Il più semplice ed il più rapido metodo ed apparecchio per la localizzazione dei corpi estranei mediante i raggi röntgen, Radiol. Med. 2:49-59, 1915.

Grier, G. W.: Roentgen examination of foreign bodies, Amer. J. Roentgen. 2:109-122, 1915.

Weber, André: Localisation des projectiles de guerre au moyen des rayons X, Paris, 1915, Le François,

Weski, Oskar: Die röntgenologische Lagebestimmung von Fremdkörpern; ihre schulgemässe Methodik dargestellt an kriegschirurgischen Material, Stuttgart, 1915, Ferdinand, Enke.

1916 Heyl, Werner: Ueber röntgenologische Lokalisation metallischer Fremdkörper, Berlin, 1916, E. Ebering.

Renard, Leon Paul Ernest: Contribution à l'étude de la localisation anatomique et repérage rigoureux des projectiles par le radio stéréometre Tauleigne-Mazo, Paris, 1916, Ollier-Henry.

1917 Beck, Emil G.: Stereo-clinic: localization of foreign bodies with stereoscopic roentgenograms, and methods of their removal, Troy, 1917, Southworth Co.

Blaine, E. S.: The caliper method of foreign body localization, Amer. J. Roentgen. 4:545-550, 1917.

Cole, Lewis G.: Localization of foreign bodies, Amer. J. Roentgen. 4:455-461, 1917.

Skinner, E. H.: The Sutton method of foreign body localization, Amer. J. Roentgen. 4:350, 1917.

Wilkins, W. A.: The localization of foreign bodies, Amer. J. Roentgen. 4:343, 1917.

1918 Bowen, David Ralph: Localization of foreign bodies, Amer. J. Roentgen. 5:59-76, 1918.

Case, James T.: A brief history of the development of foreign body localization by means of the X-ray, Amer. J. Roentgen. 5:113-124, 1918.

Lilienfeld, Leon: Methodik der Fremdkörperlokalisation, In Holzknecht: Röntgenologie, 1918, pp. 139-341.

1919 Gage, Harold: X-ray observations for foreign bodies and their localization, London, 1919.

1920 Case, James Thomas: Localization and extraction of foreign bodies under x-ray control, Oxford Loose-Leaf Surg. 5:449-488, 1920.

1921 de Abreu, Manoel D.: La localisation et l'extraction des corps étrangers par la double projection, Paris, 1921, Bourse de commerce.

1932 Lewis, Raymond: A roentgenographic study of glass and its visibility as a foreign body, Amer. J. Roentgen. 27:853-857, 1932.

1934 Thompson, Bazil: The localization of foreign bodies with the roentgenoscope, Amer. J. Roentgen. 32:412-413, 1934.

1935 Béclère, Henri: La radiographie sur films cintrés pour la recherche des corps étrangers du genou, Presse Méd. 43:1839-1845, 1935.

Kimble, H. E.: Un método mecano simplificado para la medicon radiografía y la localizacion, Rev. Rad. Fis. 2:20-28, 1935. Taken from Radiology 24:39-46, 1935.

1936 Lea, Paul: Localization of a foreign body with x-ray, Xray Techn. 7:150-152, 1936.

Schmitz, Ewald: Die röntgenologische Festellung von Fremdkörpern, Bonn, 1936, A. Brand.

1937 Ulrich, K.: Zur Splitterlokalisation im Rücken, Röntgenpraxis 9:770-773, 1937.

1938 Reid, E. K., and others: Foreign body localization in military roentgenology, Radiology 31:567-583, 1938.

1939 Brailsford, James F.: Simple radiographic method for the localization of foreign bodies, Brit. J. Radiol. 12:65-75, 1939.

Clark, K. C.: Radiographic depth localization of foreign bodies, Radiography 5:195-211, 1939.

Roberts, R. I.: Visualization of non-metallic foreign bodies, Brit. J. Radiol. 12:680-684, 1939.

1940 Clark, K. C.: Localization of a metallic foreign body in the buttock, Radiography 6:105-106, 1940.

Sayman, Ismet: A new method for localization of foreign bodies, Radiology 35:87-88, 1940.

Watson, W.: Simple triangulation and localization, Radiography 6:107-109, 1940.

1941 Westermark, Nils: A simple method of localizing foreign bodies, Acta Radiol. 22:490-492, 1941.

1942 DeLorimier, Alfred A.: Foreign body localization as provided with the United States army table unit, Am. J. Roentgen. 47:307-313, 1942.

1946 Mannheimer, B.: Visualization of foreign bodies of low radio-opacity, Brit. J. Radiol. 19:469-470, 1946.

Rudisill, Hilljer, Jr.: Foreign bodies other than those in the eye, In Pillmore, G. U., editor: Clinical radiology, Philadelphia, 1946, F. A. Davis Co., vol. 2, pp. 644-677.

1948 Hassel, M. K., and Wilson, E. J.: Foreign body localization—double parallel film method, Xray Techn. 19:227-229, 1948.

ROENTGEN EXPOSURE TECHNIQUES

1896 MacIntyre, John: X-ray demonstration with special reference to the soft tissues, Brit. Med. J. 1:750, 1094, 1896.

1926 Files, Glenn W.: The relation, radiographically, of Kv. P. to time or exposure, Radiology 7:255, 1926.

1927 Bronkhorst, W.: Kontrast und Schärfe im Röntgenbild, Leipzig, 1927, Georg Thieme.

1930 Files, Glenn W.: Soft tissue differentiation, Xray Techn. 1:65-69, 1930.

1931 Bouwers, A.: Ueber die Technik der Momentaufnahmen, Acta Radiol. 12:175-182, 1931.

Laurell, Hugo: Eine Methode, beim Röntgenphotographieren den grösseren Teil der Schädlichen Sekundärstrahlung auszuschalten, Acta Radiol. 12:574-579, 1931.

1932 Bassett, Clara: Soft tissue differentiation, Xray Techn. 4:59-61, 1932.

Hunsberger, Harvey S.: Adaption of techniques to individual cases, Radiology 18:320-323, 1932.

1933 Loughery, Thomas P., and Stecher, Wm. R.: Useful procedures in radiologic practice, Radiology 20:225-230, 1933.

Newman, Herbert: Relation of kilovolts to thickness of part; X-ray technic, Xray Techn. 5:21-26, 1933.

Wey, C., Warren, S. R., and O'Neill, D. B.: Scientific control of radiographic results, Radiology 21:546-555, 1933.

1934 Benassi, Enrico: Realazione sui nuovi mezzi di contrasto in radiologia, Atti XI Congr. Ital. Rad. Med. 11:1934.

Fuchs, Arthur W.: Radiography of the entire body, Radiogr. Clin. Photogr. 10:9-14, 1934.

Kirkin, B. R.: Old principles and new radiography, Xray Techn. 6:56-62, 1934.

1935 Files, Glenn W.: La diferenciación e tejidos blandos, Rev. Rad. Fis. 4:38-49, 1935.

Files, Glenn W.: Maximum tissue differentiation, Xray Techn. 7:17-24, 1935.

1936 Carty, John R.: Soft tissue roentgenography, Amer. J. Roentgen. 35:474-484, 1936.

Carty, John R.: Roentgenographic diagnosis of soft tissue tumors excluding the breast, Amer. J. Roentgen. 36:932-935, 1936.

Franke, Heinrich: Ein röntgen-photographisches Verfahren zur gleichzeitigen Darstellung der Weichteile und Knochenpartien des Profilschädels, Röntgenpraxis 8:43-46, 1936.

Fuchs, Arthur W.: A radiographic view-finder, Radiogr. Clin. Photogr. 12:2-7, 1936.

Gratz, C. M.: Air injections of the fascial spaces; new method of soft tissue roentgenography, Amer. J. Roentgen. 35:750-751, 1936.

Lingeman, L. R.: Infection of soft tissues by gas-producing organisms; early recognition by roentgenogram, New York J. Med. 36:259-263, 1936.

1937 Files, Glenn W.: Non-screen procedure with Potter-Bucky diaphragm, Radiology 29:582-595, 1937.

Zintheo, Clarence J.: The specification of roentgenographic technique, Amer. J. Roentgen. 38:352-361, 1937.

Zintheo, Clarence J.: Transferring of x-ray technic from one laboratory to another, Xray Techn. 9:77-81, 114, 1937.

1938 Bettelheim, Frederick: Concerning roentgenographic details, Amer. J. Roentgen. 40:401-404, 1938.

Carty, John R.: Some important considerations in roentgenographic demonstration of tissues, normal and pathological, having a relatively low differential absorption, Radiology 30:417-419, 1938.

Fuchs, Arthur W.: Higher kilovoltage technic with high-definition screens, Radiogr. Clin. Photogr. 14:2-8, 1938.

Hötterman, Carl: Die Augenlieder im Röntgenbild, Röntgenpraxis 10:377-384, 1938.

1939 Files, Glenn W.: Estudios recientes relativos a la manera de mejorar el detalle radiografico, Rev. Rad. Fis. 6:28-33, 1939.

Files, Glenn W.: Factores que influyen en la nitidez de detalle o definición; efecto del área focal del tubo de rayos X en la nitidez de detalle, Rev. Rad. Fis. 6:284-296, 1939.

1940 Allen, P. E., and Calder, H. W.: Soft tissue radiography, Brit. J. Radiol. 13:422-427, 1940.

Fuchs, Arthur W.: Balance in radiographic image, Xray Techn. 12:81-84, 118, 1940.

Hulpien, Esther: X-ray technic charts, Xray Techn. 11:224-226, 1940.

Melter, C. B.: Technic of soft tissue radiography, Xray Techn 11:229, 1940.

Newey, M.: Soft tissue radiography, Radiography 6:29-40, 1940.

1941 Lingley, J. R., and Elliott, W. J.: Soft tissue roentgenography, In Golden, Ross: Diagnostic roentgenology, New York, 1941, Thos. Nelson & Sons, vol. 2, pp. 1097-1121.

Meloy, G. J.: Roentgenologic examination of the soft tissues Amer. J. Roentgen. 46:189-196, 1941.

1942 Cahoon, John B., Jr.: Uses of opaque plastic filters in radiography of the lateral lumbodorsal spine, lateral cervicodorsal spine, and cases of suspected placenta previa, Xray Techn. 13:242-243, 246, 1942.

Doyle, Margaret: Hundred factors in high-class radiography, Radiology 8:12-16, 1942.

Gould, D. R.: In defence of orthodox radiography; a consideration of the total tissue differentiation, Radiology 8:78-79, 1942.

Jaffke, Ruth C.: Tissue thickness measurements technique, Xray Techn. 13:150-152, 180, 1942.

Lewis, Raymond W.: Roentgenographic soft tissue study in orthopedic hospital, Amer. J. Roentgen. 48:634-642, 1942.

1943 Davis, F. G., and Fagen, Morton: Factores que influyen en la densidad y en el contraste de la radiografía, Rev. Rad. Fis. 10:88-90, 1943.

Mahoney, H. O., and Thomas, J. B.: Factores que influyen en la densidad y en el contraste de la radiografía; la opacidad de los tejidos, Rev. Rad. Fis. 10:37-39, 1943.

1944 Altman, William S.: The advantage of increased filtration, Amer. J. Roentgen. 52:344, 1944.

Brill, Edith: Close-range radiography, Xray Techn. 16:97-100, 1944.

1945 Arendt, Julian: Close range technic in diagnostic roentgenology, Radiology 44:177-180, 1945.

Champness, L. J.: Variations of routine techniques, Radiography 11:17-20, 1945.

Dawdy, Edith B.: Consideration of distance as a technical factor, Xray Techn. 16:131-133, 1945.

Henderson, Ethel: Helpful aids in chest work, Xray Techn. 16:196-198, 1945.

Holly, E. W.: Balsawood accessory for chest radiography, Radiogr. Clin. Photogr. 21:38-39, 1945.

1946 Alexander, Sidney: A simple method of radiography of chests which presents marked variations in density, Xray Techn. 18:57-61, 1946.

Carty, John Russell: Soft tissue radiography 2:619-632. In Pillmore, G. U., editor: Clinical radiology, Philadelphia, 1946, F. A. Davis Co., vol. 2, pp. 619-632.

1947 Alexander, Sidney: A simple method for roentgenography of the chest presenting marked variations in density, Amer. J. Roentgen. 57:532-535, 1947.

Avery, Gail: Changing extremity technique to compensate for aluminum filter, Xray Techn. 19:24-27, 37, 1947.

Bannen, J. E.: Radiographic technique and its relationship to pathology and injury, Radiography 13:28-31, 1947.

Guyant, Maude: Roentgenograms of surgical and post mortem specimens, Xray Techn. 18:164-165, 1947.

Hulbert, M. H. E.: Radiography as an aid to dose control in the radium treatment of the cervix, J. Obstet. Gynec. Brit. Emp. 54:137, 1947.

Lingley, James R., and Elliott, William J.: Soft tissue roentgenography. In Golden, Ross, editor: Diagnostic roentgenology, ed. 3, New York, 1947, Thos. Nelson & Sons, vol. 2, pp. 1097-1121.

Piatrowski, Brother Dominic: Double tilt technique, Xray Techn. 18:286-288, 1947.

Torp, Inex M.: Problems of mass chest x-ray in industry, Xray Techn. 18:216-219, 1947.

1948 Alexander, Sidney: Fundamentals of soft tissue radiography, Xray Techn. 19:174-179, 205, 1948.

Terzo, Charles: Long scale radiography, Roentgenography, pp. 17, 21, 1948.

1951 Pearson, G. R.: Radiographic projection studies, Xray Techn. 23:1-9, 1951.

Updegrave, W. J.: Higher fidelity in intraoral roentgenography, J. Amer. Dent. Ass. 62:1-8, 1951.

1952 Gilardoni, A., and Schwarz, G. S.: Magnification of radiographic images in clinical roentgenology and its present day limit, Radiology 59:866-878, 1952.

1954 Lofstrom, J. E., and Warren, C. R.: Magnification techniques in radiography: their practical value, Xray Techn. 26:161-165, 1954.

1958 Fuchs, Arthur W.: Principles of radiographic exposure and processing, ed. 2, Springfield, Ill., 1958, Charles C Thomas, Publisher.

1961 Cahoon, J. B., Jr.: Radiographic technique: its origin, concept, practical application and evaluation of radiation dosage, Xray Techn. 32:354-364, 1961.

Mahoney, G. J., and Rule, I.: The design of optical

density filters for long film radiography of the lower extremities, Xray Techn. 33:103-105, 1961.

1962 Isard, H. J., Ostrum, B. J., and Cullinan, J. E.: Magnification roentgenography, Med. Radiogr. Photogr. 38:92-109, 1962.

Morgan, J. A.: The art and science of medical radiography, St. Louis, 1962, Catholic Hospital Association.

1963 Agnesia, Sister Mary: A wide-angle rib technique, Xray Techn. 34:289-290, 1963.

Berlin, H. S., and others: Wide-angle roentgenography, Amer. J. Roentgen. 90:189-197, 1963.

1964 Horenstein, R., and others: The subtraction method, Acta Radiol. Diagn. 2:264-272, 1964.

1965 Cahoon, John B., Jr.: Formulating x-ray technics, ed. 6, Durham, N. C., 1965, Duke University Press.

Chynn, Kuo-York: Simplified subtraction technique, Amer. J. Roentgen. 95:970-975, 1965.

1966 Greissberger, H.: Wedge-shaped filters for improved radiography of the thoracic vertebrae and the foot, Med. Radiogr. Photogr. 42:6-8, 1966.

STEREOSCOPY

1930 Wilsey, R. B.: Identification of right and left eye radiographs of a stereoscopic pair, Radiogr. Clin. Photogr. 6:2-5, 1930.

1932 Kelly, James F.: Stereoscopy, Xray Techn. 3:93-98, 133-139, 1932.

Sweany, Henry C., and Martinson, William: A note on the principles of stereoroentgenography, Xray Techn. 3:140-144, 1932.

Wilsey, R. B., and Fuchs, Arthur W.: Stereoradiography, Radiogr. Clin. Photogr. 8:2-8, 1932.

Wilsey, R. B.: Stereoradiography and distortion, Radiogr. Clin. Photogr. 8:2-5, 1932.

1933 Jarre, H. A., and Teschendorf, O. E. W.: Roentgenstereoscopy, Radiology 21:139-155, 1933.

Wilsey, R. B.: Stereoradiography, Xray Techn. 5:4-9, 1933.

1934 Gianturco, Cesare: Un metodo di radiografia stereoscopica con l'uso di una sola film; l'applicazione in radioscopia stereoscopica, Ann. Rad. Fis. Med. 8:311-313, 1934.

USEFUL MOVEMENT IN RADIOGRAPHY

1929 Ottonello, Pietro: Nuevo método para la radiografía de la columna cervical completa en proyección sagital ventro-dorsal, Anal. Radiol. (Havana) 1:57-58, 1929.

1937 Barsóny, T., and Winkler, K.: Die "elective" Profilaufnahme der Brustwirbelsäule, Röntgenpraxis 9:9, 1937.

Jönsson, Gunnar: Method of obtaining structural pictures of the sternum, Acta Radiol. 18:336-340, 1937.

1938 Barsóny, T., and Winkler, K.: Beiträge zur Röntgenologie der Wirbelsäule; "Gasfreie" Aufnahmen durch Atmung, Röntgenpraxis 10:384-390, 1938.

Weiser, Martin: "Tomographie" ohne Tomographen, Röntgenpraxis 10:28, 1938.

1939 Bloom, Arthur R.: A new technic of taking roentgenographs of the upper ribs, Radiology 33:648-649, 1939.

1942 Holly, Elmer W.: Some radiographic technics in which movement is utilized, Radiogr. Clin. Photogr. 18:78-83, 1942.

CONTRAST MEDIA

1897 Williams, Francis H.: A study of the adaptation of the x-rays to medicine, Reports of the Boston City Hospital, Jan., 1897.

1898 Cannon, W. B.: Movements of the stomach studied by means of the roentgen ray, Amer. J. Physiol. 1:359-382, 1898.

1910 Bachem, C., and Günther, H.: Bariumsulfat als schattenbildendes Kontrastmittel bei Röntgenuntersuchungen, Ztschr. Röntgenk. Radiumforsch. 12:369, 1910.

1918 Cameron, Donald F.: Sodium and potassium iodides in roentgenography, J.A.M.A. 70:1516, 1918.

Dandy, Walter E.: Ventriculography following the injection of air into the cerebral ventricles, Ann. Surg. 68:5-11, 1918.

Weld, E. H.: The use of sodium bromide in radiography, J.A.M.A. 71:1111-1112, 1918.

1919 Dandy, Walter E.: Roentgenography of the brain after the injection of air into the spinal canal, Ann. Surg. 70:397-403, 1919.

1920 Schanz, Robert T.: Iodid and bromid pastes as used in roentgenography, J.A.M.A. 74:316, 1920.

1922 Sicard, J. A., and Forestier, J.: Méthode générale d'exploration radiologique par l'huile iodée (Lipiodol), Bull. Soc. Méd. Hôp. Paris 46:463-469, 1922.

1923 Rowntree, L. G., Sutherland, C. G., Osborne, E. D., and Scholl, A. J., Jr.: Roentgenography of the urinary tract during excretion of sodium iodid, J.A.M.A. 80:368-373, 1923.

1924 Graham, E. A., and Cole, W. H.: Roentgenologic examination of gall bladder, new method utilizing intravenous injection of tetrabromphenolphthalein, Ann. Surg. 80:473-477, 1924.

1925 Graham, E. A., Cole, W. H., and Copher, G. H.: Cholecystography: the use of sodium tetraiodophenolphthalein, J.A.M.A. 84:1175-1177, 1925.

1926 Sicard, J. A., and Forestier, J. E.: Radiological exploration with iodized oil, Brit. J. Radiol. 31:239, 1926.

1927 Levyn, L., and Aaron, H. H.: Cholecytography by oral administration of sodium tetraiodophenolphthalein, Amer. J. Roentgen. 18:557-559, 1927.

1928 Levyn, L., and Aaron, H. H.: Simplified method of oral cholecystography, New York J. Med. 28:264, 1928.
    Odin, and Rundstrom: Iodized oils, Acta Radiol. 7(supp.): 1928.

1929 Radt, Paul: Eine Methode zur röntgenologischen Kontrastdarstellung vom Milz und Leber, Klin. Wschr. 8:2128, 1929.
    Roseno, A., and Jephins, H.: Intravenous pyelography, Fortschr. Roentgenstr. 39:859-863, 1929. Abst.: Amer. J. Roentgen. 22:685-686, 1929.
    Swick, M.: Darstellung der Niere und Harnwege im Röntgenbild durch intravenose Einbringung eines neuen Kontraststoffes, des Uroselectans, Klin. Wschr. 8:2087-2089, 1929. Abst.: Amer. J. Roentgen. 23:686-687, 1930.

1930 Swick, M.: Intravenous urography by means of the sodium salt 5-iodo-2-pyradon-N-acetic acid, J.A.M.A. 95:1403, 1930.

1933 Swick, M.: Excretion urography with particular reference to newly developed compound: sodium orthoiodohippurate, J.A.M.A. 101:1843, 1933.

1934 Egas Moniz, A. C.: L'angiographie cérébrale: Ses applications et résultats en anatomie, physiologie et clinique, Paris, 1934, Masson & Cie.

1938 Green, Alfred B.: The chemistry of contrast media used in radiography, Xray Techn. 9:231-237, 1938.
    Robb, G. P., and Steinberg, I.: Practical method of visualization of chambers of the heart, the pulmonary circulation, and the great blood vessels in man, J. Clin. Invest. 17:507, 1938.

1939 Robb, G. P., and Steinberg, I.: Visualization of the chambers of the heart, the pulmonary circulation, and the great blood vessels in man, Amer. J. Roentgen. 41:1-18, 1939.

1940 Alexander, O. M.: The use of differential media in radiography, Radiography 6:121-138, 1940.
    Dohrn, Max, and Diedrich, P.: Ein neues Röntgenkontrastmittel der Gallenblase, Deutsch. Med. Wschr. 66:1133-1134, 1940.
    Lauer-Schmaltz, W.: Erfahrungen über perorale Cholezystographie mit dem neuen Kontrastmittel Biliselectan, München. Med. Wschr. 87:1139, 1940.

1941 Anderson, H. T.: The use of iodized oil in roentgenography, Amer. J. Roentgen 46:362, 1941.
    Rating, B.: Ueber ein neues Kontrastmittel zur Röntgendarstellung der Gallenblase (Biliselectan), Fortschr. Roentgenstr. 63:99-110, 1941.

1942 Modell, W.: Pharmacology of beta (3, 5 di-iodo-4-hydroxy phenyl) alpha phenyl propionic acid, J. Lab. Clin. Med. 27:1376-1384, 1942.

1943 Einsel, I. H., and Einsel, T. H.: Gall bladder visualization with beta (3, 5 di-iodo-4-hydroxy-phenyl) alpha-phenyl-propionic acid (Priodax), Amer. J. Dig. Dis. 10:206-208, 1943.
    Marshall, William A.: Some observations on Priodax, Amer. J. Roentgen. 50:680-682, 1943.
    Wasch, M. G.: A new medium for gall bladder visualization, Amer. J. Roentgen. 50:677-679, 1943.

1944 Hefke, H. W.: Cholecystography with Priodax: a report on 600 examinations, Radiology 42:233, 1944.
    Ochsner, H. C.: A new cholecystographic preparation, Amer. J. Roentgen. 51:326-327, 1944.
    Ramsay, G. H., French, J. D., and Strain, W. H.: Iodinated organic compounds as contrast media for radiographic diagnoses. IV. Pantopaque myelography, Radiology 43:236-240, 1944.
    Ramsay, G. H., and Strain, W. H.: Pantopaque: a new contrast medium for myelography, Radiogr. Clin. Photogr. 20:25-33, 1944.

1945 Rigler, Leo G.: The development of roentgen diagnosis, Radiology 45:467-502, 1945.

1946 Epstein, B. S., Natelson, S., and Kramer, B.: A new series of radiopaque compounds, Amer. J. Roentgen. 56:201-207, 1946.

1947 Unfug, George A.: A comparative clinical investigation of cholecystographic preparations, Radiology 46:489-495, 1947.

1952 Eubank, M. C.: Properties and uses of contrast media, Xray Techn. 23:255-264, 1952.

1953 Okel, E.: Opaque media, Xray Techn. 24:337-350, 1953.

1958 Garinkel, B., and Furst, N. J.: Simultaneous roentgen examination of the urinary and biliary tracts with Duografin, Radiology 70:243-245, 1958.

1962 Sanen, F. J.: Considerations of cholecystographic contrast media, Amer. J. Roentgen. 88:797-802, 1962.

1964 Pattinson, J. N.: Iodine compounds in the alimentary tract, Radiography 30:103-109, 1964.
    Strain, W. H., Rogoff, S. M., Greenlaw, R. H., Johnston, R. M., Huegin, F., and Berliner, W. P.: Radiologic diagnostic agents: a compilation, Med. Radiogr. Photogr. 40(supp.):1-110, 1964.

1966 Sheradi, William H.: Clinical problems and toxicity of contrast agents, Amer. J. Roentgen. 97:762-771, 1966.

Index

A

Abdomen
  anatomy
    Addison's planes, 541
    habitus, 542, 543
    surface markings, 541
  body positions and specialized procedures, 590-593
  examination before urinary system radiography, 695
  radiography
    air studies, exposure decrease for, 593
    anteroposterior projection, 588
    artificial pneumoperitoneum, 592
    exposure technique, 587
    fistulae and sinuses, 591
    fluid level (positions for), 590
    free air (positions for), 590
    immobilization, 587
    lateral projection, 589
    pneumoradiography, 592-593
    preparation, 586
  scout film, cholegraphy, 601
Abel, Martin S., 228
Abo, Stanley, 570
Acetabulum; see also Hip
  anatomy, 176, 177, 179
  radiography
    posterior oblique (Teufel), 200
    superoinferior (Dunlap, Swanson, and Penner), 201
Acromioclavicular articulation
  anatomy, 120
  radiography
    anteroposterior and lateral projections (Alexander), 137
    bilateral frontal projection (Pearson), 136
Adamson, D. L., 753
Addison, Christopher, 541
Adenoids
  anatomy, 528
  hypertrophy, examination, 530
Adrenal glands
  anatomy, 678
  retroperitoneal pneumoradiography, 696-697
Air enema, administration, 668
Akerlund, A., 611
Albers-Schönberg positions
  atlas and axis, 220
  temporomandibular joints, 483
Albrecht, L. F., 186
Alexander, J. H., 785
Alexander, O. M., positions for acromioclavicular articulations, 137
Alexander, S., position for optic foramen, 357
Alimentary canal
  anatomy, 578, 579-581
  exposure time for radiography, 631

Alimentary canal—cont'd
  radiation protection, 631
  radiologic apparatus, 629
  radiologic examinations, 626
Altman, W. S., 666
Altschul, Walter, 337, 483
Alveolar process, radiography, 459, 460
Amphiarthrosis, 24
Anatomic
  position, 23
  projections and depressions, 25
Anatomy
  general, 20-24
  specific; see under regional headings
  terms, 25
Andrén, L., 116
Angiocardiography, 834-835
Angiography
  cerebral
    anterior circulation projections, 814-817
    chart, 805
    circulation time, 810
    definition and use, 806
    equipment and preparation, 811
    injection sites, 808-809
    positions, 812, 813
    posterior circulation projections, 818-819
    radiation protection, 812
  contrast media, 832
  equipment, 832-833
  purpose, 831
  team, 833
  terminology, 830
  visceral and peripheral, 830-838
Ankle
  anatomy, 62
  radiography, 88-91
    anteroposterior, 88
    lateral, 89
    lateromedial, 89
    mediolateral, 89
    oblique, 90
    stress studies, anteroposterior, 91
Anterior pelvic bones; see Pelvic bones
Antra
  anatomy, 421
  radiography
    Granger 23-degree position, 436
    Granger 107-degree position, 437
    posteroanterior, 430-431
Antral floor, relationship of teeth to, inferosuperior oblique projection (Law), 433
Aortography, 594, 830, 836, 837
Apex, pulmonary; see Pulmonary apices

Apophysial joints, positions for
  cervical, 211
  lumbar, 215
  lumbar-lumbosacral, 254-256
  thoracic, 213
Arcelin position, petrous portion, 404
Arm, anatomy, 31
Arteries of brain, anatomy, 806-807
Arteriography
  definition, 830
  peripheral, 838
  visceral, 836-837
Arthrography, contrast, 114
  of knee
    horizontal ray method, 116, 117
    vertical ray method, 115
Aseptic technique, 6
Atlas
  anatomy, 210
  and axis
    anteroposterior projection (open-mouth), 220
    lateral projection, 225
  and odontoid process
    posteroanterior (Judd), 223
    semiaxial projection (Jackson), 222
Attic-aditus-antral areas
  anatomy, 322
  radiography, 400-402, 406, 407
Auditory ossicles
  anatomy, 323
  radiography, 400-402
Axilla, lymphography, 844
Axis
  anatomy, 211
  and atlas
    anteroposterior projection (open-mouth), 220
    lateral projection, 225

B

Badgley, C. E., 72, 187
Baker, D. H., 690
Bakes, F. P., 530
Ball, Robert P.
  pelvimetry method, 762-765
  posture of ankle for anteroposterior projection, 88
Barium enema apparatus, disposable, 670-671
  standard, 659
Barium sulfate
  as contrast medium, 626
  inspissation in colon, 627
  for large intestine examination, 656
  mixture for gastrointestinal series, 635
  preparations for esophageal examination, 632
  for small intestine examination, 652
  suspension, preparation, 660
Barnes, A. C., 715
Barsony, T., 232, 558
Beam, x-ray, delimitation of, 13
Bean, Bert C., intracerebral circulation chart, 805
Beath, T., 81
Béclère position, intercondyloid fossa, 100
Benassi positions
  liver, 596
  spleen, 597
Berdon, W. E., 690
Berens, D. L., 125
Berkebile, R. D., 186
Berlin, H. S., 172
Bertel position, inferior orbital fissure, 361
Bertelson, T. I., 364
Bibliography
  Volume I, 289-309
  Volume II, 513-526
  Volume III, 845-878
Bicipital groove
  anatomy, 123
  position for, 130

Bile ducts
  anatomy, 584
  extrahepatic, oblique projection, 616
Biliary tract
  anatomy, 584
  cholangiography
    operative, 618-619
    percutaneous transhepatic, 617
    postoperative, 620-621
  cholegraphy, 598-611; *see also* Cholegraphy
Billing, L., 665
Biologic effects of ionizing radiation, 14-15
Blackett, Charles W., 126
Blackett-Healy positions
  subscapularis insertion, 127
  teres minor insertion, 126
Bladder, urinary; *see* Urinary bladder
Blood circulation, 823-827
Blood vessels of brain, 806-807
Blood-vascular system, anatomy, 823-827
Bloom, Arthur R. (rib technique), 167
Bodily habitus, 542-543
Body
  cavities, 540-543
  planes, 23
  positions, 25
    in rib examinations, 165
    in skull radiography, 330-331
Bolus injection nephrotomography, 685, 698-699
Bone, long; *see* Long bone
Bones, 20, 21
  of cranium and face, anatomy, 312-326
  of lower extremities, anatomy, 60-63
Bony thorax, anatomy and positioning, 151-173
Boreau, J., 720, 721
Boylston, B. F., cervical vertebrae, functional studies, oblique
    position, 233
Braasch, W. P., 705
Brailsford, J. F., 658, 660
Brain
  anatomy, 774-777
  blood vessels of, anatomy, 806-807
  radiography
    angiography, 805-819
    pneumoencephalography, 786-794
    pneumography, 778-785
    pneumoventriculography, 790-794
Breast
  anatomy, 724
  radiography; *see* Mammography
  tissue variations, 725
Breathing instructions, radiography of thoracic viscera, 552
Bridenbaugh, R. B., 594
Bridgman, C. F., 44
Broden positions, subtalar joint, 84, 85
Broderick, T. F., 188
Bronchi, primary, anatomy, 546, 547
Bronchography, 572-575
Buetti, C., 218
Bullitt position
  mastoid, lateral, 386-387
  temporomandibular joints, lateral, 387
Burman, M., 39, 41
Bursae, anatomy, 24, 123
Buzaid, L. L., 801

C

Cahoon, John B., 753, 756
Cahoon, John B., Jr., 11
Cahoon position, temporal styloid process, 411
Calatroni, C. J., 715
Calcaneus (os calcis)
  anatomy, 61
  "coalition view," 81
  dorsoplantar projection, 81
  lateral projection, 75
  plantodorsal projection, 80

Caldwell, C. W., Jr., femoral neck, anteroposterior and inferosuperior projection, 194, 195
Caldwell, Eugene W., position for paranasal sinuses, 426-427
Caldwell-Moloy method of pelvioradiography, 768-771
Cameron, M. F., 753
Camp, J. D., 12
  epiphyseal chart, 21
Camp-Coventry position for intercondyloid fossa, 98, 99
Camp-Gianturco position for optic foramen, 356
Campoy, F., 690
Cardona, G., 116
Carelli, H. H., 696
Carpal
  boss, position for, 33
  bridge, position for, 46
  canal, position for, 45
Carpometacarpal joint, first, radiography, 39
Carter, F. R., 617
Casey, W. C., 699
Casualty patients, radiography of ribs, 165
Cathartics in preparation for diagnostic enema, 658
Causton position, sesamoids, 69
Central nervous system
  anatomy, 774-777
  radiography, 778-819
Central ray, direction of, 12
Cephalometry
  Ball method, 762-765
  purpose, 752
Cerebral
  angiography, 805-819
  pneumography, 778-785
  ventricles
    anatomy, 776, 777
    radiography, 778-794
Cervical
  diskography, 802
  intervertebral foramina; see Intervertebral foramina
  vertebrae; see under Vertebrae
Cervicothoracic region
  lateral projections
    Pawlow, 238
    Twining, 239
  spinous processes, 231
Chamberlain, W. Edward, 260, 579
  measurement of differences of leg length, 112, 113
  positions for sacroiliac joints, 260-261
Chassard-Lapiné position
  pelvimetry, 772
  pelvis and hip joints, 188
  rectosigmoid, 667
Chaussé positions
  jugular foramina, 416
  petrous portions, 405, 406, 407
Chest; see Thoracic viscera
Child, C. G., portal venography, 594
Cholangiography, 598, 604
  operative (or immediate), 618-619
  percutaneous transhepatic, 617
  postoperative, 620-621
Cholecystocholangiography, simultaneous, and urography, 624
Cholecystography, 598, 604
Choledochography, 619
Cholegraphy
  abdomen, scout film, 601
  fatty meal, 603
  instructions to patient, 600
  intestinal tract preparation, 602
  intravenous, 606-611
  media, 598, 599
  oral, 604-605, 608-611
  preliminary diet, 602
  purpose and route, 598
  simultaneous, and urography, 624-625
  untoward side reactions to iodinated media, 600
Cieszynski, Anton, Law of Isometry, 497
Cilley, Earl I. L. (epiphyseal chart), 21
Cimmino, C. V., 667

Circulation
  blood, 825-827
  intracerebral, chart, 805
Circulatory system, anatomy, 823-827
Cisternal puncture in myelography, 799
Clavicle
  anatomy, 120
  radiography
    axial projections, 139-142
    posteroanterior projection, 138
    Quesada method, right angle projections, 143
Cleaves position
  femoral neck, inferosuperior ("frog" position), 184-185
  shoulder (rolled-film axial projection), 131
Cleft palate studies, position for, 530
Clemett, A. R., 623
Clinical history needed by technologist, 5
Clinoids
  anatomy, 317
  anterior, radiography, 349, 350, 358
    eccentric-angle parieto-orbital (Lysholm), 358
  posterior, radiography, 347, 348, 349, 350
Cloward, R. B., 801
Clubfoot, positions for
  dorsoplantar (Kite), 78, 79
  lateral (Marique), 79
  suroplantar (Kandel), 79
Coalition, tarsal, position for, calcaneotalar, 81
Coccyx
  anatomy, 217
  radiography
    frontal projection, 262
    lateral projection, 263
Coe, Fred O., 750
  cephalopelvimetry, posturing exact lateral, 760
Colcher-Sussman method of pelvimetry, 766-767
Cole, W. H., 598
Colon; see also Intestine, large
  insufflated, radiography, 669
  opacified radiography, 664-667
Colonna position, hip injury, view of acetabulum, 199
Colostomy
  diagnostic enema studies via, 672-675
Comberg, W., localization of foreign bodies within orbit or eye, 365, 373-375
Compere, W. E., 402
Composite projection, foot, 77
Conchae, nasal, anatomy, 325
Contrast
  arthrography, 114-117
  infusion method, retrograde cystography, 712-713
  injection method
    female cystourethrography, 714
    retrograde cystography, 710-711
  instillation in bronchography, methods, 574-575
  media, 626-628
    in angiography, 832
    for female genital examinations, 742
    for large intestine examination, 656-657
    in lymphography, 839
    for myelography, 796
    in retrograde urography, lower urinary tracts, 708
    in urography, 688-689
Converse, J. M., 351
Cooper, F. W., Jr., 673
Copher, G. H., 598
Coracoid process
  anatomy, 121
  inferosuperior projection, 128
Corbin technique, wide-angle frontal projection of ribs, 172
Cornea, anatomy, 362
Costal joints
  anatomy of, 164, 212, 213
  radiography, 173
Coventry, M. B., 81, 98
Cranial base, radiography
  axiolateral (Lysholm), 343
  full basal (submentovertical) projection (Schüller), 340-342

Cranial bones, anatomy
  ethmoid, 315
  frontal, 314
  occipital, 318
  parietals, 316
  sphenoid, 317
  temporals, 320-321
Cranium
  anatomy, 312-323, 328, 329
  localization points and planes, 327
  radiography
    anteroposterior (Grashey), 336-338
    lateral, 332-333
    nuchofrontal (Haas), 339
    occiptofrontal (Valdini), 344-345
    posteroanterior, 334-335
Cross, F. S., 674
Cross, K. Stuart, paranasal sinuses, erect position, 423
Cross, L. C., middle ear projection variations, 402
Curcio, Barbara M., 725
Cushing, Harvey, 391
Cystography
  procedures, 686
  retrograde
    contrast infusion method, 712-713
    contrast injection method, 710-711
Cystourethrography
  female
    contrast injection method, 714
    metallic bead chain method, 715
  male, 716

D

Dacryocystography, 376, 377
Dandy, Walter E., 778, 795
Danelius-Miller modification of Lorenz position, femoral
    neck, 190-191
Dann, D. S., 750
Daub, H. P., 715
Davis, Dorothy W., 222
Davis, L. A., 78
de Abreu, J., tomographic studies of ear, 393
de Abreu, M., orbital emphysema, 364
Dean, A. L., Jr., 712
Decubitus
  position, chest, 570, 571
  radiographic projections, 25
Deglutition, studies during, 531, 532, 533
de Lambert, R. M., 569
Delano, P. J., 753
Delimitation of x-ray beam, 13
de Moor, J., 554
Dental
  arch
    anatomy, 494; *see also* Teeth
    radiography, 458, 461
  equipment, 498
  radiography, 496-511
    aseptic technique, 501
    periapical projections, 500-509
Depressions, anatomic, 25
De Santis, V., 753
Diagnosis and technologist, 5
Diaphragm
  anatomy, 165
  respiratory excursion, 165
Diaphragmatic hernias, anteroposterior projections, 646-647
Diarthrosis, 24
Digestive system
  anatomy, 578-585
  radiography, 586-587
Disinfectant solutions, 7
Diskography
  cervical, 802
  lumbar, 803-804
  terminology and use, 801
Doehner, G. A., 594
Donaldson, S. W., 187

Dooley, E. A., femoral neck, anteroposterior and inferosu-
    perior projections, 194, 195
Dorland, P., 228
Dorsum sellae
  anatomy, 317
  radiography, 347, 348, 349, 350
Dose, radiation, 15
Doub, H. P., 72
Doubilet, H., 623
Double-contrast arthrography of knee, 116, 117
Dreyfuss, J. R., 670
Dubilier, W., Jr., 364, 698
Ductus deferens, anatomy, 719
Duncan, William, intervertebral disks, position for, 257
Dunlap, Swanson, and Penner position, acetabula, superio-
    inferior projections, 201
Duodenum
  anatomy, 580
  radiography
    anteroposterior, 646-647
    gastrointestinal series, 637
    lateral, 645
    oblique, 644
    posteroanterior, 642-643
Dye substance, in lymphography, 839

E

Ear
  anatomy, 322-323
  radiography, occipitofrontal (Valdini), 344-345
  tomographic studies, 393
Egan, R. L., 727
Egas Moniz, A. C., 806, 810
Egbert, E. W., 88
Eiselberg, A., 556
Ejaculatory duct, anatomy, 719
Elbow
  anatomy; *see* Upper extremity
  radiography
    anteroposterior, 48
    anteroposterior, partial flexion, 50
    frontal, acute flexion, 51
    lateral, 49
    oblique, 48
    Pierquin position, axial view, olecranon, 54, 55
    radial head, axial view, 53
    radial head, lateromedial rotation, 52
    Schmitt method, 52
    Viehweger position, axial, medial epicondyle, 54, 55
Electrokymography, 554
Elkin, M., 667, 704, 705
Elstrom, E. R., 362
Emmett, J. L., 705
Enema
  air, administration, 668
  apparatus, barium, description and cleansing method, 659
  cleansing, 8, 658
  diagnostic, 656-663
  opaque, administration, 662-663
  studies via colostomies, 672-675
Enterostomy, 672
Epididymis, anatomy, 718
Epididymography, 720
Epiphyseal chart, 21
Epps, R. G., 569
Epstein, B. S., 537, 632
Equipment
  in angiography, 832-833
  for dental radiography, 498
  for gravid uterus examination, 752
  for urinary system procedures, 693
Eraso, S. T., position, jugular foramina, 414
Ernst, R., 554
Esophagus
  anatomy, 550
  examination procedure, 626
  exposure time, 631
  radiography, 632, 633

Ethics in roentgenography, 5
Ethmoid bone, anatomy, 315
Ethmoid sinuses
    anatomy, 420
    radiography
        (anterior) Granger 23-degree position, 436
        (anterior) posteroanterior (Caldwell), 426-427
        oblique (Rhese), 432
        (posterior) Granger 107-degree position, 437
        posteroanterior, 430-431
Etter, L. E., middle ear projection variations, 402
Ettinger, Alice, 611, 667
Evans, J. A., 364
    nephrotomography, 698, 699
    percutaneous transhepatic cholangiography, 617
    splenoportal venography, 594
Examination
    initial, 5
    procedure
        gastrointestinal tract, 636-637
        mammography, 728-729
Examining room
    preparation
        for alimentary tract examination, 629-630
        for bronchography, 573
        in cerebral angiography, 811
        for cerebral pneumography, 781
        for myelography, 796
        for pelvic pneumography, 746
    radiographic, care of, 6
Excretory urography, 686, 687, 689, 701
Exposure technique
    adaptation of, 11
    cerebral pneumography, 781
    dental radiography, 498
    foundation, 11
    mammography, 727
    urograms, 693
Exposure time, alimentary tract examination, 631
Extremity
    lower; *see* Lower extremity
    upper; *see* Upper extremity
Eye
    anatomy, 362-364
    localization of foreign bodies
        film quality, 365
        modified Waters position, 367
        parallax motion method, 369
        Pfeiffer-Comberg method, 373-375
        preliminary examination, 366-367
        Sweet method, 370-372
        Vogt bone-free projections, 368
Eyeball, anatomy, 362-364

F

Facial bones
    anatomy, 324-326
    radiography, 440-483
        facial profile, 441
        inferosuperior anteroposterior, 443
        inferosuperior oblique (Law), 445
        lateral, 440
        nasal bones, 446-449
        oblique, 444
        parietoacanthial (Waters), 442
        zygomatic arches, 450-457
Facial profile, relationship of bony and soft tissue contours, 441
Fallopian tubes, anatomy, 737
Fasano, C., 351
Fatty meal, 603
Feet, lymphatic injection, 841
Feist-Mankin position, tarsus and subtalar joint, 82
Female patient
    gravid
        cephalometry, pelvimetry and, 762-765
        fetography, 754-755
        pelvic outlet radiography, 772
        pelvioradiography, 768-771

Female patient — cont'd
    gravid—cont'd
        placentography, 756-757
        radiologic examinations, protection, equipment, and preparations, 752-753
        roentgen pelvimetry, 758-767
    nongravid
        hysterosalpingography, 744-745
        pelvic pneumography, 746-749
        radiologic investigations, preparations and precautions, 742-743
        vaginography, 750-751
Female reproductive system, anatomy and positioning, 735-772
Femora, upper, and pelvic girdle, radiography, 182-183
Femoral head
    anatomy, 177
    dislocation, positions
        anteroposterior (Martz-Taylor), 183
        oblique (Urist), 198
Femoral neck
    anatomy, 177, 178
    radiography
        anteroposterior (Dooley, Caldwell, and Glass method), 194
        bilateral inferosuperior (Cleaves), 184-185
        inferosuperior (Danelius-Miller modification of Lorenz position), 190-191
        inferosuperior (Dooley, Caldwell, and Glass method), 195
        mediolateral (Johnson), 193
        superoinferior projection (Leonard-George), 192
Femur
    anatomy
        lower end, 63
        upper end, 177-178
    radiography
        anteroposterior, 106, 182-183
        lateral, 107
Ferguson, A. B., positions
    lumbosacral region examination, 252
    scoliosis, 266-267
Fertilization, 739, 740, 741
Fetography
    posteroanterior projection, 754-755
    purpose and use, 752
Fibula, anatomy, 62
Film
    dental, handling and mounting, 500
    placement, 12
    quality
        for gravid uterus examination, 752
        for urograms, 693
    retention, dental, 499
Fine, A., 359
Fingers
    anatomy, 28
    radiography
        lateral, 37
        posteroanterior, 36
        thumb, 38
Fiolle, J., 33
Fischer, D. L., 186
Fisk position, bicipital groove, 130
Flecker, H., 423
Fleischner position, lungs, posteroanterior lordotic projection, 568
Fletcher, G. H., 666
Florence, T. J., 699
Focal-film distance, 13
Foegelle, E. F., 649
Fontanels, anatomy, 312
Foot
    anatomy, 60, 61
    radiography, 70-77
        dorsoplantar, 70
        lateral, 74, 75
        longitudinal arch, weight-bearing, 76, 77
        oblique medial and lateral, 72
        oblique plantodorsal, 71, 73
        sesamoids; *see* Sesamoids

Forearm
  anatomy, 29-30
  radiography, 47, 50, 51
Foreign bodies within orbit or eye, localization, 365-375
Forestier, J., 795
Foundation exposure technique, 11
Fractures of labyrinth, demonstration by Chaussé procedure, 405
Freemond, A., 364
Freiberger, Robert H., contrast arthrography, 114, 115, 116, 117
Frémont, J., 228
Friedman position, lateral hip, 196
Frontal bone, anatomy, 314
Frontal sinuses
  anatomy, 420
  radiography
    Granger 23-degree position, 436
    oblique (Rhese), 432
    posteroanterior (Caldwell), 426-427
Fuchs, Arthur W.
  positions
    odontoid process, anteroposterior, 221
    temporal styloid, 410, 413
    thoracic vertebrae, 241, 244
    zygomatic arches, semiaxial oblique, 454
  radiographic view-finder, 553
Funderburk, W. W., 729
Funke, Thomas, 148

G

Gallbladder
  anatomy, 584
  radiography
    cholegraphy, 610-611
    lateral decubitus, 615
    lordotic, 615
    oblique, 614
    posteroanterior, 612-613
Gamble, Felton O., 76
Garrett, R., 727
Gas
  insufflation
    perirenal, 696
    retroperitoneal, 685
  myelography, 795, 796, 800
Gastrointestinal
  intubation, 654-655
  motility studies, 650-651
  series, procedure, 634-637
  tract, radiography
    esophagus, 633
    stomach and duodenum, 642-647
  tract, serial and mucosal studies, 638-640
Gaynor-Hart position for carpal canal, 45
Genetic effects of ionizing radiation, 15
Genital organs, female, 736-739
George, A. W., 220
George and Leonard position, femoral neck, 192
Geraghty, J. A., 691
Gersh, W., 41
Gershon-Cohen, J., 726, 727
Gianturco, C., sinus device, 390
Gill, Gerald G., spot scanography, 111
Gillespie, J. B., 658
Gladiolus, anatomy, 153
Glass, G. A., femoral neck, anteroposterior and inferosuperior projections, 194, 195
Glenn, F., 617
Glenohumeral joint, semiaxial anteroposterior projection, 135
Glenoid fossa
  anatomy, 121
  radiography, 129
Glossary of anatomical and medical terms, 271-287
Golden, Ross, 654, 762, 765
Gonads, radiation received by, table, 16
Goodwin, W. E., 699
Gordon, S. S., 642

Goree, John A., 333
Govoni, A., 658, 660
Graham, E. A., 598
Grandy method, cervical vertebrae, lateral projection, 230
Granger positions
  mastoid, lateral, 384-385
  paranasal sinuses, 436, 437
  sella turcica, 350
Grashey positions
  cranium, anteroposterior, 336-338
  foot, oblique plantodorsal, 71
  glenoid fossa, 129
Gravid female patient; *see* Female patient, gravid
Greisheimer, Esther M., 827
Greitz, T., 810, 813
Gugliantini, P., 642
Guglielmo, J., 648
Gunson method, deglutition studies of pharynx, 532-533
Gynecography, 746

H

Haas, Ludwig
  cranium, nuchofrontal, 336
  sella, nuchofrontal, 339, 348
Haas position, petrous portions, semiaxial posteroanterior, 394
Habitus, bodily
  asthenic, 543
  hypersthenic, 542
  hyposthenic, 543
  sthenic, 543
Hampton, A. O., 634
Hand
  anatomy, 28-29
  lymphatic injection, 844
  radiography
    lateral, in extension, 34
    lateral, in flexion, 33
    oblique, 35
    posteroanterior, 32
Handel, J., 704
Harris, R. I., 81
Hart position for carpal canal, 45
Hatt, W. S., 78
Hays, Mark A., 623
Healy positions, shoulder, 126, 127
Heart; *see also* Thoracic viscera
  anatomy, 546, 823-827
  radiography
    anteroposterior, 567
    lateral, 562-563
    oblique, 564, 565, 566
    posteroanterior, 560-561
Henschen, F., position for mastoid and petrous regions, 390-391
Hermann, P., 720, 721
Hernias
  diaphragmatic, anteroposterior projections, 646-647
  hiatal, minimal, radiography, 648, 649
Herrmann, E., 224
Hiatal hernias, minimal, radiography
  Sommer-Foegelle method, 649
  Wolf method, 648
Hickey positions
  lateral hip, 197
  mastoid process, anterior tangenital, 388
Hickey, Preston M., orthoroentgenography, 109
Hip
  anatomy, 176, 177, 179
  radiography; *see also* Femoral neck
    anteroposterior, 189
    inferosuperior (Friedman), 196
    posterior oblique (Hsieh), 198
    posterolateral (Lilienfeld), 199
Hip joint
  anatomy, 179
  radiography
    Lauenstein and Hickey projections, 197
    semiaxial (Chassard-Lapiné), 188

Hirtz, E. J., position for cranial base, 397
Hodes, P. J., 364, 401, 555
Hodgkinson, C. P., 715
Hoen, Thomas, 257
Holly, E. W.
  positions for
    head of radius, 50
    tarsophalangeal sesamoids, 68
  utilization of movement, 156
Holman, C. B., 12
Holmblad, Edward C.
  position for intercondylar fossa, 101
  posterior oblique positions for knee, 96
Holzknecht, weight-bearing position for os calcis, 81
Hope, J. W., 690
Horizontal ray method, contrast arthrography of knee, 116, 117
Hough position, sphenoid strut, 359
Hsieh position, hip, posterior oblique projection, 198
Hubeny, M. J., 753
Humerus
  anatomy, 31, 122
  radiography, 50, 51, 54, 55, 56, 57, 58
    anteroposterior and lateral, 57
    frontal and lateral, 56
    transthoracic lateral, 58
Hunsberger, W. G., 187
Hunziker, R. J., 8
Hyoid bone, anatomy, 326
Hypoglossal canal, anterior profile projection, Miller position, 418
Hysterosalpingography, 742, 744, 745

I
Identification markers, 12
Iglauer, S., 492
Ilium
  anatomy, 176
  radiography, 206
Implantation, 740
Infraspinatus insertion
  anatomy, 121, 122, 123
  radiography, 125
Infusion nephrotomography and nephropyelography, 700-701
Injection sites and supplies in lymphography, 840
Instillation, contrast, methods, 574-575
Intercondyloid fossa
  radiography
    Béclère position, 100
    Camp-Coventry position, 98, 99
    Holmblad position, 101
Interproximal projections, teeth, 510-511
Intervertebral disks, lumbar, weight-bearing flexion and extension studies (Duncan-Hoen method), 257
Intervertebral foramina
  anatomy, 212
  positions for cervical, 212, 232-234
    lumbar, 215, 253
    thoracic, 213
Intestinal tract preparation
  for cholegraphy, 602
  for diagnostic enema studies, 658
  for enema studies via colostomy, 672
  for female genital examinations, 742
  for visualization of urinary system, 690-693
Intestine
  large
    air enema, 668
    anatomy, 580-581
    colostomies, enema studies via, 672-675
    contrast enema, 651
    diagnostic enema studies, examination procedures, 656-663, 670-671
    double contrast enema, 656, 657
    insufflated colon, radiography, 669
    opacified colon, radiography, 664-667
  small
    anatomy, 580

Intestine—cont'd
  small—cont'd
    exposure time, 631
    intubation examination procedures, 654-655
    oral methods of examination, 652-653
Intraglottic instillation, 574
Intratracheal intubation, 574
Intubation, gastrointestinal, 654-655
Iodinated contrast media, 627-628
  untoward side effects, 689
Ionizing radiation, 14-17
Ischium, anatomy, 177
Isherwood positions, subtalar joint, 86, 87
Isolation technique, 7
Isometry, Law of, 497

J
Jackson position for atlas and odontoid process, 222
Jacots, Lewis, 227
Jacobson, H. G., 46, 172, 621
Jagailoux, S., 720, 721
James, D. F., 698
Jawetz, E., 659, 670
Jepkins, H., 689
Johnson position, femoral neck, 193
Johnston, J. D. H., 785
Joint hip, anatomy, 179
Joints
  anatomy, 24
  apophysial; *see* Apophysial
  sternoclavicular; *see* Sternoclavicular
  vertebral, anatomy, 209
Jones position (elbow in flexion), 51
Judd position, atlas and odontoid process, 223
Jugular foramina
  anatomy, 318
  radiography
    subbasal (Eraso), 414
    subbasal (Kemp Harper), 415
    transmandibular (Porcher), 417
    transoral (Chaussé II), 416

K
Kancel, B., position for clubfoot, 78
Kasabach, H. H., position for odontoid process, 224
Kaufman, S. A., 660
Kelly, W. T., 715
Kemp Harper, R. A., 839
  position, jugular foramina, 415
Kidneys
  anatomy, 678-681
  radiography, 684, 685
  retroperitoneal pneumoradiography, 696-697
Killian, C. H., 362
Killoran, P. J., 116
Kinmonth, J. B., 839
Kirdani, M. A., 418
Kirklin, B. R., 611
Kisch, Eugen, 196
Kite, J. H., position for clubfoot, 78, 79
Kjellberg, S. R., 568
Knee
  anatomy, 63
  contrast arthrography, 115, 116, 117
  radiography
    anteroposterior, 94
    lateral, 95
    oblique, 96, 97
Kohana, A., 715
Kohen, R., 659
Kohler, R., 593
Koppenstein, E., 232, 558
Kovács, Ákos, position for last lumbar intervertebral foramina, 253
Krecel, R. A., 532
Kretschmer, H. L., differentiation of ureteral stone (shift technique), 707
Kuchendorf position, patella, 103

Kühne and Plageman, radiography of mastoid process, 381
Kurzbauer position, sternoclavicular articulation, 163
Kurzbauer, Robert, position for sternoclavicular articulation, 163
Kymography, 554

L

Labyrinth fractures, demonstration by Chaussé procedure, 405
Lacrimal
  bones, anatomy, 324
  gland, anatomy, 376
Lambie, R. W., 750, 751
Lange, Sidney, 382
Lapiné and Chassard position
  pelvic outlet, 772
  pelvis and hip joints, 188
Laquerrière-Pierquin position
  for distal humerus and olecranon process, 54, 55
  for scapular spine, 148
Larkin, J. C., position for petrous portions, 399
Larynx
  anatomy, 528, 529
  methods of examination, 530-531
  radiography
    anteroposterior projection, 534-535
    lateral position, 536-537
Lattimer, J. K., 712
Lauenstein projection, hip joint, 197
Lauge-Hansen, N., posture of ankle for anteroposterior, 88
Law of Isometry, 497
Law positions
  facial bones, 445
  mastoids, lateral, 382
  paranasal sinuses, 433
Lawrence positions
  inferosuperior axial projection, shoulder joint, 133
  transthoracic lateral humerus, 58
Lee, R. S., 749
Leg
  anatomy, 62
  length, measurement of differences, 112, 113
  radiography
    anteroposterior, 92
    lateral, 93
    oblique, 93
Lentino, W., 46
Leonard-George position, femoral neck, 192
Levene, G., 660
Lewis position, sesamoids, 68
Lewis, Raymond W., 68
Lifting and handling patients, 10-11
Lilienfeld positions
  anterior pelvic bones, axial, 205
  calcaneotalar coalition, 81
  posterolateral hip, 199
  scapula, 147
Lindblom, K.
  diskography, 801
  gallbladder, axial projection, 611, 615
  percutaneous renal puncture, 699
Lindblom positions, lungs, anteroposterior lordotic projections, 569
Lindgren, E., 813
Liver
  anatomy, 582-584
  radiography
    anteroposterior, 595
    posteroanterior (Benassi), 596
    specialized procedures, 594
Loading of long cassettes, 108
Localization
  of foreign bodies within orbit or eye, 365-375
  of joints for long bone measurement, 108
Lockie, L. M., 125
Löw-Beer position, petrous portions, 408
Long bone measurement
  orthoroentgenographic method, 109
  radiography, preparation for, 108

Long bone measurement—cont'd
  slit scanography, 110
  spot scanography, 111
Lorenz positions
  femoral neck, Danelius-Miller modification, 190-191
  scapula, 147
Lower extremity
  anatomy, 60-63
  lymphography, 843
  radiography, 64-117
Lubetsky, H. W., 46
Luckett, W. H., 336
Lumbar
  diskography, 803-804
  intervertebral foramina, last, oblique semiaxial projection (Kovács), 253
  puncture in myelography, 798
  vertebrae; see under Vertebrae
Lumbar-lumbosacral
  apophysial joints, oblique projections, 254-256
  vertebrae; see under Vertebrae
Lumbosacral junction
  anatomy, 208, 216
  localized lateral projection, 252
  and sacroiliac joints, frontal projections, 248-249
Lungs
  anatomy, 548-549
  radiography
    anteroposterior, 567
    apices, 557, 558, 559
    bronchography, 572-575
    Fleischner position for interlobar effusions, 568
    frontal projection for fluid level, lateral decubitus, 570
    lateral, 562-563
    lateral projections for fluid levels, ventral or dorsal decubitus, 571
    Lindblom position for interlobal effusions, 569
    lordotic projections, 568, 569
    oblique, 564, 565, 566
    posteroanterior, 560-561
Lymphatic
  injection
    of feet, 841
    of hand, 844
  system, anatomy, 829
Lymphography
  contrast media and dye substance, 839
  iliopelvic-abdominoaortic region, 842
  injections, 840, 841, 844
  lower extremity, 843
  terminology and purpose, 839
  thoracic duct, 843
Lysholm positions
  cranial base, axiolateral, 343
  mastoid and petrous positions, 390-391
  optic foramen, superior orbital fissure, and anterior clinoid process, 358
  petrous portions, parietotemporal, 409

M

Magnusson, W., 586, 690
Mahoney, H. O., 428
Male reproductive system, anatomy and positioning, 717-722
Mammography
  axillary projection, 733
  craniocaudal projection, 731
  examination procedures, 728-729
  exposure techniques, 727
  history and use, 726
  mediolateral projections, 732
  routine positions, 730-733
Mandible
  anatomy, 326, 494, 495, 496
  radiography
    axiolateral, 464-469
    body and dental arch, inferosuperior, 461
    posteroanterior and semiaxial, 470-471

Mandible—cont'd
    radiography—cont'd
        submentovertical, 475
        verticosubmental, 474
Mandibular rami, radiography
    axiolateral, 465, 467, 469
    posteroanterior and semiaxial, 472-473
Mandibular symphysis, radiography
    axiolateral, 465, 466, 468
    oblique inferosuperior (intraoral), 462
    superoinferior (extraoral), 463
Mankin, H. J., 82
Manubrium, anatomy, 152, 153
Marinot, J., 611
Marique, Pierre, position for clubfoot, 79
Martz, C. D., 183
Mastography, 726
Mastoid process
    anatomy of, 321
    radiography, 378, 379, 380, 381
        anterior tangential (Hickey), 388
        lateral projections
            Bullitt, 386-387
            Granger, 384-385
            Law, 382
            part-angulation, 383
        posterior tangential, 389
        semiaxial lateral (Henschen, Schüller, and Lysholm)
            390-391
Mauton, R., 670
Maxillae
    anatomy, 324, 494, 495, 496
    radiography, 458-460
Maxillary sinuses
    anatomy, 421
    radiography, parietoacanthial (Waters), 428-429
Maximum permissible dose, 15
May position, zygomatic arches, 455
Mayer position, petrous portions, 400-402
Mazujian, Mary, 145
McBride, Earl, 43
McClure, R. D., 594
McCormack, K. R., 659, 670
McCoy, C. B., 712
McGann, Margaret J., plesiosectional tomography, 393
McLaughlin, H. L., 145
McLaughlin, J. S., 727
Meares, B. M., 333
Mediastinal structures; *see also* Thoracic viscera
    anatomy, 550
Mediastinum
    anatomy, 546
    superior, lateral projection, 556
Meese, T., position for sacroiliac joints, 248
Meniscus
    anatomy, 24
    lateral, radiography, 117
Meniscus medial, radiography, 116
Metallic bead chain method, female cystourethrography, 715
Metatarsophalangeal; *see* Sesamoids
Metatarsus, anatomy, 61
Meyers, P. H., 659, 670
Michaelis rhomboid, 759
Milk ducts, radiography, 729
Miller and Danelius modification of Lorenz position, femoral
    neck, 190-191
Miller, G. A., 658
Miller position, hypoglossal canal, 418
Miller-Abbott tube study, 654, 655
Mills, Walter R., 542
Millwee, Robert H., slit scanography, 110
Mirizzi, P. L., 618
Moloy, Howard C., method of pelvimetry, 768-771
Monitoring, personnel, 16
Monteith, J. C., 698
Moody, R. O., 579
Moore, G. E., portal venography, 594
Motion, its control, 8

Mouth
    anatomy, 486-487
    radiography; *see* Salivary glands; Teeth
Mucklow, E. H., 658, 660
Mujahed, Z., 617
Mulholland, J. H., 623
Murphy, J. T., 670
Muscles
    involuntary 9
    voluntary, 9
Myelography
    contrast media and preparation, 796
    examination procedure, 797
    gas, 800
    opaque, 798-799
    terminology, 795

N
Nasal bones
    anatomy, 324, 325
    radiography
        axial, 448-449
        lateral, 446-447
Nasal sinuses; *see* Paranasal sinuses
Nasolacrimal drainage system, 376-377
Nathan, M. H., 659
Navicular or scaphoid; *see also* Wrist
    positions for, 41, 42, 43, 44
Neck, anterior part
    anatomy, 528-529
    examination methods, 530-531
    radiography, 534-537
Nephron, anatomy, 680
Nephropyelography, infusion, 700-701
Nephotomography
    bolus injection, 685, 698-699
    infusion, 685, 700-701
    procedures, 685
Nervous system; *see* Central nervous system
Nice, C. M., 670
Nölke positions, sacral canal and sacroiliac joints, 264-265
Nucleography, 801

O
Occipital bone, anatomy, 318
Occipitocervical articulations
    oblique anteroposterior projection, 218
    posteroanterior projection, 219
Odontoid process
    anatomy, 211
    radiography
        anteroposterior (Fuchs), 221
        oblique (Kasabach), 224
        oblique anteroposterior, 218
        posteroanterior (Judd), 223
        semiaxial (Jackson), 222
O'Hara, A. E., 530
Olecranon process, radiography, 54, 55
Olnick, H. M., 698
Opaque myelography, 795, 796, 798, 799
Operating room, 7
Operative pancreatography, 622-623
Oppenheimer, A., 665, 666
Oppenheimer positions
    cervical vertebrae, intervertebral foramina, 235
    thoracic vertebrae, 242, 244
Optic foramen
    anatomy, 317
    radiography
        eccentric-angle parieto-orbital (Lysholm), 358
        orbitoparietal (Alexander), 357
        orbitoparietal (Rhese), 353
        parieto-orbital (Camp-Gianturco), 356
        parieto-orbital (Pfeiffer), 354-355
        parieto-orbital (Rhese), 352
Orbit
    anatomy, 351
    blowout fractures, radiography, 351
    localization of foreign bodies, 365-375

Orbital fissures
  anatomy, 351
  inferior, radiography
    posteroanterior (Bertel), 361
  superior, radiography
    eccentric-angle parieto-orbital (Lysholm), 358
    posteroanterior projection, 360
Orbital pneumotomography, 364
Orbital region, diagram, 363
Orthoroentgenographic method, long bone measurement, 109
Os calcis; *see* Calcaneus
Osborne, E. D., 689
O'Sullivan, W. D., 594
Ottonello method, cervical vertebrae, 227
Ovaries, anatomy, 736
Oviducts
  anatomy, 737
  radiologic investigations, 744
Owen, G. R., 401, 402

P

Palate
  hard
    anatomy, 486
    radiography, 458, 459, 460
  soft
    anatomy and positioning, 527-537
    lateral position, 536-537
    methods of examination, 530-531
Palatine bones, anatomy, 325
Palm, anatomy, 28
Pancoast, H. K., 222, 225
Pancreas
  anatomy, 585
  operative pancreatography, 622-623
  position for retrogastric soft tissues, 641
Pancreaticograms, 633
Pancreatography, operative, 622-623
Parallax motion method, localization of foreign bodies within orbit or eye, 369
Paranasal sinuses
  anatomy, 314, 315, 317, 420-421
  radiography
    Granger 23-degree for frontals, anterior ethmoids, and antra, 436
    Granger 107-degree for sphenoids, posterior ethmoids, and antra, 437
    inferosuperior oblique for relationship of teeth to antral floor (Law), 433
    lateral, 424-425
    oblique for ethmoids, frontals, and sphenoids (Rhese), 432
    parietoacanthial for maxillary (Waters), 428-429
    position, 423
    posteroanterior for frontals and anterior ethmoids (Caldwell), 426-427
    posteroanterior for sphenoids, ethmoids, and antra, 430-431
    semiaxial transoral for sphenoids (Pirie), 435
    technique, 422
    verticosubmental for sphenoids (Schüller), 434
Parietal bones, anatomy, 316
Parma position, temporomandibular articulations, 478
Parotid gland
  anatomy, 488
  radiography
    lateral, 492
    tangential, 490-491
Patella
  anatomy, 63
  radiography, 102-105
    axial (Settegast position), 104, 105
    posteroanterior, 102
    superoinferior (Kuchendorf position), 103
Patients
  dress, ornaments, surgical dressings, 10
  lifting and handling, 10-11
  preparation; *see* Preparation
  protection, 17

Pawlow position, cervicothoracic region, lateral projection, 238
Payne, M. A., 594
Pearson position, acromioclavicular joints, 136
Pelvic
  bones, anterior, radiography
    axial (Lilienfeld), 205
    posteroanterior, 203
    semiaxial (Staunig), 204
    semiaxial anteroposterior (Taylor), 202
  girdle
    anatomy, 180-181
    and upper femora, radiography, 182-183
  inlet, external landmarks, 759
  outlet, superoinferior projection, Chassard-Lapiné position, 772
  pneumography, 742, 744, 746-749
Pelvimetry
  Ball method, 762-765
  breathing instructions, 753
  Colcher-Sussman method, 766-767
  posturing of exact lateral, 760
  purpose, 752
  Thoms method, 758-761
Pelvioradiography, Caldwell-Moloy method, 768-771
Pelvis; *see also* Pelvic girdle
  anatomy, 176-181
  radiography
    lateral, 186-187
    semiaxial (Chassard-Lapiné), 188
Pelvocalyceal system
  anatomy, 681
  retrograde urography, 706-707
Pendergrass, E. P., 222, 225, 401
Pendergrass, R. C., 673
Penner, R. S., 201
Percutaneous cricothyroid instillation, 575
Periapical
  films, 498-499
  projections, teeth, 497-509
Peripheral arteriography and venography, 838
Perirenal pneumoradiography, 696
Peristalsis, 581
Peritoneum, anatomy, 578
Personnel monitoring, 16
Petrous portion
  anatomy, 320, 321
  radiography
    anterior profile (Arcelin), 404
    anteroposterior half-axial, 392-393
    Chaussé procedure for demonstration of fractures of labyrinth, 405
    Chaussé III position for attic-aditus-antral areas, 406
    half-axial oblique (Mayer), 400-402
    occipitofrontal (Valdini), 395
    parietotemporal (Löw-Beer), 408
    parietotemporal (Lysholm), 409
    posterior profile (Stenvers), 403
    Sansregret modification of Chaussé III position, 407
    semiaxial lateral (Henschen, Schüller, and Lysholm), 390-391
    semiaxial posteroanterior (Haas), 394
    subbasal (submentovertical), 396-398
    subbasal (verticosubmental) (Larkin), 399
Pfeiffer, R. L.
  localization of foreign bodies within orbit or eye, 365, 373-375
  position for optic foramen. 354-355
Pfeiffer, W., 341
Phalanges of foot, anatomy, 60
Pharynx
  anatomy, 528
  deglutition studies, 532-533
  methods of examination, 530-531
  radiography
    anteroposterior projection, 534-535
    lateral position, 536-537
Pierquin position
  olecranon process, 54, 55
  scapular spine, 148

Pirie position, paranasal sinuses, 435
Placenta previa, 741, 752, 756
Placentography
    anteroposterior, 757
    breathing instruction, 753
    lateral, 756
    purpose, 752
Planes
    of abdomen, 541
    of body, 23
Plesiosectional tomography, 393
Pleura
    anatomy, 548, 549
    radiography, 570, 571
Pneumocystography, 688
Pneumoencephalography
    brow-down position, 793
    brow-up position, 790-791
    fractional injection method, upright studies, 786-789
    injection procedures, 779-780
    lateral with head in extension, 792
    recumbent lateral positions, 794
    terminology, 778
    tomograms in, 784, 785
Pneumography
    cerebral
        angulation of central ray, 784
        head positioning, 782
        injection procedures, 779-780
        patient care, preparation of room, and exposure technique, 781
        projections and positions, 784, 785
        terminology, 778
    pelvic
        examination procedure, 748-749
        examining room preparation, 746
        preliminary film, 747
        purpose, 742, 744
Pneumoperitoneum, 592, 593, 594, 748
Pneumoradiography
    abdominal, 592-593
    of kidneys and adrenals, 696-697
Pneumothoraces, small, position for, 570
Pneumotomography, orbital, 364
Pneumoventriculography
    brow-down position, 793
    brow-up position, 790-791
    injection procedures, 779-780
    lateral with head in extension, 792
    recumbent lateral positions, 794
    terminology, 778
Pochaczevsky, R., 671
Poliaka, A., 715
Poppel, M. H., 46
    biplane projections for retrogastric tissues, 641
    pancreatography, 623
    wide-angle roentgenography, 172
Porcher position, jugular foramina, 417
Porot, J., 417
Portal venography, 594
Positioning patient and part for long bone measurement, 108
Positioning, structural relationship in, 9
Positions, body, 25
Preexposure instructions, 11
Preliminary steps in roentgenography, 4-13
Preparation
    instructions, 10
    of patient
        for diagnostic enema, 660-661
        for enema studies via colostomy, 675
        for gastrointestinal series, 635
        for myelography, 796
Presacral pneumoradiography, 696
Procedure book, 8
Projections, anatomic, 25
Prostate
    anatomy, 683, 719

Prostate—cont'd
    radiography, 722
    retrograde urography, 708-709
Prostatography, 722
Protection, radiation; *see* Radiation protection
Pterygoid processes, anatomy, 317
Pubis
    anatomy, 177
    radiography, 202, 203, 204, 205
Pulmonary apices
    anatomy, 548
    radiography
        anteroposterior, 559
        posteroanterior, 558
        transshoulder lateral, 557
Puncture, spinal, in myelography, 780, 798, 799
Pyelography
    excretory, ureteric compression, 694
    intravenous, 702-705
    percutaneous anterograde, 699
    procedures 686

Q

Quesada, Fortunato, clavicle right-angle projections, 143

R

Raap, Gerard, 188, 667
Radiation
    beam, delimitation of, 13
    dose, 15
    protection
        alimentary tract examination, 631
        cerebral angiography, 812
        dental radiography, 498
        gravid female patient, 752
        ionizing radiation, 14-17
        long bone measurement, 108
        thoracic viscera radiography, 553
        urinary system radiography, 695
    received by gonads, table, 16
Radiograph, standpoints of study, 5
Radiographic room, care of, 6
Radiography, dental, precautions, 16
Radiologic apparatus, alimentary tract examination, 629
Radiologist, protection of, 15-17
Randall, P., 530
Raper, Howard R., 510
Rasomoff, H. L., 785
Rea, C. E., 586
Reay, E. R., 705
Rectal tube insertion for barium enema, 661
Rectosigmoid, radiography, 664, 665, 666, 667
References; *see* Bibliography
Reflux method of operative pancreatography, 623
Renal
    parenchyma
        bolus injection nephrotomography, 685, 698-699
        infusion nephrotomography and nephropyelography, 700-701
    puncture, percutaneous, 685, 699
    tubules, anatomy, 680, 681
Reproductive system
    female
        anatomy, 736-741
        radiography; *see* Female patient
    male
        anatomy 718-719
        radiography, 720-722
Respiration
    in gravid uterus examinations, 753
    in urinary system radiography, 695
Respiratory
    excursion
        diaphragm, 165
        ribs, 164
    system; *see also* Thoracic viscera
        anatomy, 546-549

Retina, anatomy, 363
Retrogastric soft tissues, biplane projections for, 641
Retrograde
    cystography; *see* Cystography, retrograde
    injections in cerebral angiography, 808, 809
    urography; *see* Urography, retrograde
Retroperitoneal
    gas insufflation, 685
    pneumoradiography, 696-697
Rhese positions
    optic foramen, 352, 353
    paranasal sinuses, oblique, 432
Ribs
    anatomy, 164-165
    radiography, 166-172
        axillary portion, oblique projections, 170, 171
        in casualty patients, 165
        costal joints, 173
        posterior, anteroposterior projection, 169
        upper anterior, posteroanterior projection, 168
        wide-angle frontal projection (Corbin technique), 172
    respiratory excursion, 164
Richards, G. E., localization of foreign bodies within orbit
        or eye, 369
Richards, M., 670
Rigler, L. G., 570
Rizzi, J., 753
Robbins, L. L., 670
Robin, P. A., 673
Robins, S. A., 666
Robinson, A. E., 333
Roentgen pelvimetry; *see* Pelvimetry
Rolleston, G. L., 705
Rosen, S. W., 746, 748, 749
Rosenberg, L. S., 659
Roseno, A., 689
Rossand, L., 417
Rossi, P., 753
Rousseau, R., 659, 670
Rousselot, L. M., splenoportal venography, 594
Rowntree, L. G., 689
Rubin, S., 750
Rubin's test, 744, 745
Ruguero, W., 729
Ruiz Rivas, M., 696
Rundle, F. F., 569
Runge, R. K., 156
Runström, Gosta, 391
Ruzicka, F. F., 594

S

Sacral canal
    anatomy, 216
    radiography
        axial (Nölke), 264-265
Sacroiliac joints
    anatomy, 176, 208, 217
    radiography
        anterior oblique, 259
        axial (Nölke), 264-265
        Chamberlain method for abnormal sacroiliac motion,
            260-261
        frontal, 248-249
        posterior oblique, 258
Sacrovertebral junction; *see* Lumbosacral junction
Sacrum
    anatomy, 216-217
    radiography
        frontal, 262
        lateral, 263
Saito, M., 593
Saleeby, G. W., 666
Salivary glands
    anatomy, 488
    radiography
        parotid and submaxillary, lateral, 492
        parotid, tangential, 490-491
        submaxillary and sublingual, 493

Salivary glands—cont'd
    sialography, 489
Salomon, A., 726
Samuel, M., position for lumbosacral joint, anteroposterior in
        flexion, 249
Sansregret, A., modification of Chaussé III position, petrous
        portions, 407
Saypol, G. M., 617
Scanography
    slit, for long bone measurement, 110
    spot, long bone measurement, 111
Scapula
    anatomy, 120-121
    radiography
        anterior oblique, 146
        anteroposterior, 144
        lateral, 145
        posterior oblique (Lorenz and Lilienfeld), 147
Scapular spine, tangential projections
    Laquerriere-Pierquin position, 148
    prone and erect positions, 149
Schaeffer, J. P., 222, 225, 401
Scheie, H. G., 364
Schein, C. J., 621
Scheller, Sven, 95
Schencker, B., 700
Schlereth, J., 658
Schmier, A. A., 41
Schmitt, H., 52
Schneider, Cathryn C., 35
Scholl, A. J., 689
Schüller positions
    cranial base (submentovertical), 340-342
    cranium (posteroanterior), 334-335
    mastoid and petrous regions, 390-391
    paranasal sinuses, sphenoid, 434
Schulz, Emil, 746, 748, 749
Schwartz, S., 704
Sciatic notches
    anatomy, 177
    radiography, 206
Sclera, anatomy, 362
Scoliosis series, Ferguson method of distinguishing deforming
        curve from compensatory curve, 266-267
Seamon, William B., contrast arthrography, 114
Segal, G., 81
Sella turcica
    anatomy, 317
    radiography
        lateral, 346
        nuchofrontal (Haas), 348
        occipitofrontal (Valdini), 344-345
        posteroanterior, 349
        posteroanterior (Granger), 350
        semiaxial anteroposterior for dorsum sellae and posterior
            clinoids, 347
Seminal ducts
    anatomy, 718
    radiography, 720-721
Seminal vesicle, anatomy, 719
Sesamoids
    anatomy, 61
    radiography
        axial (Lewis position), 68
        lateromedial (Causton position), 69
Settegast position, patella, 104, 105
Sgalitzer, D. M., 556
Shehadi, William H.
    intravenous cholegraphy, 606
    iodinated contrast media, 627
    protection against ionizing radiation, 14-17
    simultaneous cholegraphy and urography, 624
    stress studies of ankle, 91
Sherman, R. S., 671, 674, 727
Shoulder
    girdle, anatomy, 120-123
    radiography
        acromioclavicular articulations, 136, 137

Shoulder—cont'd
  radiography—cont'd
    anteroposterior projections, 124, 125
    bicipital groove (Fisk), 130
    clavicle; *see* Clavicle
    coracoid process, 128
    glenohumeral joint, semiaxial anteroposterior projec-
      tion, 135
    glenoid fossa (Grashey), 129
    horizontal transaxilla projection, 134
    inferosuperior axial projection (Lawrence), 133
    infraspinatous insertion, 125
    rolled-film axial (Cleaves), 131
    scapula; *see* Scapula
    subacromial space (Berens and Lockie), 125
    subscapularis insertion (Blackett-Healy), 127
    superoinferior axial projection, 132
    teres minor insertion (Blackett-Healy), 126
Shoulder joint
  anatomy, 123
  radiography, 132-134
Sialography, 489
Sicard, J. A., 795
Siler, W. M., 727
Sinberg, S. E., 41
Sinuses; *see* Paranasal sinuses
Skeleton, 20-22
Skull
  anatomy, 312-313
    atypical, 328
    basic localization points and planes, 327
    cranium, 312-323
    face, 324-326
  body posture in radiography, 330-331
  radiography, 327-331; *see also* specific regions
Slit scanography for long bone measurement, 110
Smith, B., 351
Smith, C. W., 729
Smith, S. P., 715
Snyder, R. E., 674, 727
Soft structures of neck, 527-537
Somatic effects of ionizing radiation, 14-15
Sommer Foegelle method, radiography of minimal hiatal
    hernias, 649
Sordelli, E., 697
Soule, A. Bradley, 8
Sphenoid bone, anatomy, 317
Sphenoid sinuses
  anatomy, 421
  radiography
    Granger 107-degree position, 437
    oblique (Rhese), 432
    posteroanterior, 430-431
    semiaxial transoral (Pirie), 435
    verticosubmental (Schüller), 434
Sphenoid strut, parieto-orbital projection (Hough), 359
Spinal fusion series
  lateral projection in flexion and extension, 269
  supine right and left bending positions, 268
Spinal puncture in myelography, 780, 798, 799
Spinous processes, cervicothoracic, radiography, 231
Spleen
  anatomy, 585
  radiography
    anteroposterior, 595
    oblique anteroposterior (Benassi), 597
    pneumoperitoneum, 594
    specialized procedures, 594
Splenoportal venography, 594
Spot scanography, long bone measurement, 111
Staunig position, anterior pelvic bones, 204
Stecher, William R., 41, 44
Steinbach, H. L., 659, 670
Stenström, B., 616
Stenvers position, petrous portion, 403
Stereoscopic examinations of mastoids, 380
Stern, H. S., 670
Stern, W. Z., 621

Sternoclavicular articulations
  anatomy, 120, 153
  radiography
    lateral (Kurzbauer), 163
    lateromedial (Zimmer), 162
    posteroanterior, 160
    unilateral, 161
Sternum
  anatomy, 152, 153
  positioning, 154
  radiography
    lateral, 158, 159, 163
    lateromedial (tube-tilt), 156-157
    oblique, 155
    thickness-tilt guide, 156
Stevens, G. M., 749
Stevens, W. E., 715
Stevenson, C. L., 649
Stewart, William H., 336
Stomach
  anatomy, 579
  exposure time, 631
  radiography
    anteroposterior, 646-647
    gastrointestinal series, 637
    lateral, 645
    oblique, 644
    posteroanterior, 642-643
  radiologic examination, 626
Stress studies of ankle joint, 91
Strickler, J. M., jugular foramina, 414, 416
Structural relationship in positioning, 9
St. Stender, H., 224
Styloid process; *see* Temporal styloid processes
Subacromial space, radiography, 125
Sublingual gland
  anatomy, 488
  radiography, 493
Submaxillary gland
  anatomy, 488
  radiography
    intraoral, 493
    lateral, 492
Subscapularis insertion
  anatomy, 120, 122, 123
  radiography, 127
Subtalar joint
  anatomy, 61
  radiography
    Isherwood positions, 86, 87
    lateromedial oblique (Feist-Mankin position), 82
    medial oblique projections, 84, 85
    middle and posterior articulations, superoinferior oblique
      lateral projection, 83
    posterior articulation (Brodens positions), 84
Supraglottic instillation, 574
Suprarenal glands; *see* Adrenal glands
Surface markings of abdomen, 541
Surgical procedures, minor, in x-ray department, 8
Sussman and Colcher method of pelvimetry, 766-767
Sutherland, C. G., 689
Sutures, 24
Swanson, A. B., 201
Sweet, W. H., localization of foreign bodies within orbit or
    eye, 365, 370-372
Swenson, Paul C., 768
Swick, M., 688
Synarthrosis, 24
Syphax, B., 729

T

Talipes; *see* Clubfoot
Tarrant position, clavicle, axial projection, 142
Tarsus
  anatomy, 61
  radiography, 80, 81, 82
Taylor, Clifford C., 183
Taylor, G. W., 839

Taylor, H. O., position, temporal styloid process, 412
Taylor, Henry K., 231, 398, 629
  position for petrous portion, 397, 398
Taylor position, anterior pelvic bones, 202
Technique
  adaptation of exposure, 11
  foundation, 11
  lifting and handling patients, 10-11
Technologist
  clinical history needed by, 5
  diagnosis and, 5
  protection of, 15-17
Teeth
  anatomy, 494-495
  examination procedure, 496-501, 510
  interproximal projections, 510-511
  Law of Isometry, 497
  periapical projections, 497-509
    bicuspid, lower, 508
    bicuspid, upper, 504
    canine, lower, 507
    canine, upper, 503
    incisor, lower, 506
    incisor, upper, 502
    molar, lower, 509
    molar, upper, 505
  radiography, 496-511
    precautions, 16
  relationship to antral floor, inferosuperior oblique projection
    (Law), 433
Templeton, A. W., 45
Templeton, F. E., 532
Temporal bones
  anatomy, 320-321
  radiography, mastoid process, 378-379
Temporal styloid processes
  anatomy, 320
  radiography
    anteroposterior (Fuchs), 410
    lateral (Fuchs), 413
    oblique anteroposterior (Wigby-Taylor), 412
    semiaxial posteroanterior (Cahoon), 411
Temporomandibular articulation
  anatomy, 326
  radiography
    inferosuperior transfacial, 482
    lateral (Bullitt), 387
    lateral (Parma), 478
    lateral transcranial, 479
    lateral transfacial (Albers-Schönberg), 483
    oblique transfacial (Zanelli), 481
    semiaxial anteroposterior, 476-477
    semiaxial transcranial, 480
Teres minor insertion
  anatomy, 121, 122, 123
  radiography, 126
Testes, anatomy, 718
Teufel position, acetabulum, 200
Thickness-tilt guide for posteroanterior sternum, 156
Thigh, anatomy, 63
Thoms, Herbert, pelvimetry method, 758-761
Thoracic duct, lymphography, 843
Thoracic vertebrae; *see under* Vertebrae
Thoracic viscera
  anatomy, 546-550
    mediastinal structures, 546, 550
    respiratory system, 546-549
  radiography
    apices, 557-559
    body positions for, 551
    body-section, 554
    breathing instructions, 552
    chest, 560-567
    equipment, specialized, 554
    esophagus, 550
    heart, 560-567
    kymography, 554
    lungs, 560-571

Thoracic viscera—cont'd
  radiography—cont'd
    part position for, 551
    radiation protection, 553
    technical procedure, 553
    trachea, 555-557
Thorax, bony
  anatomy, 152-154, 164-165
  radiography
    costal joints, 173
    ribs, 166-172
    sternoclavicular joints, 160-163
    sternum, 154-159
Thorbyarnarson, B., 617
Throat structures; *see* Neck
Thumb, radiography, 38
Thymus gland
  anatomy, 550
  radiography
    lateral, 556
    posteroanterior, 561
Thyroid gland
  anatomy, 528
  radiography
    lateral, 556
    posteroanterior, 561
Tibia, anatomy, 62
Titterington position, zygomatic arches, 451
Toes
  anatomy, 60
  radiography
    dorsoplantar, 65
    frontal, 64, 65
    lateral, 66, 67
    oblique, 66
    plantodorsal, 64
Tomographic studies
  of ear, 393
  of pharynx and larynx, 530
Tomography in pneumoencephalography, 784, 785
Tongue, anatomy, 487
Tonsils, anatomy, 528
Towne, E. B., 337
Trachea
  anatomy, 529, 546
  radiography
    anteroposterior, 555
    lateral, 556, 557
Transduodenal pancreatography, 623
Tuberculum sellae
  anatomy, 317
  radiography, 347, 349, 350
Tuberosities, greater and lesser, anatomy, 122
Twining, E. W., positions
  cervicothoracic spine, 239
  trachea and pulmonary apex, 557

U

Ulna, anatomy, 29, 30
Unger, S. M., 172
Upper extremity
  anatomy, 28-31
  lymphography, 844
  radiography, 32-58
Ureteric compression, 694
Ureters
  anatomy, 678, 681, 682
  Kretschmer shift in radiography, 707
  retrograde urography, 706-707, 708-709
Urethra
  anatomy, 683
  retrograde urography, 708-709
Urinary bladder
  anatomy, 678, 682
  radiography, 684, 702
  retrograde urography, 708-709

Urinary system
  anatomy, 678-683
  radiography
    equipment, film quality, and exposure technique, 693
    intestinal tract preparation, 690-693
    motion control, 694
    preliminary examination, 695
    procedures, 684-687
    radiation protection, 695
    respiration, 695
    ureteric compression, 694
Urinary tract, simultaneous cholegraphy and urography, 624-625
Urist, M. R., position for fracture-dislocation of hip, 198
Urograms, film quality and exposure technique, 693
Urography
  contrast media, 688-689
  excretory, 686, 687, 689, 701
  procedures, 686
  retrograde, 686, 687, 688
    pelvocalyceal system and ureters, 706-707
    urinary bladder, lower ureters, urethra, and prostate, 708-709
  simultaneous cholegraphy and, 624-625
Uterine tubes, anatomy, 737
Uterus
  anatomy, 738-739
  gravid, radiologic examinations, 752
  radiologic investigations, 744
Uvula, anatomy, 486

V

Vagina, anatomy, 739
Vaginography, 750-751
  purpose, 742
Valdini positions
  cranium, sella turcica, and ear, 344-345
  petrous portions, 395
Valsalva maneuver, 530
Valvassori, G. E., 418
Van Nuys, R. G., 579
Vasselle, B., 720, 721
Vaughan, C. E., 753
Vaughan, W. H., 81
Velum, anatomy, 486
Venography
  definition, 830
  peripheral, 838
  portal and splenoportal, 594
Ventilation, 6
Ventricular system
  anatomy, 776, 777
  radiography, 778-794
Vertebrae, anatomy, 208, 209, 210, 211
Vertebrae, cervical
  anatomy, 210-212
  radiography
    adaptation of positions to severely injured patient, 236-237
    anteroposterior and oblique anteroposterior, 237
    anteroposterior (Ottonello method), 227
    flexion-extension studies, 231
    intervertebral foramina (Oppenheimer), 235
    lateral, 231, 236
    lateral (Grandy), 230
    lower, anteroposterior projection, 226
    and upper thoracic vertebrae, vertebral arch projections, 228-229
Vertebrae, lumbar
  anatomy, 214-215
  radiography, intervertebral disks (Duncan-Hoen method), 257
Vertebrae, lumbar-lumbosacral
  frontal projections, 246-247
  lateral projections, 250-251
Vertebrae, thoracic
  anatomy, 212-213
  radiography
    anteroposterior, 240-241

Vertebrae, thoracic—cont'd
  radiography—cont'd
    apophysial articulations, oblique projection, 244-245
    lateral, 242-243
    upper, and cervical vertebrae, vertebral arch projections, 228-229
Vertebral
  arch, anatomy, 209
  column
    anatomy, 208-217
    radiography; see specific region
Vertical ray method, contrast arthrography of knee, 115
Vesiculography, 720
Viehweger, G., medial epicondyle, axial projection for, 54, 55
Vik, Frances L., 579
Visceral arteriography, 836-837
Vogt bone-free projections, localization of foreign bodies within orbit or eye, 367
Vomer, anatomy, 325
von Gal, H., 364
Voorhis, Mary W., 148

W

Wagner, F. B., 535
Wangensteen, O. H., 586
Warner, F., lumbosacral joint, anteroposterior in flexion, 249
Warren, J. V., 698
Waters, Charles A., positions
  facial bones, 442
  paranasal sinuses, 428-429
Waters position, modified, localization of foreign bodies within orbit or eye, 367
Weaver, R. T., 753
Weens, H. S., 698, 699
Wehlin, L., 116
Weigen, J. F., 749
Whelan, Frank J., lateral decubitus position for gallbladder, 615
Wickbom, I., 699
Wide-angle roentgenography, Corbin technique, 172
Wigby-Taylor position, temporal styloid process, 412
Williams, A. Justin, position for costal joints, 173
Wilson, Hugh M., 758
Wolf, B. S., hiatal hernias, 648
Wrist
  anatomy, 29
  radiography, 40-46
    anteroposterior, 40
    carpal canal (Gaynor-Hart), 45
    frontal projections, 40
    lateral, 41
    navicular (Stecher), 44
    oblique, 43
    posteroanterior, 40
    radial flexion, 42
    ulnar flexion, 42

Z

Zanelli position, temporomandibular articulations, 471, 481
Zeides des Plantes, B. G., 785
Zim, I. D., 45
Zimmer positions
  sternoclavicular joints, 162
  sternum, 154
  zygomatic arches
    axial transoral, 453
    oblique lateral, 457
Zizmor, J.
  petrous portions, 402
  radiographs of blowout fractures of orbit, 351
Zones of abdomen, 541
Zygapophyses, anatomy, 210
Zygomas, anatomy, 325
Zygomatic arches
  anatomy, 320

Zygomatic arches—cont'd
  radiography
    axial (submentovertical), 450
    axial oblique, 452
    axial transoral (Zimmer), 453
    oblique lateral (Zimmer), 457

Zygomatic arches—cont'd
  radiography—cont'd
    semiaxial anteroposterior, 456
    semiaxial oblique (Fuchs), 454
    semiaxial oblique (May), 455
    semiaxial (superoinferior) projection (Titterington), 451

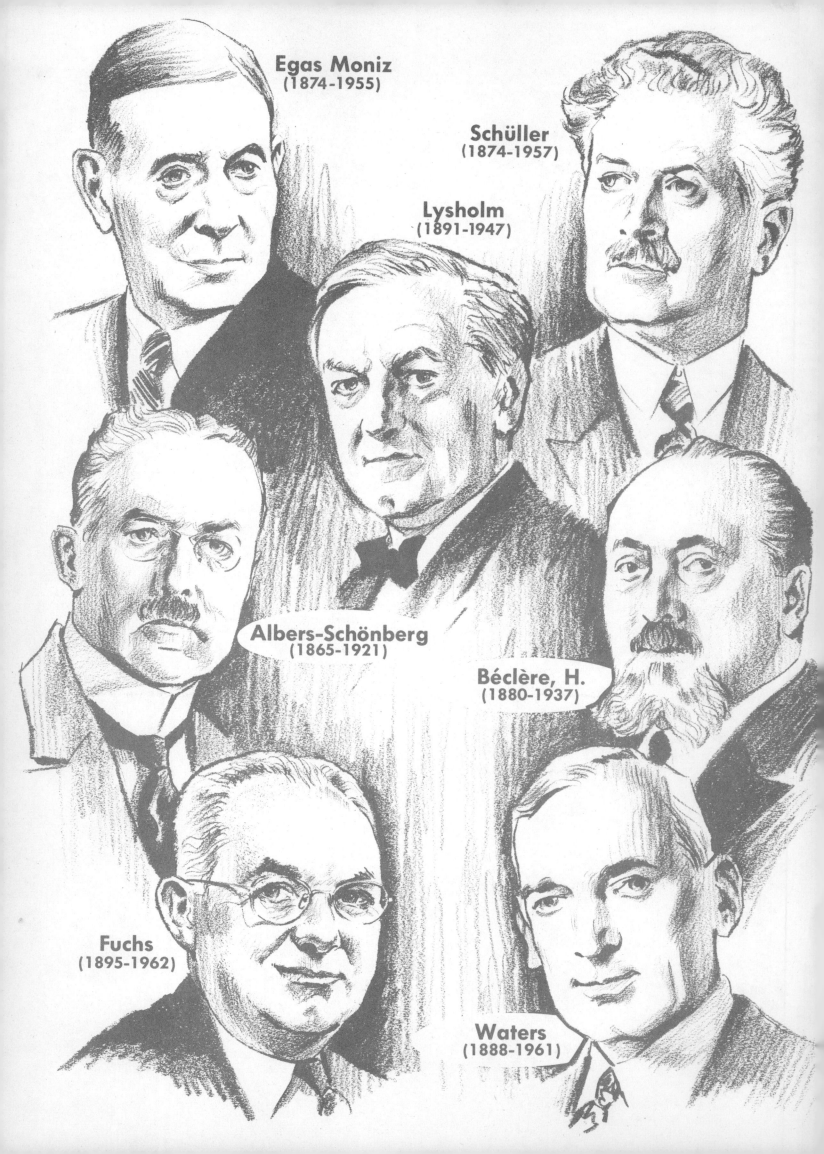

Egas Moniz
(1874-1955)

Schüller
(1874-1957)

Lysholm
(1891-1947)

Albers-Schönberg
(1865-1921)

Béclère, H.
(1880-1937)

Fuchs
(1895-1962)

Waters
(1888-1961)